T0406504

Bioinspired Approaches for Human-Centric Technologies

Roberto Cingolani
Editor

Bioinspired Approaches for Human-Centric Technologies

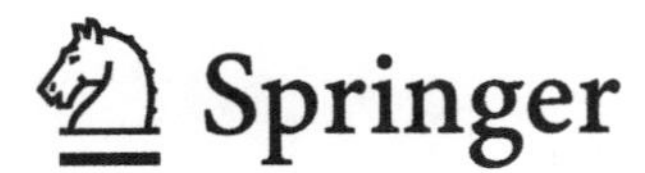

Editor
Roberto Cingolani
Istituto Italiano di Tecnologia
Genoa
Italy

ISBN 978-3-319-04923-6 ISBN 978-3-319-04924-3 (eBook)
DOI 10.1007/978-3-319-04924-3
Springer Cham Heidelberg New York Dordrecht London

Library of Congress Control Number: 2014940930

Printed on acid-free paper

Springer is part of Springer Science+Business Media (www.springer.com)

Contents

List of Contributors

Maria Rosa Antognazza Center for Nanoscience and Technology, Istituto Italiano di Tecnologia, Milan, Italy

John Assad Central Research Laboratory, Istituto Italiano di Tecnologia, Genova, Italy

Athanassia Athanassiou Central Research Laboratory, Istituto Italiano di Tecnologia, Genova, Italy

Andrea Barberis Central Research Laboratory, Istituto Italiano di Tecnologia, Genova, Italy

Gabriel Baud-Bovy Central Research Laboratory, Istituto Italiano di Tecnologia, Genova, Italy

Ilker Bayer Central Research Laboratory, Istituto Italiano di Tecnologia, Genova, Italy

Lucia Beccai Center for Micro-Biorobotics, Istituto Italiano di Tecnologia, Pisa, Italy

Fabio Benfenati Central Research Laboratory, Istituto Italiano di Tecnologia, Genova, Italy

Luca Berdondini Central Research Laboratory, Istituto Italiano di Tecnologia, Genova, Italy

Darwin G. Caldwell Central Research Laboratory, Istituto Italiano di Tecnologia, Genova, Italy

Laura Cancedda Central Research Laboratory, Istituto Italiano di Tecnologia, Genova, Italy

Massimo De Vittorio Center for Biomolecular Nanotechnology, Istituto Italiano di Tecnologia, Lecce, Italy

Francesco DeAngelis Central Research Laboratory, Istituto Italiano di Tecnologia, Genova, Italy

Alberto Diaspro Central Research Laboratory, Istituto Italiano di Tecnologia, Genova, Italy

Michele Dipalo Central Research Laboratory, Istituto Italiano di Tecnologia, Genova, Italy

Tommaso Fellin Central Research Laboratory, Istituto Italiano di Tecnologia, Genova, Italy

Despina Fragouli Central Research Laboratory, Istituto Italiano di Tecnologia, Genova, Italy

Guglielmo Lanzani Center for Nanoscience and Technology, Istituto Italiano di Tecnologia, Milan, Italy

Alessandro Maccione Central Research Laboratory, Istituto Italiano di Tecnologia, Genova, Italy

Liberato Manna Central Research Laboratory, Istituto Italiano di Tecnologia, Genova, Italy

Virgilio Mattoli Center for Micro-Biorobotics, Istituto Italiano di Tecnologia, Pisa, Italy

Barbara Mazzolai Center for Micro-Biorobotics, Istituto Italiano di Tecnologia, Pisa, Italy

Giorgio Metta Central Research Laboratory, Istituto Italiano di Tecnologia, Genova, Italy

Vishwanathan Mohan Central Research Laboratory, Istituto Italiano di Tecnologia, Genova, Italy

Pietro Morasso Central Research Laboratory, Istituto Italiano di Tecnologia, Genova, Italy

Lorenzo Natale Central Research Laboratory, Istituto Italiano di Tecnologia, Genova, Italy

Paolo Netti Center for Advanced Biomaterials for Health Care, Istituto Italiano di Tecnologia, Napoli, Italy

Francesco Nori Central Research Laboratory, Istituto Italiano di Tecnologia, Genova, Italy

Stefano Panzeri Center for Neuroscience and Cognitive Systems, Istituto Italiano di Tecnologia, Rovereto, Italy

Teresa Pellegrino Central Research Laboratory, Istituto Italiano di Tecnologia, Genova, Italy

Simona Petroni Center for Biomolecular Nanotechnology, Istituto Italiano di Tecnologia, Lecce, Italy

Pier Paolo Pompa Central for Biomolecular Nanotechnology, Istituto Italiano di Tecnologia, Lecce, Italy

Alessandra Quarta National Nanotechnology Laboratory of CNR-NANO, Lecce, Italy

Loris Rizzello Central for Biomolecular Nanotechnology, Istituto Italiano di Tecnologia, Lecce, Italy

Francesco Rizzi Center for Biomolecular Nanotechnology, Istituto Italiano di Tecnologia, Lecce, Italy

Giulio Sandini Central Research Laboratory, Istituto Italiano di Tecnologia, Genova, Italy

Alessandra Sciutti Central Research Laboratory, Istituto Italiano di Tecnologia, Genova, Italy

Claudio Semini Central Research Laboratory, Istituto Italiano di Tecnologia, Genova, Italy

Leonardo Sileo Central Research Laboratory, Istituto Italiano di Tecnologia, Genova, Italy

Edoardo Sinibaldi Center for Micro-Biorobotics, Istituto Italiano di Tecnologia, Pisa, Italy

Nikos Tsagarakis Central Research Laboratory, Istituto Italiano di Tecnologia, Genova, Italy

Introduction

Most living things are constituted by hardly a dozen types of atoms (primarily C, H, O, N, and few metals). Despite the fact that nature makes available more than 100 atoms to build our world, evolution has selected these atomic species and has optimized their organization to create living organisms and organic systems according to minimal energy requirements and highest stability and adaptability. Therefore, biodiversity, expressed by macroscopic differences among species and organic materials, relies primarily on the way few atoms are arranged together—i.e., by their collective architecture—rather than by the atoms themselves. A good representative example is the one of carbon that can generate many materials depending on its aggregation symmetry (graphene, diamond, graphite, coal, etc.). The same atom combined in diverse ways with H and O (both in terms of number of atoms and molecular architecture) generates the majority of the common organic molecules.

Therefore, any living system is characterized by the type and number of atoms of which is composed, with its complexity to be defined by the architecture of its atomic ensemble, a product of the optimization accomplished by evolution. This is exemplified in the left column of Fig. 1, where complex systems built by evolution over three billion years are increasingly demonstrated. The less complex and relatively small atomic *ensembles*, such as antibodies and proteins, are primarily capable of biochemical interactions. With increasing size and complexity, nature has introduced some biomechanical capabilities, in the form of cilia, tails, legs, arms, etc., so that mechanical work could be produced by larger systems. This is true not only for microorganisms and animals but even for plants whose roots move and grow following chemical and mechanical force gradients. Biomechanics and production of mechanical work thus become more and more important with increasing size and complexity. Movement implies higher-level interactions, so that cognition comes into play for most complex organisms like big animals and humans. Biochemistry, biomechanics, and cognitions thus follow the pipeline of complexity, i.e., the size and the architectural design of the different species, as schematically depicted in the left column of Fig. 1.

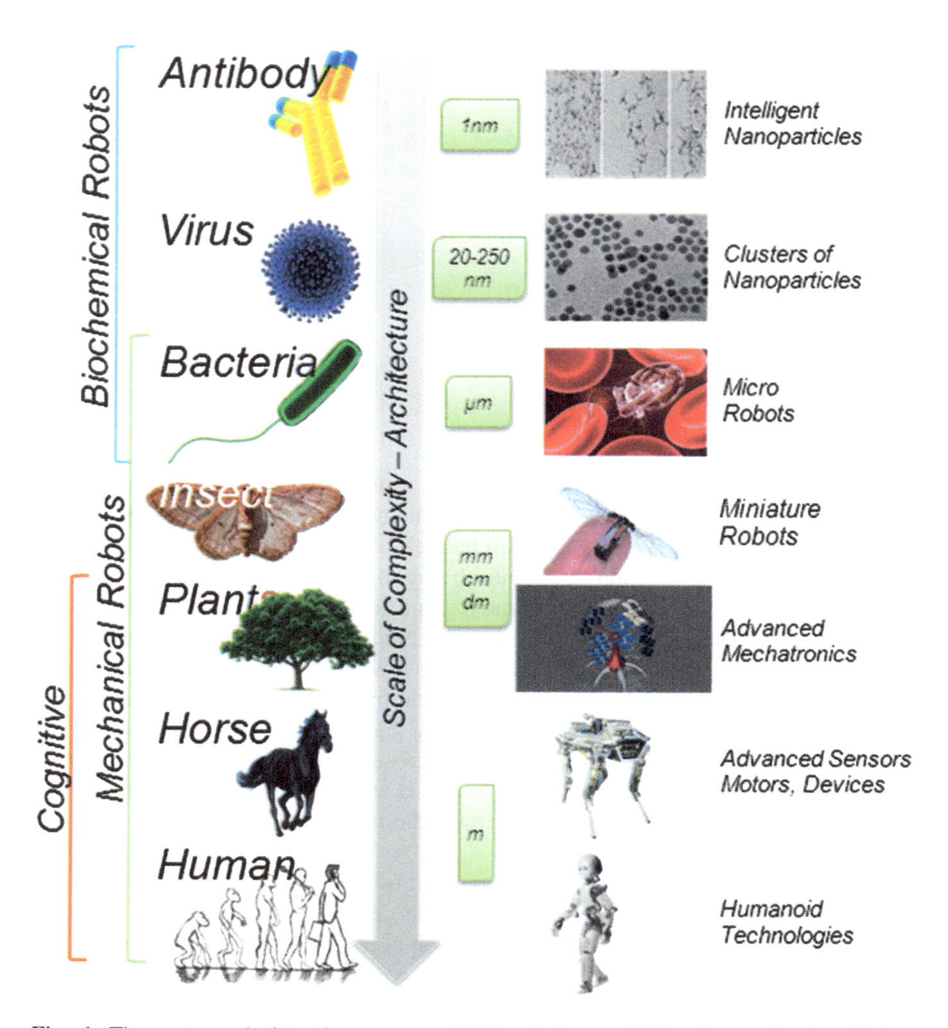

Fig. 1 The cartoon depicts the concept of "Translating evolution into technology." The *left column* highlights the evolution of biological entities of increasing complexity, as indicated by the *arrow*. The *right column* displays the corresponding bio-inspired systems. In both cases, one has to deal with architectures of increasing complexity, in which function and size are connected: smaller entities (from nanometers to micrometers) primarily operate via biochemical interactions. With increasing size and complexity, measurable work is produced so that ciliae, muscles, legs, and wings, appear and biomechanics becomes increasingly important. For most complex architectures, social behaviors emerge, which are connected to brain and cognition

Such an *architectural* vision of nature was made possible only due to nanotechnology, a unifying discipline that studies the formation and differentiation of complex systems in a bottom-up fashion, from molecules to humans. Nanotechnology, creating a common background for all other disciplines (from biology to robotics), gave the possibility, apart from studying and understanding the living

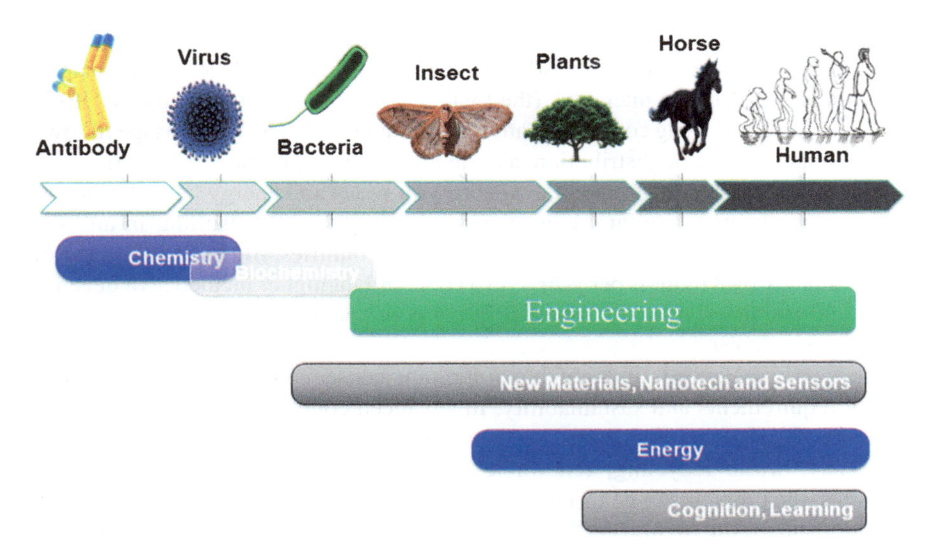

Fig. 2 The figure exemplifies the concept of converging sciences and interdisciplinary technology development. Most modern disciplines intersect and follow the evolutionary pathway discussed in this book

systems, also to create novel architectures, depicted in the right column of Fig. 1 spanning from nanoparticles, to sensors and robots, that mimic the designs and functionalities emerged from the natural evolution.

In this way, the boundaries between the long-standing separated disciplines of physics, chemistry, biology, medicine, and engineering are fading away. This separation is somewhat an artifact created by mankind to order and classify apparently different phenomena and systems. Physics, chemistry, and biology explain most of the interactions and processes that rule the formation of complex systems at the microscopic level and in turn provide the basic knowledge for medicine and engineering to describe macroscopic properties of both living and nonliving systems. This is exemplified in Fig. 2 where conventional disciplines are mapped onto the same evolutionary pathway of Fig. 1. It appears quite clearly that most modern disciplines intersect and follow the evolutionary pathway.

Most importantly, Fig. 2 gives a clear indication about the development that science and technology will have to pursue in the next years in order to produce sustainable solutions to mankind's problems: (1) technological disciplines will become *convergent*, i.e., more and more cross-disciplinary and (2) bio-inspired approaches dictated by natural evolution need to be adopted by technology, to develop efficient and sustainable tools.

This is the focus of the book, in which we revisit traditionally differentiated scientific fields in the light of a more unified, *evolutionistic*, vision of technology. In order for such vision to be effective to solve real problems of humans, it is however important to identify the main needs of future generations. Presently, our planet experiences a strong unbalancement of resource distribution. Approximately, 20 % of the population employs about 80 % of the total energy produced in the planet, despite that the "energy intensity" (the total energy consumption per unit GDP) is much higher in emerging countries than in Europe and the USA. Water usage follows approximately the same distribution, as water and energy production are intimately related. Countries having efficient availability of water and energy have developed advanced economies, welfare, education, and health system resulting in an ever increasing life expectancy. Today in the advanced countries, life expectancy grows approximately by 3 months per year with a concomitant higher incidence of degenerative and oncologic diseases, whereas in the poor countries, it stays constant or it grows much slower.

Such an unbalanced situation has important consequences on future technological requirements and sustainability. In advanced countries, the challenges will be personalized care for oncology and heart diseases, neurodegeneration and aging of society, waste recycling, renewable energy sources, etc. In less developed countries, the problems to be faced will be totally different: spanning from shortage of water and food to the need of welfare and health care. Surely, aging and degenerative diseases of the richer countries will not be relevant problems in countries where lack of primary resources, education, and health infrastructures prevent long-life expectancy.

Such a situation very likely will become more and more difficult, primarily because the planet population is steadily increasing—forecast nine billion people in about 30 years—and some large countries with emerging markets are growing faster than countries with already consolidated economies. This means that not only natural global resources will be increasingly limited but even their distribution among consolidated and emerging economies will become more problematic.

Interestingly, this has to do with the practically parasitic role of humans in the natural system. Mankind basically consumes natural resources without returning anything to the planet. The increase of users leads to a faster consumption of our environmental supplies, whereas the unbalanced distribution of resources among humans leads to societal differences at planetary level, which in turn inevitably have strong impact on the mankind equilibrium. The thermodynamic equivalent of such a situation could be an off-equilibrium isolated system such as a bottle full of water in which only a small portion of the water is hot while the rest is cold. The second principle of thermodynamics, as well as reasonable social considerations, suggests that progressively the temperature will get uniform throughout the bottle. The small portion of warmer molecules must release its excess energy to the other molecules. Unfortunately, thermodynamic equilibrium is easily reached in a population of H_2O molecules, whereas it is extremely difficult to be reached in a planetary population.

Development of science and technology is the way of choice to accomplish a peaceful and sustainable balancing of resources and wealth among people, keeping in mind that the different scenarios existing today will require completely different approaches and solutions to different problems. For instance, in advanced countries, it will be necessary to develop technologies (1) to improve diagnostic and therapy for cancer, heart diseases, and degenerative diseases; (2) to guarantee a sustainable aging in long-living populations; (3) to improve resource utilization, prime matter exploitation, and material recycling; (4) to make materials and infrastructures environmentally sustainable; and (5) to develop new (renewable) energy sources. In less developed countries, it will be a priority to develop technology (1) to improve food and water quality; (2) to improve health, prevention, and diagnostic; (3) to increase resource availability and reduce cost and environmental impact of industrial products; and (4) to build sustainable infrastructures.

In both cases, however, a strong and innovative knowledge has to be shared among traditionally noncommunicating scientific and technological fields. Most of the above problems have to do with natural systems and resources, and consequently it is very likely that science will have to copy nature, translating evolution into new sustainable, bio-inspired technologies.

The book follows the cartoon of Fig. 1 to propose such a development scenario. A new *class* of bio-inspired artificial devices, including diagnostic and therapeutic microdevices, nanoscale-engineered multifunctional materials, and robots inspired by plants, animals, and humans, are introduced to face problems spanning from personalized therapy to assistance to elder people. These technologies can only be developed by a synergistic approach of different disciplines, including material science and nanotechnology, biology, medicine, engineering, and brain science. Ultimately, the target is to develop materials and systems very similar to natural entities which operate inside, aside, or outside the human body to help humans in their daily life. The contents of the book are the following:

Chapter 1 introduces the concept of theranostics, i.e., a combination of tools combining diagnostic and therapy which is ultimately inspired by the natural operation of antibodies. Nanotechnology is developing new promising materials for fighting cancer and other important diseases at cellular level. Magnetic, semiconductors, and metal nanocrystals, consisting of crystalline clusters of atoms (from few atoms up to several tens of atoms), are some of the nanomaterials that are currently exploited as nano-heating probes for hyperthermia triggered by an external radiofrequency source. This offers the great advantage to generate a heat gradient only in the proximity of the place where the nanoparticles are accumulated and thus to specifically kill cells to whom these particles are associated (for instance, a tumor mass). The same types of nanoparticles can be also used as chemotherapeutic delivery tools operating via a triggered drug release mechanisms, as the heat produced by the nanoparticles could additionally induce the controlled release of drug molecules (either chemotherapeutic agents or short oligonucleotides) associated to the nanoparticle. Particularly, interesting is the association of nanocrystals with thermo-responsive polymers: this particular class of polymers can change their conformation upon a temperature transition; when increasing the temperature above a defined threshold, the polymer structure undergoes from a stretched to a coiled configuration. If nanocrystals capable of eliciting hyperthermia are encapsulated in these polymers, together with other payloads, the heat released by them will cause mechanical shrinking of the polymer and subsequent release of the payload. Moreover, some nanomaterials can be also applied as imaging probes in diagnostic applications. Magnetic nanoparticles indeed can be employed as contrast agents in molecular resonance imaging (MRI), while semiconductor nanocrystals can be used as optical probes when excited by the light. In all these biomedical applications, specific delivery based on active targeting toward antibody–antigen coupling is always desired. In this way, accumulation toward the target in cancer therapy is ensured, so that the total dose of the nano-therapeutic agents is reduced and the side effects are minimized. Additionally, nonspecific distribution in imaging applications is also avoided, thus making the imaging technique more sensitive.

Chapter 2 deals with the development of new technologies to produce artificial tissues starting from nano-engineered scaffolds onto which cell cultures are grown. A vast range of biocompatible, bioinert polymers are already used as implants in the human body in order to mimic the activity of a body part. The recent challenge though for the research in this field is to develop biodegradable scaffolds where specific cells can grow, adhere, proliferate, get vascularized, and eventually develop a tissue. Next generation of scaffolds requires the encoding of complex arrays of biofunctional signals to control and guide cellular events and tissue remodeling. Novel concepts in bioactive material design exploit nanometric control of structural and functional features to rule the spatiotemporal molecular regulatory program and the three-dimensional architecture of the native extracellular matrix. Although these materials are a first attempt to mimic the complex and dynamic microenvironment presented in vivo, an increased symbiosis among material engineering, micro- and nanotechnology, drug delivery, and cell or molecular biology is needed to fabricate biomaterials that encode the whole array of bio-signals to guide and control developmental processes in tissue- and organ-specific differentiation and morphogenesis. A representative target of such research is damaged skin healing and regeneration. There are already numerous wound dressings in the market, each one tackling diverse types of wounds, acute or chronic. These dressings can be passive (i.e., gauzes), interactive (like foams and gels that promote the healing being oxygen and water vapor permeable and bacteria resistant), and active (alginates, chitosan, and hydrocolloids that deliver substances accelerating the healing process). Lately, active nanocomposite dressings containing silver or other antimicrobial agents are also being developed. The majority of these research efforts are concentrated to hydrogel-type materials and nanofibrous, especially electrospun, materials that have a big potentiality as active wound dressings, providing new possibilities for the wound-healing market.

Chapter 3 introduces the concept of bio-hybrid interfaces, in which a soft polymeric prosthesis comes into direct contact with a biological tissue. The background knowledge of such technology traces back to the plastic optoelectronics, including light-emitting diodes, transistors, and photovoltaic cells based on conductive, photovoltaic, and piezoelectric soft materials. As compared to inorganic semiconductors, organic materials offer attractive characteristics in terms of mechanical properties, possibility of chemical engineering, and ease of processing, transparency, and flexibility. The drawback of such materials is the reduced electronic mobility and poor environmental instability, which might reduce their applicability in optoelectronic market, but it turns out to be potentially less detrimental for biointerfaced devices. Polymers are also suited for in vivo applications by virtue of their superior biocompatibility and adaptability to work at the interface with living tissues. At the macroscopic level, the soft surface of polymer thin films represents an ideal substrate to grow cells for in vitro studies as well as for in vivo applications. At a submicroscopic level, the polymers' softness finds an explanation in their peculiar conjugated structure, constituted by alternating single and double carbon bonds, which is indeed very similar to the structure found in many biological molecules (the retinal molecule, for instance). Moreover, conducting and semiconducting polymers offer the unique capability of mixed electronic conduction and ionic conduction, opening thus a new communication channel for interacting with the living matter. Material science has also developed piezoelectric and flexoelectric polymeric materials, in which a polarization charge, i.e., a current, can be generated under mechanical stress, like bending, pressure, or shear. These polymers are excellent candidates to replace natural mechanoreceptors which make skin, ears, and proximity sensors of animals (hair cells or stereocilia) so effective. The chapter thus overviews the applications of such multifunctional polymeric materials to biomedical engineering, neurotechnology, and life sciences. A few representative examples of evolutionary concepts translated into technology will be presented, including an all-organic artificial retinal prosthesis, artificial hair cells for flow sensors in underwater life, and "active" adaptable hair cells for acoustic prosthetics (hair cells for hearing and vestibular prosthetics). In some cases, their performances outperform those reported so far by adopting standard, inorganic technologies and have already reached the necessary development for preclinical and clinical application.

Chapter 4 gets the inspiration from the vegetal world. In contrast to common sense, plants have fantastic biomechanical capabilities through the specialized growth and motion of their roots. Roots are complex biomechanical systems integrating a network of sensors (humidity, softness, salinity, acidity, etc.) at the tip of a protrusion whose growth is fed by the plant. The root guarantees stability to the plant and feeding, and there is no mechanical/artificial counterpart of such a fantastic system in the technology landscape. Evolution has developed the capability of plants to manage a large amount of information (which is primarily obtained from the soil) to survive in any condition, avoiding dangers even if they cannot move quickly within the soil. Obviously, learning how to penetrate and explore soil as well as to maintain good performance in terms of energy efficiency for a mechanical system is a technological challenge which might be essential, for instance, for satellites landing on the surface of planets or for agronomy studies. Again biomimetics is the approach of choice to study plants and to transfer their properties into artificial systems and robots. The chapter follows this track, describing some of the main characteristics of plants, specifically their roots, and focusing on the natural strategies that plant roots use to penetrate soil. Then the problem of elongation is faced, discussing the elongation of the root tip apex from an engineering perspective and providing insight into the pressure required for the root to move forward. Finally, we introduce the Plantoid, a robot developed at the Istituto

Italiano di Tecnologia for environmental exploration and monitoring, which mimics the root behavior, thanks to a distributed sensing network and an intelligent actuation system. The chapter is concluded with a discussion of the active mechanism in plant movements based on an analytical approach to a bio-inspired osmotic system.

Chapter 5 deals with the transfer of advanced biomechanical ability to artificial systems such as robots imitating humans (humanoids) and four-legged animals (animaloids) to let them move appropriately in the surrounding environment. The world is a complex, unstructured, cluttered, and dynamically changing environment through which humans and animals move with consummate ease, adapting to changing environments, terrains, and challenges. Wheeled robots are increasingly able to work in some of these terrains, particularly those that have naturally or artificially smoothed surfaces, but there are, and will continue to be, many scenarios where only human-/animallike levels of agility, compliance, dexterity, robustness, reliability, and movement/locomotion will be effective. These domains will create new opportunities for legged locomotion (both bipedal and quadrupedal), but these new challenges will demand increased functionality in the legged robots, moving from the current domain dominated by simple walking and balance maintenance, to address key whole-body interaction issues during physical contact with humans, other robots, and the environment. Robots imitating humans (humanoids) and animals (animaloids) must employ multiple adaptive locomotion strategies which allow them to move like naturally evolved living systems, namely they have to walk on smooth, undulating, and cluttered surfaces; climb steps and stairs; crawl on two, three, or four limbs; use external supports to assist and augment locomotion (handrails, crutches, desks, walls, etc.), maneuver through small, cramped, and confined spaces; grasp and manipulate objects while moving; jump to reach or catch an object, etc. Legged robots can dramatically increase the range of terrains and situations in which an autonomous machine can be useful. The actions outlined above are crucial as we seek to develop robots to operate in such unstructured environments that have not been specifically built for the usage of machines. It is in these environments that legged robots will have particular advantages. Throughout the chapter, we will present the different strategies of biomechanics and mechatronics developed at the Istituto Italiano di Tecnologia to accomplish natural movement in prototype robotic platforms named CoMan (Compliant Man) and HyQ (Hydraulic Quadruped).

Chapter 6 introduces the concept of humanoids which move and interact with the environment. A humanlike behavior not only requires biomechanical characteristics as close as possible to those of human beings but also a very advanced sensory-motor coordination capable of processing a multitude of sensory inputs (vision, hearing, etc.) and to elaborate strategies to move and interact with the external world. Evolution has suitably developed our senses and our computational capability to process in real time the sensory stimulations and has also developed massive and parallel computational strategies to learn from experience and to anticipate situations through the brain. For an artificial humanoid, such capabilities are very difficult to imitate and reproduce. There are essentially three problems:

(1) the sensitivity, dynamical range, and integration of human senses (tactile, vision, hearing) are still quite difficult to reproduce artificially; (2) the fast elaboration of large data set of sensory input is a tremendous computational task, which is hard to accomplish with an electronic computer whose power consumption is orders of magnitude higher than that of a living brain; and (3) the surrounding environment and the situations change continuously in a random way requiring very fast adaptability. In this chapter, we consider a variety of basic sensorimotor coordination problems which are typically encountered in the domain of humanoid robotics. Despite these difficulties, humanoid robots are becoming increasingly complex, and, to a certain extent, they can now imitate human behavior. All the discussions will be developed around the humanoid platform *iCub*, a humanoid robot platform shaped as a three-and-half-year-old child, developed by the Istituto Italiano di Tecnologia.

One of the greatest challenges in designing controllers for humanoid robots is the implementation of interfaces that allow humans to collaborate, communicate, and teach robots as naturally and efficiently as they would with other human beings. This line of inquiry follows a twofold approach by drawing on our knowledge of natural cognition and, simultaneously, by instantiating plausible models of cognitive skills on humanoid robots. The hallmark of cognition, according, e.g., to developmental psychologists, is the ability to predict the functional behavior of the environment and its interaction with the body, simulating and evaluating the possible outcomes of actions before they are actually executed. In the brain, this is thought to happen through the activation of appropriate sensorimotor schemas that effectively function to couple sensory and motor signals leading to efficient action execution. Force and impedance control, impact-free motion strategies, whole-body coordination during physical interaction with the environment, point-to-point reaching movement, and finally grasping and manipulating visually identified objects are the main problems featured by this chapter.

Chapter 7 goes beyond machines and summarizes the fundamental properties of the nervous system, which confer living organisms the ability to perceive and appropriately respond to external signals. Such a basic view is the starting point of any attempt to translate the microscopic operation principles of the brain into a future machine. At any given moment, a multitude of different stimuli are received, processed, and integrated by the brain. The correct handling of this huge amount of information requires the coordination of extraordinary number of different events at both cellular and network levels. The basis of this extremely complex regulation lays on synapses, the specific contact sites between neurons. At the presynaptic level, electrical stimuli are translated into chemical signals, i.e., the release of neurotransmitters, which are recognized and translated into an appropriate biological response (either electrical or metabolic or both) at the postsynaptic level. The combined action of synapses acting in distinct brain areas is ultimately responsible for the generation and shaping of higher brain functions such as learning and memory. The molecular mechanisms modulating synaptic function have been the subject of intense investigation since the earliest days of modern neuroscience. Initially, synapses were thought to be "static" structures where presynaptic stimuli are linearly converted into neurotransmitter release and action potentials. This idea has now been substituted by a more modern view, whereby synapses represent extremely dynamic sites whose activity can be modified by a vast array of signals coming from the presynaptic, postsynaptic, and extracellular compartments, as well as by the previous history of the neuron. This new view of synaptic functioning has been obtained by the application of novel advanced techniques that allow interrogating the synapses in live neurons under various environmental conditions. Among these are patch-clamp electrophysiology, dynamic electron microscopy, and innovative imaging and optogenetic techniques coupled with high-resolution and super-resolution live imaging approaches.

Chapter 8 treats the problem of motor control and motor cognition in humanoid robots. The abundance of new behavioral, neurophysiological, and computational approaches makes the present understanding quite complicated, by "flooding" researchers with frequently incompatible evidences, loosing view of the overall picture. The chapter revises well-known notions, like synergy formation, equilibrium point hypothesis, and body schema, in order to *reuse* them in a larger context, focused on whole-body actions; this context, typical of humanoid robotics, stresses the need of efficient computational architectures, capable to defeat the curse of dimensionality determined by the frightening "trinity": complex body + complex brain + complex (partly unknown) environment. The idea is to organize the computational process in a local to global manner, grounding it on emerging studies in different areas of neuroscience, while keeping in mind that motor cognition and motor control are inseparable twins, linked through a common body/body schema. The long-term goal is to make a humanoid robot like iCub capable of "cumulatively learning." A humanoid robot should mirror both the complexity of the human form and the brain that drives it to exhibit equally complex and often creative behaviors! This requires to emulate the gradual process of infant "cognitive development" in order to investigate the underlying interplay among multiple sensory, motor, and cognitive processes in the framework of an integrated system: a coherent, purposive system that emerges from a persistent flux of fragmented, partially inconsistent episodes in which the human/humanoid perceives, acts, learns, remembers, forgets, reasons, makes mistakes, introspects, etc. We aim at linking such a model-building approach with emerging trends in neuroscience, taking into account that one of the fundamental challenges today is to "causally and computationally" correlate the incredibly complex behavior of animals to the equally complex activity in their brains. This requires to build a shared computational/neural basis for "execution, imagination, and understanding" of action while taking into account recent findings from the field of "connectomics," which addresses the large-scale organization of the cerebral cortex and the discovery of the "default mode network" of the brain. We will particularly focus, in the near future, on the organization of memory instead of "learning" per se because this helps understanding development from a more "holistic" viewpoint that is not restricted to "isolated tasks" or "experiments." Computationally, this results in the so-called *DARWIN* architecture (see http://www.darwin-project.eu), which should lead toward novel nonlinear, non-Turing computational machinery based on quasi-physical, nondigital interactions grounded in the biology of the brain.

Chapter 9 deals with implicit communication in human–robot cooperative actions, which rely on subtle cues about the body and the movement of partners. Many human activities are performed in groups and require that the individuals in the group coordinate their actions. For example, carrying bulky objects, dancing, handshaking, and musicians playing together in an orchestra are examples of joint actions. A crucial aspect of joint action is that it requires that the partners share information and communicate to update the information in order to be able to coordinate their actions. The chapter describes research that analyzes whether and under which conditions a robotic device can trigger this form of covert communication with a human partner. It also focuses on physical interaction with robots, a crucial form of interaction in many types of joint action. It presents work done to develop novel compliant actuation technologies that aim at facilitating physical interaction between a robot and a person, and it illustrates the importance of being able to read the state of the partners in the context of robot-assisted rehabilitation of the upper limb. A characteristic of the research on human-robot interaction presented in this chapter is to be closely inspired by our current understanding of the human sensory, motor, and cognitive systems. As a matter of fact, a deep understanding of humans' body and mind appears crucial to develop machines and robots, whether they have a humanoid appearance or not, that can interact closely and cooperate with humans.

Finally, Chap. 10 presents a glimpse of the multidisciplinary approaches that scientists are applying to the fundamental challenge of understanding neural circuits and computations and illustrates how advanced technology and analysis are driving discovery in neuroscience. Examples include novel optical methods to probe neural circuits and subcellular elements, innovative micro- and nanoscale devices to measure electrical and chemical signaling by neurons, and advanced analytical techniques to make sense of the dizzying multi-scale complexity of the brain. The overarching view is that the brain overcomes the limitations of its biological hardware by the brilliance of its *architecture*. If we could develop the right tools to deduce that architecture, we could begin to meaningfully mimic the functionality of the brain.

The central nervous system of mammals is among the most elaborate structures in nature. For example, the cerebral cortex, which is involved in perception, motor control, attention, and memory, is organized in horizontal layers, each of astonishing complexity. One cubic millimeter of mammalian neocortex contains about 100,000 neurons. Each neuron receives on the order of 20,000 synapses and communicates with tens to hundreds of other cells in an extraordinarily complex and highly interwoven cellular network. Moreover, neurons are remarkably diverse in terms of their morphology, electrical properties, connectivity, and neurotransmitter phenotype. The entire brain system is a strongly interconnected three-dimensional architecture exploiting ionic conduction in a water-rich environment. This is just the opposite to silicon-based computation, in which two-dimensional arrays of billions of transistors are interconnected to the nearest neighbors only and communicate through electrons in a solid (metallic or semiconducting) medium. Given this daunting complexity, the cellular and network mechanisms generating higher brain functions are still poorly understood. There are immense challenges in elucidating how information coming from the outside world is encoded in the form of electrical signals in neurons and how activities in cellular subpopulations and networks give rise to sensation, perception, memory, and complex behaviors. To address these fundamental issues—with an eye toward ultimately developing brain-mimetic artificial devices—we envision at least three essential experimental and technical tasks. First, we need to generate high-resolution maps of the electrical activity of large numbers of cells within the intact brain during complex behavior. Although this is a *correlative* analysis, it provides the initial information about *where* and *when* electrical activities are generated during specific behaviors and *what* information these activities carry. Second, we need to *causally* test the role of identified neurons in specific brain circuits and the role of specific brain circuits in behaviors. By using various types of cell-type-specific actuators, it is now possible to generate or suppress electrical activity in identified neurons and thus to test their necessity and sufficiency for a given behavior in living organisms. Third, because so much of the adaptability and plasticity of the brain appears to reside in synapses, we need to better characterize synaptic mechanisms and dynamics over broad timescales. All these goals require the development of innovative new experimental tools. Finally, collecting the experimental data is only the initial step: mathematical models are needed to truly "understand" brain function, to integrate descriptions at different levels of experimental inquiry, to reduce dimensionality, to devise testable hypotheses, and ultimately to provide the essential computational framework for brain-mimetic artificial devices.

In conclusion, we try to give a unified description of traditionally independent technologies. Material science and nanotechnology provide multifunctional materials and molecular-scale engines of transformation to create complex entities to be used both in living and artificial systems. Electronics and engineering add mechanical and computational capability to these entities, which in turn provide intelligence and enable interaction between humans and machines. Cognition, social behavior, and other higher-level capabilities can be accomplished by imitating human brain processes. In a few words, the fantastic nexus between the body, brain, and mind that evolution has developed over billions of years is the inspiring masterpiece of science.

This book reflects the cross-disciplinary vision of the scientific plan of the Istituto Italiano di Tecnologia (http://www.iit.it). The multidisciplinary effort of about 1,000 scientists operating at IIT in 17 different fields is strongly acknowledged.

Genoa, Italy Roberto Cingolani

Chapter 1
Antibody-Functionalized Inorganic NPs: Mimicking Nature for Targeted Diagnosis and Therapy

Alessandra Quarta, Liberato Manna, and Teresa Pellegrino

1.1 Introduction

Starting from raw materials, nature has developed macro- and nanoscale systems in which multiple processes, controllable at molecular level, are integrated into highly sophisticated and functional solutions. Understanding how these subunits assemble at different levels of complexity, and how this translates in the ability to perform specific functions, has inspired the development of artificial nanomaterials which mimic the naturally occurring processes. This is of particular relevance when such artificial nano-objects are engineered to be biologically active and thus mimicking some protein functions.

Antibodies are proteins that are naturally produced by the immune system of a guest organism, as a consequence of the biological response to identify and recognize extracellular ligands, called antigens, present on the surface of invader organisms or cells (such as viruses, bacteria, tumor cells), and subsequently to promote the immune response of the guest organism as a defense mechanism. Thanks to the unique affinity between the antibody and the antigen, which is often compared to that of a lock/key couple, the interaction of antibodies toward their corresponding targets is highly specific even at very low concentration of antigen expression. Once the antibody–antigen pair is activated, this stimulates the immune response, as demonstrated for antibodies that are specific toward the cell targets overexpressed in many different diseases.

As an effort toward mimicking these natural defense mechanisms and thanks to the research and development of monoclonal antibodies, in the last 30 years, many antibody-based formulations have been approved as immunotherapeutic agents to

A. Quarta
National Nanotechnology Laboratory of CNR-NANO, Lecce, Italy

L. Manna • T. Pellegrino (✉)
Central Research Laboratory, Istituto Italiano di Tecnologia, Genova, Italy
e-mail: teresa.pellegrino@iit.it

R. Cingolani (ed.), *Bioinspired Approaches for Human-Centric Technologies*,
DOI 10.1007/978-3-319-04924-3_1, © Springer International Publishing Switzerland 2014

cure many diseases. These range from the more conventional ones, like rheumatoid arthritis, to different types of cancers, to more specialized pathologies (e.g., the so-called rare diseases) (Chan and Carter 2010).

In the cancer field, monoclonal antibodies directed against clinically validated tumor targets, such as tumor necrosis factors (TNF), or against human epidermal growth factors overexpressed in certain types of tumors (such as lung and colon cancer to cite only some examples) have been successfully proven to block tumor growth (Dougan and Dranoff 2009). In the last 20 years, antibodies have been exploited not only to promote the immune response but also as the Trojan horses to deliver radionuclides in radio-immunotherapy: synergic effects due to the combination of radiotherapy with immunotherapy have improved the patient survival in specific cancer types (Waldmann 2003).

Nanotechnology is now developing new promising materials for fighting cancer (Nie et al. 2007). Among the proposed treatments that make use of inorganic nanoparticles, we mention, for example, hyperthermia, which is based on the local temperature increase directly to the tumor area. Even in this form of therapy, the inspiration comes from nature: fever is indeed a body defense mechanism that weakens bacteria and viruses and activates the immune response. Likewise, in case of "artificially induced hyperthermia," the generated heat will preferentially kill tumor cells, which are more vulnerable than healthy cells to stress conditions, and at the same time it should also activate the immune response. Magnetic, semiconductor and metal nanocrystals, consisting of crystalline clusters of atoms (from few atoms up to several tens of atoms), are some of the nanomaterials which are currently exploited as nano-heating probes for hyperthermia (Cherukuri et al. 2010; Kumar and Mohammad 2011). These nanocrystals can be truly defined as a new generation of "nanoimplants" for hyperthermia, as they have the unique advantage of being actuated by a specific external source. This could be a radio frequency, in the cases of magnetic nanoparticles, or a laser, in the case of plasmonic and semiconductor nanoparticles. This offers the great advantage to generate a heat gradient only in the proximity of the place where the nanoparticles are accumulated and thus to specifically kill cells with whom these particles are associated (for instance, a tumor mass). Moreover, their external activation can allow the personalization of the treatment, for example, through multiple applications depending on the specific clinical case. The same types of nanoparticles can be also used as chemotherapeutic delivery tools operating via a triggered drug release mechanisms, since the heat produced by the nanoparticles could additionally induce the controlled release of drug molecules (either chemotherapeutic agents or short oligonucleotides) associated to the nanoparticle.

Particularly interesting is the association of nanocrystals with thermo-responsive polymers: this unique class of polymers can change their conformation as a result of temperature variation; when increasing the temperature above a defined threshold, the polymer structure undergoes a transition from a stretched to a coiled configuration. If nanocrystals capable of eliciting hyperthermia are encapsulated in these polymers, together with other payloads, the heat released by them will cause mechanical shrinkage of the polymer and subsequent release of the payload.

Alternatively, the presence of thermolabile molecules (i.e., azo or peroxide groups, which can be decomposed above a certain temperature), placed in between the nanoparticle surface and the drug molecule, can promote the release "on demand" of the drug agents, as soon as sufficient heat is generated locally, i.e., at the nanoparticle surface. Moreover, some nanomaterials can be also applied as imaging probes in diagnostic applications (Sun et al. 2008; Corot et al. 2006; Michalet et al. 2005). Magnetic nanoparticles indeed can be employed as contrast agents in molecular resonance imaging (MRI), while semiconductor nanocrystals can be used as optical probes when excited by the light.

In all these biomedical applications, specific delivery based on active targeting toward antibody–antigen coupling is always desired. In this way, accumulation toward the target in cancer therapy is ensured, so that the total dose of the nano-therapeutic agents is reduced and the side effects are minimized. Additionally, nonspecific distribution in imaging applications is also avoided, thus making the imaging technique more sensitive.

Nanotechnology is already taking advantages of the monoclonal antibody therapy, as documented by the increasing number of works in literature on antibody-nanoparticle (Anb-NP) formulations. Merging such inorganic nanomaterials with antibodies will contribute to the development of intelligent multifunctional nano-therapeutic and nano-diagnostic tools that are more specific toward their targets than the corresponding nonfunctionalized nanoparticles.

In this chapter, we will provide an overview of the current state of the art in the preparation of antibody-functionalized nanocrystals and their application in the biomedical fields. This will include the critical steps related to the preparation of antibody–nanoparticle conjugates via different binding chemistries. Many aspects of the chemistry of conjugation between the surface of the nanocrystals and the antibodies have been understood in detail, and a considerable amount of work has tackled the challenge of synthesizing antibody–nanoparticle conjugates while maintaining the high specificity, avidity, and targeting performances. The results of these efforts have led to fabrication of new multifunctional imaging, sensing, and therapeutic tools. At the current state of the art, antibodies have been extensively exploited as shuttles for carrying chemotherapeutic agents or radioisotope drugs directly to the tumor, and many of these products have already reached the clinic. However, in the case of inorganic nanoparticles functionalized with antibodies, formulations are still in a preclinical stage. Some selected examples of in vivo applications of antibody-functionalized nanocrystals will be additionally provided, together with our considerations on the critical issues to be taken into account when using such nano-formulations.

1.2 The Antibodies: Structure, Bioactivity, and Their Employment

During the course of evolution, nature has developed immunoglobulins as part of the defense machinery, the so-called humoral response, against foreign bodies, cells, and molecules. Immunoglobulins, also known as antibodies, are complex proteins produced and secreted by specialized cells of the immune system, the lymphocyte B, in response to the interaction with an antigen. In mammals, there are five different classes of immunoglobulins (IgM, IgG, IgA, IgD, and IgE), each of them having a distinct role in the immune response and a different functional location. The IgGs are the most abundant antibodies circulating in the serum, and indeed they are the most studied and exploited in research and clinic. IgG antibodies are glycoproteins with a mass of approximately 150 kDa and having a typical Y-shaped conformation (Fig. 1.1). They consist of two identical functional subunits, each of them made of two polypeptide chains, the heavy chain (50 kDa) and the light chain (25 kDa). The two subunits are linked together through disulfide bonds at the so-called hinge region. Also the two chains of each subunit are connected by a S–S bond (Davies et al. 1990).

Both the heavy and the light chains consist of a variable region at the N-terminal domain and of a constant region, at the carboxyl terminus. The constant region of the heavy chain is approximately three times longer than that of the light chain, while the variable regions of both chains have similar lengths. The two domains contribute to the functionality of the antibody: the constant region of the heavy chain is the effector domain which binds to the complement proteins and regulates the immune response through the activation of the complement cascade, while the variable domains are devoted to recognize and bind the antigen with high affinity. Thanks to the high variability of this region, it has been estimated that about ten billion different antibodies can be generated and thus an unlimited number of antigens can be recognized (Amit et al. 1986).

Each antibody can bind two antigen molecules, which precisely fit in the pocket formed by the variable regions of each subunit. The process of recognition of an antigen is generally depicted as a "lock/key" system, but the binding strength of the antibody–antigen complex may greatly vary. Antigen binding is mediated by hydrophobic interactions, hydrogen bonds, and ionic interactions. Affinity and specificity are the two parameters that describe respectively the strength of the interaction and the ability of an antibody to discriminate between two different antigens (Poljak 1991).

Starting from the 1970s and then in the following decades, new technologies have been developed for the production and the engineering of large amounts of antibodies (Maynard and Georgiou 2000). The advent of the hybridoma technology first enabled the preparation of murine monoclonal antibodies, i.e., antibodies that recognize a specific epitope of the antigen. The technique is called "hybridoma" because it is based on the fusion of two cell populations. The first is a lymphocyte B which produces a specific antibody and has been extracted from a mouse injected

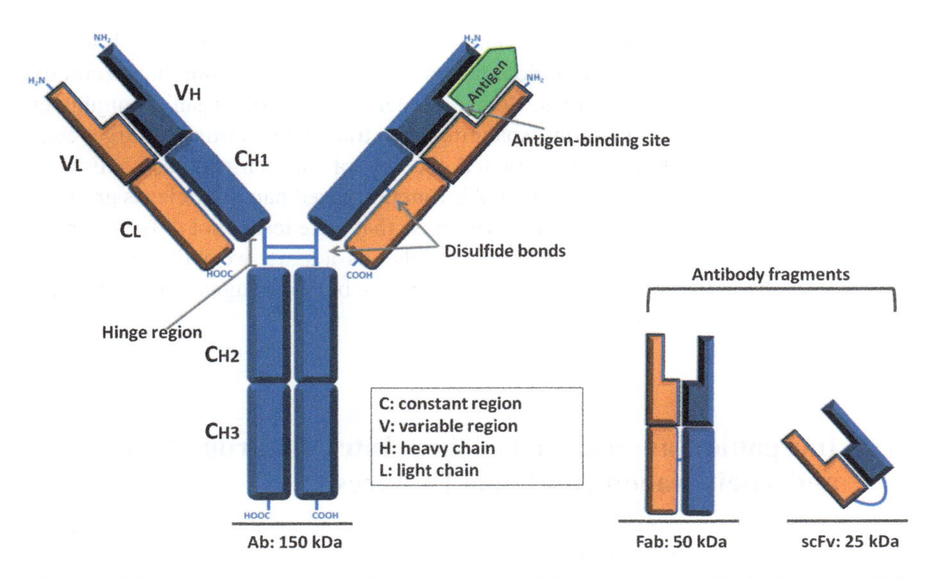

Fig. 1.1 Schematic showing the antibody structure and the functional antibody fragments (Fab and scFv) commonly used for the bioengineering of inorganic nanoparticles

with the correspondent antigen. The second population is a long-lived cancerous immune cell called myeloma cell. The fused hybrid cells possess the advantages of the starting populations, i.e., they are able to produce large amounts of antibodies and to grow continually in vitro (Kohler and Milstein 1975). Then the recombinant technologies, such as cloning, phage display, and the generation of transgenic mice, took a step forward and led to the development of humanized and fully human antibodies. This reduced or definitely canceled the main limitations to the use of murine antibodies on humans due to activation of the host immune response and rapid clearance. Both cloning and phage display are techniques that use PCR (polymerase chain reaction) and virus vectors for the rapid selection and production of the desired antibodies (Baca et al. 1997), while the transgenic technology allows to insert "foreign" DNA sequences into the mice genome. Transgenic mice are generally used as models of human diseases or for the production of human proteins (Bruggemann and Taussig 1997).

Furthermore, functional antibody fragments are genetically engineered, such as fragment antigen binding (Fab) and single-chain variable fragment (scFv), to cite some examples (Hudson and Souriau 2003; Batra et al. 2002). These technical advances have started a revolution in the antibody-based applications, opening new opportunities for their use in diagnosis and therapy (Waldmann 2003). Today, antibodies are extensively used in diagnostic assays and in the biosensor area, and their therapeutic potential has recently emerged in the treatment of several diseases, such as autoimmune diseases and cancer (Adams and Weiner 2005).

Moreover, the ability of the antibodies to bind to the target antigen with high affinity has fostered their use as targeting agents for the specific delivery of drugs or drug carriers and for the targeted imaging of cells through antibody anchored to imaging tools. Also inorganic colloidal nanoparticles benefited from the specificity and biofunctionality of antibodies. So far, a plethora of bioinorganic conjugates were implemented for applications, spanning from tracking to sorting of target cells and from controlled delivery to targeted therapy of antigen-expressing tissues. Since the number of works dealing with Ab-functionalized nanoparticles is growing exponentially, we will limit our analysis to those that were tested not only in vitro in cell culture but also in vivo on animal models. As a start, we will give a brief overview of the inorganic nanomaterials which have been conjugated to antibodies, highlighting their intrinsic properties.

1.3 Inorganic Nanomaterials: Their Intrinsic Properties and Their Nanometer Scale Features

Is it has been extensively documented that, when the size of a given material is reduced to the nanometer scale, its intrinsic properties can be drastically modified and new physical properties can arise, which can be exploited for several applications (Lu et al. 2007; Parak et al. 2004; Daniel and Astruc 2004). In this respect, colloidal nanocrystals, synthesized directly in the liquid phase, are unique sets of samples: they couple the advantage of being made of a core of one or more inorganic materials of controllable size and shape, which guarantees their structural stability and resistance to degradation, with the additional feature of being coated by a monolayer shell of organic passivating ligands, which ensures their solubility in a variety of solvents and is at the basis of their ease of processability, as if they were standard macromolecules (Talapin et al. 2010). Recent work on inorganic nanocrystals of magnetic, semiconducting, and metallic materials has uncovered several perspectives in nanomedicine (Gao et al. 2009; Junghanns and Muller 2008; Smith et al. 2008; Zrazhevskiy et al. 2010). One of the first proposed applications of nanocrystals was that of fluorescent labeling: semiconductor nanocrystals of several materials exhibit size-dependent fluorescence in a narrow range of wavelengths, which can be indeed finely tuned by adjusting the size of the crystals. As opposed to the more traditional organic fluorescent tags, nanocrystals offer the advantages of much higher robustness to degradation and the possibility that several nanocrystals of different sizes can be excited at once, that is, with a single exciting radiation, each nanocrystal size emitting light of a different color. This has had a strong impact on multiplexing analysis. Also, depending on the material of choice, such size-dependent tunability can span the visible range or the near-infrared range; therefore, different types of applications can be targeted. Recently, the development of Cd-free nanocrystals of binary, ternary, and quaternary semiconductors has allowed both enlargement of the spectral window covered by these materials and a sensible reduction of their toxicity (Talapin et al. 2010; Rosenthal et al. 2011).

Magnetic nanocrystals on the other hand, below a certain size, exhibit an interesting behavior known as superparamagnetism: this can be defined as the absence of coercivity and remanent magnetization in particles that still maintain a considerable amount of polarizable spins under the effect of an external magnetic field. This property is particularly appealing for biomedical applications if the particles are superparamagnetic at the body temperature. Among these materials, iron oxide nanoparticles (IONPs) have been synthesized extensively and studied in great detail and have been proposed as nanocarriers in drug delivery and as contrast agents in magnetic resonance imaging (MRI). In addition to these applications, IONPs have been exploited as heating probes in hyperthermia treatments: the heat generated by the magnetic nanocrystals when they are subjected to an appropriate alternating magnetic field can induce the selective death of tumor cells, since these are more sensitive to heat than healthy cells (Figuerola et al. 2010).

Heat treatment can also be elicited by means different than the magnetic hyperthermia, for example, via excitation of plasmonic modes in metal nanoparticles. In this respect, several noble metal nanoparticles, for example, gold, are characterized by size-dependent adsorption/scattering of light, due to excitation of surface plasmon resonance modes. Due to these properties, gold nanoparticles have been investigated as bio-imaging tools for the colorimetric detection of analytes. On the other hand, metallic nanoparticles too can generate heat, in this case when excited with a laser of appropriate energy, such that, for example, it is resonant to a surface plasmon mode. Gold nanorods, nanocages, nanostars, or even nanostructures containing multiple spherical gold and/or silver nanoparticles within their structures have been exploited for the photothermal ablation of tumors (Huang et al. 2006; O'Neal et al. 2004; Skrabalak et al. 2008). Recent developments in this direction include the use of nanoparticles of degenerately doped semiconductors, which likewise exhibit localized surface plasmon modes as in noble metals, but their fabrication costs are comparatively much lower.

In addition to the inorganic nanocrystals just mentioned, also carbon nanotubes, graphene, and combinations of these materials with metallic or semiconductor nanocrystals have been recently studied intensively for what concerns their potential biomedical applications, not only for detection, imaging, and drug delivery but also for tissue regeneration (Liu et al. 2009; Zhang and Webster 2009; Schrand et al. 2009). It is also worth to mention lanthanide-doped rare-earth nanoparticles that are emerging as alternative diagnostic tools (Shen et al. 2013; Mader et al. 2010). In these materials, the possibility to change the doping elements hosted in the rare-earth matrix allows the development of different functional nanoparticles, such as fluorescent upconverting probes (for instance, when the nanocrystals are doped with Yb and Er) (Wang et al. 2009) or MRI probes (when the nanocrystals are doped with Gd) (Aime et al. 2009). The term upconversion is referred to the effect by which low-energy near-infrared radiation (NIR) is converted to higher-energy light by sequential multiphoton NIR absorption and subsequent emission of light at shorter wavelength (Haase and Schaefer 2011). This phenomenon has gained great attention in the bio-imaging field, where the search for probes that adsorb in regions where tissues show poor absorption, and emit in the visible range, is still challenging (Mader et al. 2010). Moreover, advances in synthetic methods and optimization of the probe design led to the generation of dual imaging nanosystems. Currently, in vivo studies are in progress to assess the potential of these materials (Park et al. 2012; Zhou et al. 2010; Ju et al. 2012; Li et al. 2009).

In nanocrystals, apart from the intrinsic size dependence of the physical properties connected with the presence of an inorganic core, many other parameters, individually or in combination, come into play in regulating their behavior when applied to biological systems. Some of these parameters, in addition to size, are shape, surface-to-volume ratio, and surface chemistry (Algar et al. 2011; Tao et al. 2008; Pankhurst et al. 2003; Papavassiliou 1979; Alivisatos 1996; Whitesides 2003). It is important to emphasize that the size of the nanocrystals is in the same range of that of many biomolecules, which permits the functionalization of their surface with a controlled number of targeting molecules: these include peptides, oligonucleotide sequences, proteins, vitamins, and others. In many cases, these molecules can be bound to the nanocrystal surface in such a way that both the number of molecules and their packing can be finely controlled, thus increasing the affinity of the nanocrystals toward their target (Hauck et al. 2008; Nel et al. 2009). This layer of organic/biomolecules bound to the surface of the nanocrystals can affect their colloidal stability to different extents in the various biological fluids, such as cellular media, serum, blood, gastric liquid, etc. Such layer can additionally help the nanocrystals to preserve their intrinsic properties, depending on the material of which they are made (fluorescence, superparamagnetism, plasmonic behavior, etc.). One additional key role often played by this layer, when it is sufficiently thick and robust, is that of minimizing the direct exposure of the nanocrystal surface to the surrounding biological environment. This can clearly reduce or even prevent the onset of adverse/side effects, for example, the leakage of toxic (or potentially toxic) metal ions from the nanocrystals (Derfus et al. 2004; Nel et al. 2006; Lewinski et al. 2008; Kirchner et al. 2005). Even more important, such coating is capable of affecting the uptake of nanocrystals by the living cells, especially if it is carefully designed for specific targeting of the cell. As an example, when IONPs are used as hyperthermia agents or as carriers for the delivery of drugs, nonspecific uptake needs to be avoided, so that the therapeutic effect is highly specific and therefore side effects and toxicity to healthy tissues are reduced as much as possible.

Specific targeting is of utmost importance for the identification of specific cellular pathways, for instance, protein signaling or vitamin and hormone trafficking toward different cellular sub-compartments. Engineered nanocrystals can also be used for detecting and sorting of specific cell types within a biological sample. For drug delivery applications, the use of antibodies could be exploited to direct the nanocontainers toward the target tumor site which overexpresses specific antigen against the antibody attached at the nanoparticle surface. The same principle is exploitable for the delivery of nano-therapeutic tools (e.g., a plasmonic or a magnetic nanoparticle) toward a tumor site or for in vivo imaging applications using MRI.

In all these cases, the main goal is to achieve specific targeting while minimizing at the same time nonspecific targeting. Properly designed conjugates/nanocrystals have been fabricated to combine the novel and fascinating properties and potential of nanoscale materials (i.e., colorimetric signature, fluorescence, plasmonic behavior, and unique features deriving from nanoscale magnetism) with biomolecules such as whole antibodies or fragments of them. This was made possible by the high versatility of the chemistry at the nanoparticle surface and by the efforts undertaken by different groups to overcome the critical issues related to the preparation of the desired antibody–nanoparticle formulations. The surface chemistry functionalization of inorganic nanoparticles is a key issue in this respect, and it will be discussed in the next paragraph.

1.4 Surface Functionalization of Inorganic Nanoparticles

Inorganic nanoparticles can be synthesized following different routes. Among the many approaches, non-hydrolytic methods (for instance, thermal decomposition of organometallic precursors in hot surfactants) or hydrolytic methods, like water-based reduction or coprecipitation, are perhaps the most suitable ones for the preparation of high-quality colloidal nanoparticles (Sun et al. 2004; Murray et al. 1993; Brust et al. 1994). Using these methods, the particles are usually coated by a layer of stabilizers: if the nanoparticles are synthesized by thermal decomposition methods, then the coating usually consists of organic surfactant molecules, whereas if the particles are synthesized in water, the coating can be represented by charged salt counterions or charged surfactants. The coating in general is weakly bound to the nanoparticle surface and can be easily replaced with other types of agents, depending on the further use that one wants to make of the particles (Neuberger et al. 2005; Hezinger et al. 2008; Chithrani and Chan 2007). In the case of nanoparticles synthesized in organic media, new ligand molecules, mono- or multidentate, might confer to the nanoparticle a different solubility from one phase to another, thus allowing the transfer from the solvent in which they have been synthesized to the aqueous media. In the case of nanoparticle prepared directly in water, ligand molecules with proper moieties that can bind the nanoparticle surface with higher affinity than the original capping molecules can be chosen. This leads to a better stabilization of the nanoparticles in water.

The ligand molecules could be also chosen to introduce at the nanoparticle surface specific functional groups needed for further functionalization with different molecules, including antibodies, antibody fragments, or peptides.

Usually, the exchanged ligands are short molecules, and upon the replacement of the original surfactant molecules at the nanoparticle surface, the final size of the nanocrystals is comparable to that of the initial ones. It is important to remark that a small particle size and the surface charge (together with other parameters) affect the cell internalization pathway, as proven by different groups (Nel et al. 2009; Delehanty et al. 2009). In most cases, the binding of the ligand to the particle surface is generally weak, leading to nanoparticle aggregation with time. Recently, however, cross-linked ligand shells have been developed to improve nanoparticle stability in water (Dubertret et al. 2002; Jiang et al. 2008). Furthermore, the specificity of the ligand units toward the different materials, of which the nanoparticles are composed, implies that different ligands are required for different types of nanoparticles. Therefore, besides its simplicity, the ligand exchange procedure cannot be considered a method of general applicability.

In the case of organic surfactant-coated nanoparticles, as, for instance, the ones synthesized by thermal decomposition methods, the encapsulation of the nanoparticles together with its original surfactant shell within amphiphilic molecules is a commonly used approach (Pellegrino et al. 2004; Lees et al. 2009; Di Corato et al. 2008; Qi and Gao 2008). In this case, the alkyl tails of the polymer interact with the alkyl tails of the surfactant molecules at the nanoparticle surface, while the hydrophilic moieties of the polymer face the polar solution, thus providing water solubility. As the interaction between the surfactant shell and the polymer is based on several hydrophobic units, multiple interactions can occur, thus enabling a stronger coating shell. In addition, since the hydrophobic interactions between the surfactant molecules and the polymer chains are nonspecific, the same polymer can be used to coat a wide variety of nanocrystals, irrespective of the type of materials of which the nanoparticles are composed. Moreover, once a procedure for linking an antibody to a certain type of nanocrystal is established, this procedure is easily extendable and applicable to a wide range of nanocrystals having different intrinsic properties but same coating shell.

Up to date, due to the different sizes, shapes, compositions, and stabilities that characterize the various types of nanoparticle that have been prepared so far, no standardized antibody linkage protocols to nanoparticles have been developed. In the next paragraph, we will summarize the different strategies reported so far to link to a nanoparticle the antibody, highlighting the important parameters that should be considered in order to have stable and still functional antibody–nanoparticle conjugates.

The nanoparticle surface plays an important role in controlling the type and number of antibody molecules which can be associated/linked to the nanoparticles. This is determined by the types of functional groups (i.e., amino, thiol, carboxyl derivates) attached at the nanoparticle surface and by their number and density. Controlling the number of functional molecules attached at the surface of the nanoparticles can allow a control over the number and distribution of functional groups and thus the subsequent ligation of controlled number of antibodies or antibody fragments.

Often, to control the number of functional groups to be introduced at the surface of nanocrystals, mixtures of different ligands, each of them bearing the desired functional groups, are simultaneously exchanged/linked at the nanoparticle surface. Depending on the initial ratio of the different ligand molecules, the percentage of the ligands that can be introduced at the nanoparticle surface and thus of the functional units associated to them can be tuned. To cite an example, if amino groups are desired at the surface, a combination of methoxy PEG-amino derivates and diamino PEG derivates has been attached simultaneously to polymer-coated nanoparticles (Sperling et al. 2006; Quarta et al. 2012). Besides the tuning of functional groups at the nanoparticle surface, many other parameters need to be considered for the linkage of antibodies to the nanoparticles, and they will be explained in depth in the next paragraph.

1.5 Surface Functionalization of Inorganic Nanoparticles with Antibodies

A fundamental requisite for all the studies is that the antibody linked to the nanoparticle surface must preserve its biofunctionality. Therefore, it is not surprising that many efforts were made in order to optimize the coupling chemistry and the binding geometry of the bionanocomplex. In general, to attach the antibodies to the nanoparticle surface, three main different strategies can be exploited: (1) the physical adsorption, (2) the covalent linkage, or (3) the use of adapter complexes that work as spacers in a sandwich configuration.

Physical Adsorption (Fig. 1.2a) The functional groups, either basic or acid, introduced at the nanoparticle surface, can drive the electrostatic interactions of the nanoparticles with suitably charged antibodies. This allows the adsorption of biomolecules at the surface of the nanoparticles at pH values that must be different from the isoelectric point of the protein (at this pH, the protein has a net charge equal to zero) and obviously of the nanoparticles. In this type of linkage, however, there is a strong dependence of the interaction on the charge, and therefore either changes in the salinity of the media or variation in pH can strongly affect the stability of the binding. Moreover, often in this configuration, the interaction of the nanoparticle with the antibody occurs on more portions of the antibody molecules, and thus the antibody rearranges in a geometry which is not the optimal configuration for promoting the further binding with the antigen (the antibody, for instance, spreads flat on the nanoparticle surface). The physical adsorption of the antibody on top of the nanoparticles can occur also via hydrophobic interactions. In this case, however, as the hydrophobic portions of the antibody are often not exposed to the environment, the native three-dimensional structure of the antibody is modified, as the antibody rearranges due to its interaction with the nanoparticle surface, with consequent loss of its biological activity (Pavlickova et al. 2004).

Covalent Linkage (Fig. 1.2b) In the covalently linkage strategy, the formation of new chemical bonds which involves the sharing of electron pairs between a functional group present on the nanoparticle and one present on the antibody is considered safer. By looking at the antibodies, different functionalities can be exploited. The choice of the functional groups present on the antibody and on the nanoparticles to be coupled together by covalently linkage can be quite broad and

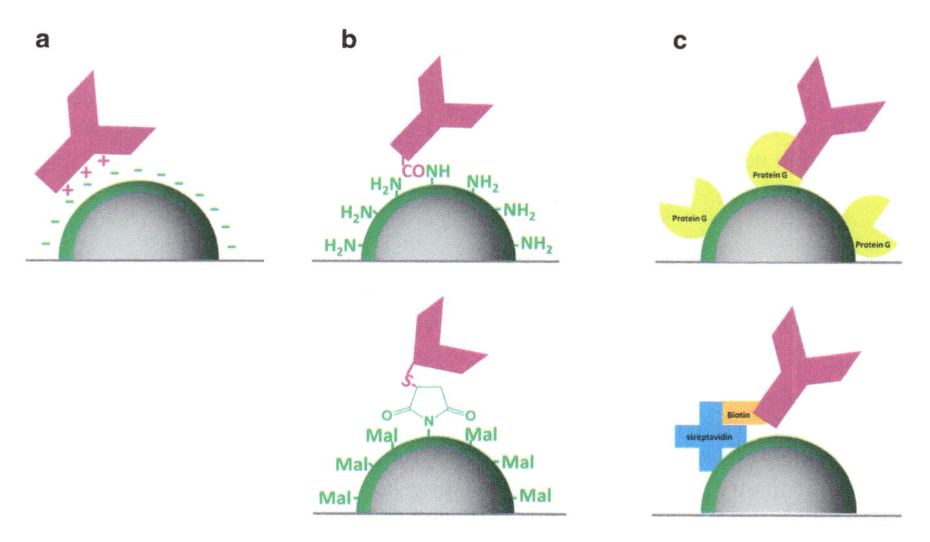

Fig. 1.2 Scheme of the possible binding strategies for the attachment of antibodies to the nanoparticle surface. (**a**) The physical adsorption, (**b**) the covalent linkage, and (**c**) the use of adapter biomolecules

should be well pondered. Usually, while the choice of the functional group on the antibody to be used for the binding to the nanoparticle is more restricted, due to the risk to compromise the binding efficiency of the antibody toward the antigen, the introduction of the proper functional group on the nanoparticle is easier and allows more freedom in the design of the functionalized nanoparticles carrying the proper binding moieties. Among the different coupling chemistries, the amino-carboxyl chemistry is considered the most used and straightforward in aqueous media.

In some works, the primary amino groups of the antibody, either the amino end groups or the ε-amino lysine present all over the antibody proteins, have been used for the coupling reaction. However, the amino-terminated groups are present in the proximity of the antigen binding sites of the antibody, and therefore they are not the most suitable choice. This is because, upon linkage to the nanoparticles, their bulky size might hinder the antigen binding site, with consequent loss of the antigen binding capacity. On the contrary, if amino-functionalized nanoparticles are used, the presence of the carboxyl-terminated functionalities on the Fc region of the antibody (see Fig. 1.1) can be exploited. The Fc region in the 3D configuration of the antibody is quite distant from the antigen binding site, and it is not involved in the binding with the antigen. To amino-bearing nanoparticles, together with the carboxyl-terminated functional group of the antibody, also carboxyl-bearing amino acid (i.e., glutamic and aspartic acid) residues of the antibody may react. However, given the bulky structure of the three-dimensional configuration of the protein, the carboxyl-terminated groups are more exposed than the carboxyl-bearing amino acids included into the antibody structure, thus allowing the attachment of the antibody to the nanoparticle on the Fc region and thus having the right orientation.

On the Fc region of the antibody, also the carbohydrate chains placed on the C2H chains can be considered as possible anchoring points for the reaction with amino- or hydrazine-functionalized nanoparticles. Indeed, upon a mild oxidation of the sugar chains, the aldehyde-activated carbohydrates can be coupled to the amino-bearing nanoparticles via condensation reaction (Puertas et al. 2010) and a further reduction step. This method however requires a modification of the antibody, but at least the coupling chemistry takes place farther away from the antigen binding site.

Among the different sites on the antibody which have been exploited for the coupling to nanoparticles, also the thiol (-SH) chemistry of the cysteine residues of the antibody protein chains can be considered suitable anchoring points. The thiol groups in a protein contribute to the ternary structure via the sulfur–sulfur (S-S) bridge formation of each of the protein subunits, and they join also the light and the heavy chains and the antibody fragments at the hinge region. The latter can be selectively cleaved to thiol groups by reducing agents such as mercaptoethanolamine or dithiothreitol and thus can be coupled to nanoparticles which carry functional groups reactive toward SH moieties (via, for instance, maleimide chemistry to cite one example). In this case however, a pre-modification of the protein is required. This type of chemistry has been shown to be suitable not only with whole antibodies but also with antibody fragments, as, for instance, the Fc or the scFc fragments (see Fig. 1.1). In one interesting study, the comparison of tumor targeting when using anti-HER2 either whole or half-chain antibody or scFv fragment targeted iron oxide nanocrystals suggested that the longer period of accumulation of the scFv-functionalized iron oxide nanocrystals makes them ideal for breast cancer. A conclusion of the work was that the advantage of using a fragment with respect to the whole antibody resides mainly in the reduced size of the final scFv-iron oxide conjugates: the smaller size and thus the better stability in physiological conditions are likely the reasons why a higher tumor targeting in vivo could be achieved (Fiandra et al. 2013).

The Use of an Adapter Complex (Fig. 1.2c) Alternatively, the antibody can be attached to the nanoparticle via spacer (bio)molecules. The most common approach is based on the use of streptavidin-biotin or avidin-biotin couple, as the binding affinities of the biotin-(strept)avidin are among the highest values known for proteins ($K = 10^{-14} \times 10^{-15}$ M). In this case, either the biotin or the streptavidin needs to be attached to the nanoparticles, and the biotin derivatization of the antibody is also required. The streptavidin can work as the bridging molecule placed in between the biotinylated nanoparticles and the biotinylated antibody (streptavidin has four binding sites for protein), or it can be directly attached to the nanoparticles and thus directly link the antibody previously modified with biotin. In both cases, a modification of the antibody with biotin is required, either to the SH chemistry of the hinge region or via the carbohydrate moieties of the Fc region (Park et al. 2011; Cho et al. 2007).

Another option for protein spacer is represented by the use of secondary antibodies. In this case, the secondary antibody (or a fragment of it) is able to recognize the Fc portion of the antibody (called the primary antibody) that is intended to be attached to the nanoparticle surface. As the interaction between the secondary and primary antibodies follows a precise orientation at the binding site, the final product could definitely maintain the right antigen binding affinity. A critical prerequisite is however that the secondary antibody (or a fragment of the secondary antibody) is attached to the nanoparticles with the proper orientation. Moreover, it must be monoclonal, which means that it can bind only one primary antibody. This avoids the aggregation at the step where the primary antibody is added. To provide some examples, proteins G and A are bacteria proteins which can bind to the Fc region of the Ig antibody. Protein A (spaBC3, about 10 kDa) is capable of capturing tightly the Fc fragment of anti-HER-2 monoclonal IgG antibody (trastuzumab) and in the optimal orientation for binding to epidermal growth factor receptor HER2 (Mazzucchelli et al. 2010).

In this respect, it is important to comment about the size of the antibody: indeed, the linkage of the nanoparticles to the whole antibody or to fragments bears advantages and disadvantages. First of all, whole antibodies have a large size, up to 15 nm in diameter, which is comparable to that of nanoparticles. And when attaching several proteins to the same nanoparticles, the stability of the bionanocomplex can be compromised. Moreover, the difference in stiffness between the hard core of the nanoparticle and a more soft one for the protein can also play a role on the stability of the final complex, especially when several flexible molecules (as antibodies) can link to the hard core of the inorganic nanoparticles, affecting the in vivo circulation and biodistribution. One recent study has investigated the role of density of antibody molecules at the nanoparticle surface on the binding toward the antigen: by increasing the number of antibody molecules, the spatial accessibility of the antigen is reduced due steric hindrance and thus results in lower affinity (Puertas et al. 2010). On the contrary, with small peptides at the surface of gold nanoparticles, a higher affinity was found toward the specific target on cells. This might be explained by the higher density of peptide molecules per nanometer squared of nanoparticle, which ensured for a multidentate binding toward their target. On the other hand, the peptides are too small to interfere with each other even when packed at the nanocrystal surface (Bartczak et al. 2011). It might be speculated that the better in vivo targeting results obtained by Prosperi for small fragments attached to the iron oxide nanoparticle, in comparison to the whole antibodies, might be related to this higher avidity of the Fc-functionalized nanoparticles (Fiandra et al. 2013).

Moreover, often it has been observed that the penetration to the tumor of the whole antibody with respect to the fragment is reduced because of its size. Fab and scFv are considerably smaller (as they have smaller molecular weight) and display almost the same affinity and specificity of the whole antibodies, thus facilitating their binding to the nanocrystal surface. On the other hand, they have reduced avidity, and the production costs are still too high.

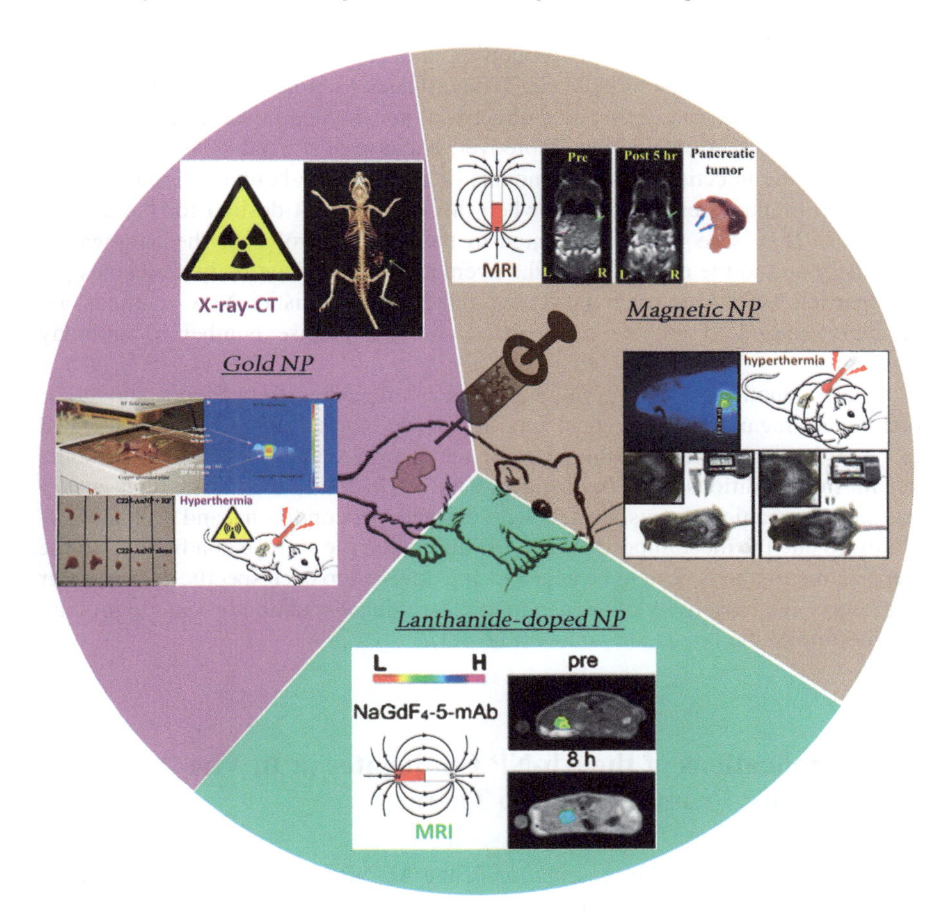

Fig. 1.3 The cartoon presents the most significant diagnostic and therapeutic applications of the antibody-nanoparticle formulations in tumor models. The image is divided into three segments, one per each type of nanoparticles, i.e., magnetic-, gold-, and lanthanide-doped nanoparticles. In the case of magnetic nanoparticles, MR imaging and magnetic hyperthermia are the most promising applications. Images of the cartoon are adapted from Yang et al. (2009) and Li et al. (2013), respectively. In the case of gold nanocrystals, imaging through X-ray-CT [image adapted from Reuveni et al. (2011)] and therapy by means of radio-frequency-mediated hyperthermia [adapted from Glazer et al. (2010)] are under investigation. Finally, lanthanide-doped nanocrystals are emerging as new MRI tools [adapted from Hou et al. (2013)]

Overall, we can summarize that, in the construction of inorganic nanoparticle antibody or antibody fragment formulations, the density and the orientation of the antibody per nanoparticles are the two main parameters which need to be controlled for achieving the optimal performance of the resulting conjugates.

An additional aspect to be considered regards the immunological compatibility between the antibody and the host organism in which the antibody (either free or bound to the nanoparticles) will be injected. Chimeric antibodies represent fusion proteins with different functional properties, and, if properly engineered, also their immune response can be modulated. Today, thanks to biotechnological advances, chimeric antibodies can be prepared directly, although the production costs for such materials are not affordable yet. Moreover, because of the native function of the antibodies, the injection of large amounts of nanoparticle-bound antibodies could trigger an immune response, even when this effect is not desired for therapeutic purposes. This issue is strictly related to the poor control over the conjugation chemistry and to the estimation of the average number of antibody molecules per nanoparticle, which is often presumed rather than realistic. New methods are certainly needed to prepare nanoparticles with a precise number of antibody molecules.

Finally, another critical point, which is often underestimated but should be mentioned, regards the biological fragility of the biomolecules. Precautions need to be undertaken when handling free or nanoparticle-bound antibodies, as some denaturing conditions need be avoided. The list includes the use of high-energy radiations, organic solvents, buffers with extreme pH conditions, and high temperatures, to cite the most important ones. Additionally, the storage conditions and the sterilization methods need to be assessed and adjusted to each specific case in order to preserve the bioactivity of the nanoparticle-conjugated antibodies and to prolong the lifetime of the bound antibodies (Fig. 1.3).

1.6 Applications of the Ab-NP Conjugates in In Vivo Studies: From Imaging to Therapy

Before proceeding with the presentation of the Ab-NP-based applicative studies, a brief premise will follow in order to frame the overview of this section. The term "in vivo" is generally referred to studies performed with living whole animals, preferably mammals, in which structure and organization of the organs, progression of diseases, and the overall response to an external treatment can be associated to those of humans. In vivo testing is a crucial and indispensable step for the validation of new pharmaceuticals and to provide new medical insights prior to clinical testing. Mice are the most commonly used animal models in research because of the low cost, ease of handling, availability, and short life, which allows to monitor the effects of a treatment on a reasonable time scale. On the other hand, cancer is certainly the most studied human disease, at both clinical and preclinical levels because of its high incidence and uncertain prognosis. Despite improved understanding of cancer biology and significant progress in detection technologies and therapeutic protocols, major concerns are due to late and invasive cancer diagnosis, poor efficacy of the therapies, and high percentage of relapse (DePinho 2000; Hahn and Weinberg 2002; Sherr 2004). Most of the current treatments cannot discriminate between tumor and healthy cells, leading to systemic toxicity and low accumulation of the treating agents at the target site.

In this context, monoclonal antibodies can bring significant benefits: the development and the engineering of antibodies that target specifically tumor biomarkers, i.e., those receptors or biomolecules which are overexpressed or expressed only at the surface of tumor cells, can greatly enhance drug delivery efficiency and thus therapeutic effectiveness. As already described in the previous sections, also inorganic nanoparticles contribute to the technological revolution that can improve cancer diagnosis and therapy. Therefore, it is not surprising that most of the recent in vivo studies performed with Ab-conjugated nanoparticles aim to evaluate their functionality and most specifically their diagnostic/therapeutic potential in rodent tumor models. In particular, these works are focused to achieve and demonstrate the three following objectives, either independently or simultaneously: (1) the targeting efficiency, (2) the diagnostic relevance, and (3) the therapeutic effect of the Ab-derived nanocomplexes.

Tumor active targeting is not straightforward and can be affected by several factors, such as the type of biomarker to target (i.e., its tumor-related specificity and the level of expression at the tumor site), the binding ability of the NP-bound antibody, the size and the stability of the nanocomplex, the type of tumor and its location, and the administration route. An interesting study on the targeting is the work of Glazer and co-workers in which gold nanoparticles were functionalized with either cetuximab or PAM4 antibodies (Glazer et al. 2010). The first is a recombinant biomolecule against the epidermal growth factor receptor (EGFR), which is overexpressed in several malignancies and is present even on healthy cells, while the second is an antibody against a specific pancreatic cancer antigen (MUC1). Mice bearing a xenograft pancreatic tumor were first injected with the Ab-NP and then exposed to radio frequencies (RF, 13.56 MHz, 600 W generator power for 10 min with an air gap of 10 cm) in order to trigger Au-mediated tumor thermal ablation. Subsequent to nanoparticles injection, RF exposure occurred one time per week. After 6 weeks of treatment, animals were sacrificed. The measurements of tumor volume showed that cetuximab-conjugated Au-NPs were more effective in tumor regression than PAM-conjugated counterparts, likely because EGFR, despite its low tumor specificity, is expressed on tumor cells at higher amounts than MUC1, thus enabling better targeting.

Interesting in vivo studies have been carried out to evaluate the effect of the tumor binding as a function of the antibody–nanoparticle molecular weights; in some cases, the whole antibody was attached to the NP and compared to the use of fragments of the same antibody. In a very recent study, for instance, the human epidermal growth factor receptor (HER2) was selected as biological target, and three anti-HER2 antibody variants were conjugated to iron oxide nanoparticles bearing a fluorescent moiety (Fiandra et al. 2013). In detail, a whole recombinant antibody, trastuzumab (TZ), a half-chain antibody (HC), and a single-chain variable fragment (scFv), respectively, were bound to the NPs in order to evaluate the effect of the antibody size on the tumor targeting ability of the whole nanocomplex. The data collected showed that NP-HC and NP-scFv were endocytosed by HER2-expressing cells faster than NP-TZ. Moreover, measurement of the NP retention time at the tumor site in breast cancer models confirmed that the two antibody variant nanocomplexes were retained for longer time and the fluorescent signal did not decrease over time, as instead occurred with the NP-TZ. This is likely due to a better and prompter interaction of the smaller nanostructures with the membrane receptor, thus resulting in a more efficient tumor targeting. The authors also claimed that the large size of the whole antibody may affect the stability of the bionanocomplex which tends to form aggregates, thus finally reducing the ability to bind the target.

In a previous work from the same group, NP-TZ were injected in tumor-bearing mice: the accumulation at the tumor site and the biodistribution were evaluated by epifluorescence, MRI, and postmortem TEM and histological analysis (Corsi et al. 2011). Remarkably, immunohistochemical analysis of extracted tumor tissues showed that NP-TZ saturated HER2 molecules on the surface, thus suggesting their exploitation as adjuvant immunotherapeutic agent in cancer treatment.

Cancer adjuvant therapy with monoclonal antibodies has been already established for several malignancies, and their combination with inorganic nanoparticles can undoubtedly enhance the potential use, enabling simultaneously targeting, imaging, and therapy. This is the encouraging perspective provided by the group of Mao, which developed iron oxide nanoparticles conjugated to an EGFRvIII deletion mutant antibody for targeting glioblastoma (Hadjipanayis et al. 2010). This variant form of the receptor is expressed in malignant gliomas but not in normal cells, thus making targeting highly selective. In order to facilitate BBB penetration, convection-enhanced delivery (CED) was applied. The results provided evidence that, once in the brain, the anti-EGFRvIII NP not only targeted cancer cells and allowed MRI contrast enhancement but most significantly elicited tumor reduction by means of EGFR signaling interruption. Indeed, the authors supposed that binding of the NP to the EGF receptor results in reduced phosphorylation of the downstream proteins and thus in apoptosis induction.

In a very recent paper, tumor regression was obtained through a more complex and promising approach, i.e., through combined magnetic hyperthermia and chemotherapy (Li et al. 2013). A multifunctional nanostructure consisting of a magnetite core loaded with the anticancer drug 5-fluorouracil (5-FU) and functionalized with anti-HER2 antibody was developed. The nanoparticles were injected either intratumorally or in the tail vein in a bladder cancer mouse model. In both cases, the combination of hyperthermia and synchronized local chemotherapy was more effective in cancer regression than the individual treatment. Although these results are extremely encouraging, it is worth to mention that the radio-frequency parameters used in this work (1.3 MHz radio frequencies and 33 kA/m magnetic field) to activate the thermal response were out of the clinical relevance range for patients. For application on humans, lower radio frequencies (within the range 80–200 KHz and maximum 30 KA/m) need to be used to prevent deleterious side effects, and therefore new nanoparticle formulations with optimal heating performance have to be prepared. Almost all the other in vivo studies performed with Ab-conjugated NPs were focused to cancer targeting, to analyze nanoparticle biodistribution and in some cases to assess cancer imaging ability, as reported in Table 1.1.

Table 1.1 Ab-conjugated nanoparticles: brief overview of the type of nanoparticles and antibodies used and their in vivo applications

Type of NP	Ab/Ab fragment	Biological target	In vivo application	Reference
Iron oxide	Trastuzumab	HER2	Targeting and imaging (by means of epifluorescene) of xenograft breast cancer Potential immunotheranostic	Corsi et al. (2011)
Iron oxide	Anti-EGFRvIII	EGFR variant III	CED-enhanced MR imaging and therapy of glioblastoma	Hadjipanayis et al. (2010)
Iron oxide	T84.1	Carcinoembryonic antigen-related cell adhesion molecule (CEACAM)	MR imaging of xenografted mouse model of cancer	Poeselt et al. (2012)
Iron oxide	A7 mAb	Colon-rectal cancer glycoprotein	MR imaging of rectal carcinoma	Toma et al. (2005)
Fe_3O_4	Anti HER2	HER2	Hyperthemia combined with drug delivery (5-fluorouracil) to non-orthotopic bladder cancer	Li et al. (2013)
Iron oxide	scFv-EGFR	EGFR	Targeted MR imaging of an orthotopic pancreatic cancer xenograft model	Yang et al. (2009)
Iron oxide	Trastuzumab half-chain anti-HER2 scFv-HER2	HER2	Targeting and imaging (by means of epifluorescene) of xenograft breast cancer	Fiandra et al. (2013)
Iron oxide	Anti HER2	HER2	Targeting of breast cancer and metastasis in transgenic mice	Kievit et al. (2012)
FePt	Anti HER2	HER2	CT and MR imaging of transplanted bladder tumor in mice	Chou et al. (2010)
Gold	Cetuximab PAM4	EGFR-1 MUC-1	RF therapy of xenograft pancreatic tumor	Glazer et al. (2010)
Gold	Cetuximab	EGFR	Targeting of orthotopic pancreatic tumor	Khan et al. (2011)
Gold	Anti HER2	HER2	CT imaging of breast tumor implanted in the mouse thigh	Hainfeld et al. (2011)
Gold	Anti EGFR	EGFR	Targeting and CT imaging of squamous cell carcinoma head and	Reuveni et al. (2011)

(continued)

Table 1.1 (continued)

Type of NP	Ab/Ab fragment	Biological target	In vivo application	Reference
			neck tumor implanted in the mouse back flank	
Gold	Anti CD4	CD4	X-ray CT imaging of mouse lymph nodes	Eck et al. (2010)
$NaGdF_4$	Anti-EGFR	EGFR	MR imaging of intraperitoneal tumor xenograft	Hou et al. (2013), Liu et al. (2013)

MRI is a noninvasive and nonionizing imaging technique, routinely used in clinic, with high anatomic resolution. Moreover, the advent of contrast agents such as iron oxide nanoparticles enabled to detect and discriminate diseased tissues from healthy ones. When the imaging probes are also specifically tailored to the target site, imaging becomes more accurate, and the signal is retained for longer time due to the specific antibody-receptor interaction (Yang et al. 2009; Poeselt et al. 2012; Kievit et al. 2012; Toma et al. 2005). Superparamagnetic iron oxide nanoparticles are known as T2 contrast agents and produce darkening of the imaged area. On the other hand, recently NaGdF4 nanoparticles have been used as T1-imaging probes, thanks to the paramagnetic nature of Gd: in this case, contrast is provided as lightening of the targeted area (Hou et al. 2013; Liu et al. 2013).

On the other hand, X-ray computed tomography (CT) is an ionizing imaging technique that uses X-rays to produce 3D anatomic information about tumor location and is considered complementary to MRI. Recently, targeted gold nanoparticles were developed as CT contrast agents to image various types of malignancies, such as squamous cell carcinoma (Reuveni et al. 2011), breast tumor (Hainfeld et al. 2011), and peripheral lymph nodes (Eck et al. 2010).

Furthermore, a contrast agent that may act as a dual imaging probe, enabling both CT and MR imaging, would bring great benefits to the diagnosis of diseases, like cancer, as it would combine the optimal bone reconstruction of CT with the soft tissue resolution of MRI. Thus, it could help to reconstruct the localization and the volume of the tumor mass with higher precision, reducing costs and time of the diagnosis. To this aim, the group of Chen developed FePt nanoparticles conjugated to anti-HER2 antibody (Chou et al. 2010). Since Pt has a high X-ray absorption coefficient, these nanoparticles were explored as dual imaging probes. The nanoparticles were injected in the tail vein of mice bearing transplanted bladder tumor. MRI and CT imaging of the tumor region were performed before and 24 h after NP injection showing a considerable enhancement of the contrast at tumor site for both imaging techniques and with enhanced contrast in both techniques for the targeted nanoprobes (Chou et al. 2010). This work represents one of the first studies in this direction, and further investigations need to be undertaken to validate such dual systems.

It is worthy of notice that EGFR is the most frequently chosen biological target, likely because it is highly expressed on the membrane of several types of cancer

(Mendelsohn and Baselga 2000), thus making the anti-EGFR Ab-conjugated nanoparticles generally exploitable in cancer diagnosis/therapy (Fiandra et al. 2013; Glazer et al. 2010; Corsi et al. 2011; Hadjipanayis et al. 2010; Li et al. 2013; Yang et al. 2009; Kievit et al. 2012; Hou et al. 2013; Reuveni et al. 2011; Hainfeld et al. 2011; Chou et al. 2010; Khan et al. 2011). On the other hand, EGFR targeting may result less selective because it is also expressed on normal cells, though at less extent. Also carcinoembryonic antigen-related cell adhesion molecule (CEACAM), colon-rectal cancer glycoprotein, and mucin 1 (MUC1) were reported as tumor-related antigens and selected as targeting molecules (Glazer et al. 2010; Poeselt et al. 2012; Toma et al. 2005). As a general remark, the ideal antigen candidate should be expressed only at the tumor site, at high amount and during all the steps of tumor growth, but so far these three points have been never satisfied, because tumor biomarkers are generally constitutive proteins whose expression becomes altered after tumor transformation but is not exclusive. Variant tumor-specific forms of these proteins also exist but are not common to all tumors, thus making their use as biomarker limited.

1.7 Fate of the Nanobioconjugate In Vivo: Immunogenicity, Toxicity, Biodegradability, and Clearance

Antibodies, both native and recombinant, are rapidly cleared by the blood flow and are not intrinsically toxic, unless they are conjugated to cytotoxic drugs for therapeutic purposes (Adams and Weiner 2005; Chari 2008).

Obviously, also the distribution and pharmacokinetic, when the antibodies are bound to the nanoparticles, are substantially different from those of the free antibodies. It was found that the distribution and pharmacokinetic are mainly guided by the inorganic core. Although antibody-tailored nanoparticles reach the target site more efficiently than the nude nanoparticles, which reduces nonspecific distribution, it is generally recognized that sequestration by the reticuloendothelial system (RES) is unavoidable when they are injected in the blood stream.

In vivo toxicity may arise after accumulation in organs, like liver, spleen, kidney, and lung, followed by the attempt to metabolize the nanoparticles and the release from the latter of toxic elements (from the core) and compounds (from the organic shell) that may trigger oxidative stress, inflammatory responses, and finally tissue damage (Soenen et al. 2011; Sharifi et al. 2012). Production of ROS and the following generation of free radicals is one of the mechanisms of nanoparticle-induced oxidative stress (Møller et al. 2010). This process can occur spontaneously in the case of metal oxide nanoparticles or after interaction with cell organelles in the case of inert materials (Xia et al. 2006).

As a general remark, the size of the whole antibody–nanoparticle, the shape, and the surface stealthiness affect the biodistribution, the circulating time of the nanoparticles, and thus the interaction with tissues and cells. On the other hand, the composition of the inorganic core and the chemistry of the coating determine the biodegradation, i.e., the products derived from the nanoparticle degradation and the eventual toxic response to these products, and thus the overall biocompatibility of the nanoparticles.

Since iron oxide nanoparticles are the model system most commonly used in biotargeting studies for either imaging or therapy, we will focus on them and on the recent findings about their behavior once injected in living animals. The biocompatibility of iron oxide nanoparticles is one of the intrinsic features which speeded up their exploitation in vivo with respect to other magnetic nanoparticles containing non-iron heavy metals (such as Pt, Co). It has been demonstrated that Fe can be metabolized by intracellular enzymatic machinery and recycled in hemoglobin and in iron transport/storage proteins, such as transferrin and ferritin (Weissleder et al. 1989; Pouliquen et al. 1991). This process has been reported in Kupffer cells, the liver macrophages devoted to filter and hold foreign bodies circulating in the blood, and can be associated to temporary stress. Indeed, measures of liver enzymes showed an increase of transaminases (Gu et al. 2012; Jain et al. 2008) soon after nanoparticle injection, likely due to oxidative stress derived from the degradation of the organic shell, that may contain surfactants and polymers. The degradation process is quite slow and also depends on the particle size: small nanoparticles (5 nm diameter) are degraded within 1 month and cleared faster than larger ones (around 20 nm). Even the spleen is involved in the degradation of the injected nanoparticles: macrophages of the red pulp internalize the nanoparticles through endocytosis and transfer them to the lysosomes where they are degraded. Magnetic measurements confirmed that Fe is converted in ionic form and loses its superparamagnetic behavior (Levy et al. 2011). Interestingly, the efficiency of the transformation process depends on the amount of nanoparticles injected and is limited by the capacity of Fe degradation. The remaining nanoparticles were stored intact into the lysosomes up to several months. Body weight measurements and histopathological analysis did not show evident signs of stress and tissue damage.

Thus, we can conclude that IONPs are well tolerated, they can be slowly degraded by the body enzymes, and temporary toxicity may derive from the organic coating. On the other hand, studies with gold nanoparticles reached controversial conclusions (Sharifi et al. 2012). Although the gold nanoparticles are largely exploited as diagnostic and therapeutic tools, few data are available about their biodegradability and biocompatibility in vivo. Furthermore, the literature data depict a fragmented view of the toxicity effects. Recent works in which mice were injected with gold nanoparticles showed that the biodistribution is size and shape dependent and most importantly provided evidence of liver and spleen sufferance (i.e., increase of the number of macrophages, inflammation, and apoptosis) (Khlebtsov and Dykman 2011). It has been also observed that several genes involved in apoptosis and in the stress response were rapidly activated soon after injection when the histopathological examinations did not indicate any pathological response. Conversely, other studies reported either no toxicity or size-dependent toxic effects. Such opposite outcomes are likely related to the testing conditions that differ not only for the type of nanoparticle used but also for the administered amount and the administration routes (Chen et al. 2009; Lasagna-Reeves et al. 2010).

In conclusion, any type of antibody–nanoparticle formulation requires a thorough and definite analysis of the health impact. It is noteworthy that cellular studies are only the first step of the safety evaluation that needs to move to animal testing to assess the effects at the whole organism level. Furthermore, standard protocols and toxicity assays should be internationally defined in order to achieve a comparable overview of the literature data and an exhaustive comprehension of the safety impact.

References

Adams GP, Weiner LM (2005) Monoclonal antibody therapy of cancer. Nat Biotechnol 23: 1147–1157. doi:10.1035/nbt1137

Aime S, Castelli DD, Crich SG, Gianolio E, Terreno E (2009) Pushing the sensitivity envelope of lanthanide-based magnetic resonance imaging (MRI) contrast agents for molecular imaging applications. Acc Chem Res 42:822–831. doi:10.1021/ar800192p

Algar WR et al (2011) The controlled display of biomolecules on nanoparticles: a challenge suited to bioorthogonal chemistry. Bioconjug Chem 22:825–858. doi:10.1021/bc200065z

Alivisatos AP (1996) Semiconductor clusters, nanocrystals, and quantum dots. Science 271: 933–937

Amit AG, Mariuzza RA, Phillips SEV, Poljak RJ (1986) 3-Dimensional structure of an antigen-antibody complex at 2.8-A resolution. Science 233:747–753. doi:10.1126/science.2426778

Baca M, Presta LG, Oconnor SJ, Wells JA (1997) Antibody humanization using monovalent phage display. J Biol Chem 272:10678–10684

Bartczak D, Sanchez-Elsner T, Louafi F, Millar TM, Kanaras AG (2011) Receptor-mediated interactions between colloidal gold nanoparticles and human umbilical vein endothelial cells. Small 7:388–394. doi:10.1002/smll.201001816

Batra SK, Jain M, Wittel UA, Chauhan SC, Colcher D (2002) Pharmacokinetics and biodistribution of genetically engineered antibodies. Curr Opin Biotechnol 13:603–608. doi:10.1016/s0958-1669(02)00352-x

Bruggemann M, Taussig MJ (1997) Production of human antibody repertoires in transgenic mice. Curr Opin Biotechnol 8:455–458. doi:10.1016/s0958-1669(97)80068-7

Brust M, Walker M, Bethell D, Schiffrin DJ, Whyman R (1994) Synthesis of thiol-derivatized gold nanoparticles in a 2-phase liquid-liquid system. J Chem Soc Chem Commun 7:801–802

Chan AC, Carter PJ (2010) Therapeutic antibodies for autoimmunity and inflammation. Nat Rev Immunol 10:301–316. doi:10.1038/nri2761

Chari RVJ (2008) Targeted cancer therapy: conferring specificity to cytotoxic drugs. Acc Chem Res 41:98–107. doi:10.1021/ar700108g

Chen Y-S, Hung Y-C, Liau I, Huang G (2009) Assessment of the in vivo toxicity of gold nanoparticles. Nanoscale Res Lett 4:858–864

Cherukuri P, Glazer ES, Curleya SA (2010) Targeted hyperthermia using metal nanoparticles. Adv Drug Deliv Rev 62:339–345. doi:10.1016/j.addr.2009.11.006

Chithrani BD, Chan WCW (2007) Elucidating the mechanism of cellular uptake and removal of protein-coated gold nanoparticles of different sizes and shapes. Nano Lett 7:1542–1550. doi:10.1021/nl070363y

Cho I-H et al (2007) Site-directed biotinylation of antibodies for controlled immobilization of solid surfaces. Anal Biochem 365:14–23. doi:10.1016/j.ab.2007.02.028
Chou S-W et al (2010) In vitro and in vivo studies of FePt nanoparticles for dual modal CT/MRI molecular imaging. J Am Chem Soc 132:13270–13278. doi:10.1021/ja1035013
Corot C, Robert P, Idee JM, Port M (2006) Recent advances in iron oxide nanocrystal technology for medical imaging. Adv Drug Deliv Rev 58:1471–1504. doi:10.1016/j.addr.2006.09.013
Corsi F et al (2011) HER2 expression in breast cancer cells is downregulated upon active targeting by antibody-engineered multifunctional nanoparticles in mice. ACS Nano 5:6383–6393. doi:10.1021/nn201570n
Daniel MC, Astruc D (2004) Gold nanoparticles: assembly, supramolecular chemistry, quantum-size-related properties, and applications toward biology, catalysis, and nanotechnology. Chem Rev 104:293–346. doi:10.1021/cr030698+
Davies DR, Padlan EA, Sheriff S (1990) Antibody-antigen complexes. Annu Rev Biochem 59: 439–473. doi:10.1146/annurev.biochem.59.1.439
Delehanty JB, Mattoussi H, Medintz IL (2009) Delivering quantum dots into cells: strategies, progress and remaining issues. Anal Bioanal Chem 393:1091–1105. doi:10.1007/s00216-008-2410-4
DePinho RA (2000) The age of cancer. Nature (London) 408:248–254. doi:10.1038/35041694
Derfus AM, Chan WCW, Bhatia SN (2004) Probing the cytotoxicity of semiconductor quantum dots. Nano Lett 4:11–18. doi:10.1021/nl0347334
Di Corato R et al (2008) Water solubilization of hydrophobic nanocrystals by means of poly (maleic anhydride-alt-1-octadecene). J Mater Chem 18:1991–1996. doi:10.1039/b717801h
Dougan M, Dranoff G (2009) Immune therapy for cancer. Annu Rev Immunol 27:83–117
Dubertret B et al (2002) In vivo imaging of quantum dots encapsulated in phospholipid micelles. Science 298:1759–1762
Eck W, Nicholson AI, Zentgraf H, Semmler W, Bartling S (2010) Anti-CD4-targeted gold nanoparticles induce specific contrast enhancement of peripheral lymph nodes in X-ray computed tomography of live mice. Nano Lett 10:2318–2322. doi:10.1021/nl101019s
Fiandra L et al (2013) Assessing the in vivo targeting efficiency of multifunctional nanoconstructs bearing antibody-derived ligands. ACS Nano 7:6092–6102. doi:10.1021/nn4018922
Figuerola A, Di Corato R, Manna L, Pellegrino T (2010) From iron oxide nanoparticles towards advanced iron-based inorganic materials designed for biomedical applications. Pharmacol Res 62:126–143
Gao JH, Gu HW, Xu B (2009) Multifunctional magnetic nanoparticles: design, synthesis, and biomedical applications. Acc Chem Res 42:1097–1107. doi:10.1021/ar9000026
Glazer ES et al (2010) Noninvasive radiofrequency field destruction of pancreatic adenocarcinoma xenografts treated with targeted gold nanoparticles. Clin Cancer Res 16:5712–5721. doi:10.1158/1078-0432.ccr-10-2055
Gu L, Fang RH, Sailor MJ, Park J-H (2012) In vivo clearance and toxicity of monodisperse iron oxide nanocrystals. ACS Nano 6:4947–4954. doi:10.1021/nn300456z
Haase M, Schaefer H (2011) Upconverting nanoparticles. Angew Chem Int Ed 50:5808–5829. doi:10.1002/anie.201005159
Hadjipanayis CG et al (2010) EGFRvIII antibody-conjugated iron oxide nanoparticles for magnetic resonance imaging-guided convection-enhanced delivery and targeted therapy of glioblastoma. Cancer Res 70:6303–6312. doi:10.1158/0008-5472.can-10-1022
Hahn WC, Weinberg RA (2002) Modelling the molecular circuitry of cancer. Nat Rev Cancer 2:331–341. doi:10.1038/nrc795
Hainfeld JF, O'Connor MJ, Dilmanian FA, Slatkin DN, Adams DJ (2011) Micro-CT enables microlocalisation and quantification of Her2-targeted gold nanoparticles within tumour regions. Br J Radiol 84:526–533. doi:10.1259/bjr/42612922
Hauck TS, Ghazani AA, Chan WCW (2008) Assessing the effect of surface chemistry on gold nanorod uptake, toxicity, and gene expression in mammalian cells. Small 4:153–159. doi:10.1002/smll.200700217

Hezinger AFE, Tessmar J, Gopferich A (2008) Polymer coating of quantum dots—a powerful tool toward diagnostics and sensorics. Eur J Pharm Biopharm 68:138–152. doi:10.1016/j.ejpb.2007.05.013

Hou Y et al (2013) NaGdF4 nanoparticle-based molecular probes for magnetic resonance imaging of intraperitoneal tumor xenografts in vivo. ACS Nano 7:330–338. doi:10.1021/nn304837c

Huang XH, El-Sayed IH, Qian W, El-Sayed MA (2006) Cancer cell imaging and photothermal therapy in the near-infrared region by using gold nanorods. J Am Chem Soc 128:2115–2120. doi:10.1021/ja057254a

Hudson PJ, Souriau C (2003) Engineered antibodies. Nat Med 9:129–134. doi:10.1038/nm0103-129

Jain TK, Reddy MK, Morales MA, Leslie-Pelecky DL, Labhasetwar V (2008) Biodistribution, clearance, and biocompatibility of iron oxide magnetic nanoparticles in rats. Mol Pharm 5:316–327. doi:10.1021/mp7001285

Jiang W, Kim BYS, Rutka JT, Chan WCW (2008) Nanoparticle-mediated cellular response is size-dependent. Nat Nanotechnol 3:145–150. doi:10.1038/nnano.2008.30

Ju Q et al (2012) Amine-functionalized lanthanide-doped KGdF4 nanocrystals as potential optical/magnetic multimodal bioprobes. J Am Chem Soc 134:1323–1330. doi:10.1021/ja2102604

Junghanns J, Muller RH (2008) Nanocrystal technology, drug delivery and clinical applications. Int J Nanomedicine 3:295–309

Khan JA et al (2011) Designing nanoconjugates to effectively target pancreatic cancer cells in vitro and in vivo. Plos One 6. doi:10.1371/journal.pone.0020347

Khlebtsov N, Dykman L (2011) Biodistribution and toxicity of engineered gold nanoparticles: a review of in vitro and in vivo studies. Chem Soc Rev 40:1647–1671. doi:10.1039/c0cs00018c

Kievit FM et al (2012) Targeting of primary breast cancers and metastases in a transgenic mouse model using rationally designed multifunctional SPIONs. ACS Nano 6:2591–2601. doi:10.1021/nn205070h

Kirchner C et al (2005) Cytotoxicity of colloidal CdSe and CdSe/ZnS nanoparticles. Nano Lett 5:331–338. doi:10.1021/nl047996m

Kohler G, Milstein C (1975) Continuous cultures of fused cells secreting antibody of predefined specificity. Nature 256:495–497. doi:10.1038/256495a0

Kumar CSSR, Mohammad F (2011) Magnetic nanomaterials for hyperthermia-based therapy and controlled drug delivery. Adv Drug Deliv Rev 63:789–808

Lasagna-Reeves C et al (2010) Bioaccumulation and toxicity of gold nanoparticles after repeated administration in mice. Biochem Biophys Res Commun 393:649–655, http://dx.doi.org/10.1016/j.bbrc.2010.02.046

Lees EE, Nguyen TL, Clayton AHA, Mulvaney P, Muir BW (2009) The preparation of colloidally stable, water-soluble, biocompatible, semiconductor nanocrystals with a small hydrodynamic diameter. ACS Nano 3:1121–1128. doi:10.1021/nn900144n

Levy M et al (2011) Long term in vivo biotransformation of iron oxide nanoparticles. Biomaterials 32:3988–3999. doi:10.1016/j.biomaterials.2011.02.031

Lewinski N, Colvin V, Drezek R (2008) Cytotoxicity of nanoparticles. Small 4:26–49. doi:10.1002/smll.200700595

Li Z, Zhang Y, Shuter B, Idris NM (2009) Hybrid lanthanide nanoparticles with paramagnetic shell coated on upconversion fluorescent nanocrystals. Langmuir 25:12015–12018. doi:10.1021/la903113u

Li T-J et al (2013) In vivo anti-cancer efficacy of magnetite nanocrystal-based system using locoregional hyperthermia combined with 5-fluorouracil chemotherapy. Biomaterials 34:7873–7883. doi:10.1016/j.biomaterials.2013.07.012

Liu Z, Tabakman S, Welsher K, Dai HJ (2009) Carbon nanotubes in biology and medicine: in vitro and in vivo detection, imaging and drug delivery. Nano Res 2:85–120. doi:10.1007/s12274-009-9009-8

Liu C et al (2013) Magnetic/upconversion fluorescent NaGdF4:Yb,Er nanoparticle-based dual-modal molecular probes for imaging tiny tumors in vivo. ACS Nano 7:7227–7240. doi:10.1021/nn4030898
Lu AH, Salabas EL, Schuth F (2007) Magnetic nanoparticles: synthesis, protection, functionalization, and application. Angew Chem Int Ed 46:1222–1244. doi:10.1002/anie.200602866
Mader HS, Kele P, Saleh SM, Wolfbeis OS (2010) Upconverting luminescent nanoparticles for use in bioconjugation and bioimaging. Curr Opin Chem Biol 14:582–596. doi:10.1016/j.cbpa.2010.08.014
Maynard J, Georgiou G (2000) Antibody engineering. Annu Rev Biomed Eng 2:339–376. doi:10.1146/annurev.bioeng.2.1.339
Mazzucchelli S et al (2010) Single-domain protein a-engineered magnetic nanoparticles: toward a universal strategy to site-specific labeling of antibodies for targeted detection of tumor cells. ACS Nano 4:5693–5702. doi:10.1021/nn101307r
Mendelsohn J, Baselga J (2000) The EGF receptor family as targets for cancer therapy. Oncogene 19:6550–6565. doi:10.1038/sj.onc.1204082
Michalet X et al (2005) Quantum dots for live cells, in vivo imaging, and diagnostics. Science 307:538–544
Møller P, Jacobsen NR, Folkmann JK, Danielsen PH, Mikkelsen L (2010) Role of oxidative damage in toxicity of particulates. Free Radic Res 44:1–46. doi:10.3109/10715760903300691
Murray CB, Norris DJ, Bawendi MG (1993) Synthesis and characterization of nearly monodisperse CdE (E = S, Se, Te) semiconductor nanocrystallites. J Am Chem Soc 115:8706–8715. doi:10.1021/ja00072a025
Nel A, Xia T, Madler L, Li N (2006) Toxic potential of materials at the nanolevel. Science 311:622–627. doi:10.1126/science.1114397
Nel AE et al (2009) Understanding biophysicochemical interactions at the nano-bio interface. Nat Mater 8:543–557. doi:10.1038/nmat2442
Neuberger T, Schopf B, Hofmann H, Hofmann M, von Rechenberg B (2005) Superparamagnetic nanoparticles for biomedical applications: possibilities and limitations of a new drug delivery system. J Magn Magn Mater 293:483–496. doi:10.1016/j.jmmm.2005.01.064
Nie S, Xing Y, Kim GJ, Simons JW (2007) Nanotechnology applications in cancer. Annu Rev Biomed Eng 9:257–288
O'Neal DP, Hirsch LR, Halas NJ, Payne JD, West JL (2004) Photo-thermal tumor ablation in mice using near infrared-absorbing nanoparticles. Cancer Lett 209:171–176. doi:10.1016/j.canlet.2004.02.004
Pankhurst QA, Connolly J, Jones SK, Dobson J (2003) Applications of magnetic nanoparticles in biomedicine. J Phys D Appl Phys 36:R167–R181
Papavassiliou GC (1979) Optical properties of small inorganic and organic metal particles. Prog Solid State Chem 12:185
Parak WJ, Manna L, Simmel FC, Gerion D, Alivisatos AP (2004) Nanoparticles—from theory to application: quantum dots. Wiley-VCH, Weinheim
Park J-W, Cho I-H, Moon DW, Paek S-H, Lee TG (2011) ToF-SIMS and PCA of surface-immobilized antibodies with different orientations. Surf Interface Anal 43:285–289. doi:10.1002/sia.3440
Park YI et al (2012) Theranostic probe based on lanthanide-doped nanoparticles for simultaneous in vivo dual-modal imaging and photodynamic therapy. Adv Mater 24:5755–5761. doi:10.1002/adma.201202433
Pavlickova P, Schneider EM, Hug H (2004) Advances in recombinant antibody microarrays. Clin Chim Acta 343:17–35. doi:10.1016/j.cccn.2004.01.009
Pellegrino T et al (2004) Hydrophobic nanocrystals coated with an amphiphilic polymer shell: a general route to water soluble nanocrystals. Nano Lett 4:703–707. doi:10.1021/nl035172j
Poeselt E et al (2012) Tailor-made quantum dot and iron oxide based contrast agents for in vitro and in vivo tumor imaging. ACS Nano 6:3346–3355. doi:10.1021/nn300365m

Poljak RJ (1991) Structure of antibodies and their complexes with antigens. Mol Immunol 28:1341–1345. doi:10.1016/0161-5890(91)90036-j

Pouliquen D, Lejeune JJ, Perdrisot R, Ermias A, Jallet P (1991) Iron-oxide nanoparticles for use as an MRI contrast agent—pharmacokinetics and metabolism. Magn Reson Imaging 9:275–283. doi:10.1016/0730-725x(91)90412-f

Puertas S et al (2010) Designing novel nano-immunoassays: antibody orientation versus sensitivity. J Phys D Appl Phys 43. doi:10.1088/0022-3727/43/47/474012

Qi LF, Gao XH (2008) Quantum dot-amphipol nanocomplex for intracellular delivery and real-time imaging of siRNA. ACS Nano 2:1403–1410. doi:10.1021/nn800280r

Quarta A, Curcio A, Kakwere H, Pellegrino T (2012) Polymer coated inorganic nanoparticles: tailoring the nanocrystal surface for designing nanoprobes with biological implications. Nanoscale 4:3319–3334. doi:10.1039/c2nr30271c

Reuveni T, Motiei M, Romman Z, Popovtzer A, Popovtzer R (2011) Targeted gold nanoparticles enable molecular CT imaging of cancer: an in vivo study. Int J Nanomedicine 6:2859–2864. doi:10.2147/ijn.s25446

Rosenthal SJ, Chang JC, Kovtun O, McBride JR, Tomlinson ID (2011) Biocompatible quantum dots for biological applications. Chem Biol 18:10–24. doi:10.1016/j.chembiol.2010.11.013

Schrand AM, Hens SAC, Shenderova OA (2009) Nanodiamond particles: properties and perspectives for bioapplications. Crit Rev Solid State Mater Sci 34:18–74. doi:10.1080/10408430902831987

Sharifi S et al (2012) Toxicity of nanomaterials. Chem Soc Rev 41:2323–2343. doi:10.1039/c1cs15188f

Shen J, Zhao L, Han G (2013) Lanthanide-doped upconverting luminescent nanoparticle platforms for optical imaging-guided drug delivery and therapy. Adv Drug Deliv Rev 65:744–755. doi:10.1016/j.addr.2012.05.007

Sherr CJ (2004) Principles of tumor suppression. Cell 116:235–246. doi:10.1016/s0092-8674(03)01075-4

Skrabalak SE et al (2008) Gold nanocages: synthesis, properties, and applications. Acc Chem Res 41:1587–1595. doi:10.1021/ar800018v

Smith AM, Duan HW, Mohs AM, Nie SM (2008) Bioconjugated quantum dots for in vivo molecular and cellular imaging. Adv Drug Deliv Rev 60:1226–1240. doi:10.1016/j.addr.2008.03.015

Soenen SJ, Rivera-Gil P, Montenegro J-M, Parak WJ, De Smedt SC (2011) Cellular toxicity of inorganic nanoparticles: common aspects and guidelines for improved nanotoxicity evaluation. Nano Today 6:446–465. doi:10.1016/j.nantod.2011.08.001

Sperling RA, Pellegrino T, Li JK, Chang WH, Parak WJ (2006) Electrophoretic separation of nanoparticles with a discrete number of functional groups. Adv Funct Mater 16:943–948. doi:10.1002/adfm.200500589

Sun SH et al (2004) Monodisperse MFe2O4 (M = Fe, Co, Mn) nanoparticles. J Am Chem Soc 126:273–279. doi:10.1021/ja0380852

Sun C, Lee JSH, Zhang MQ (2008) Magnetic nanoparticles in MR imaging and drug delivery. Adv Drug Deliv Rev 60:1252–1265. doi:10.1016/j.addr.2008.03.018

Talapin DV, Lee JS, Kovalenko MV, Shevchenko EV (2010) Prospects of colloidal nanocrystals for electronic and optoelectronic applications. Chem Rev 110:389–458. doi:10.1021/cr900137k

Tao AR, Habas S, Yang PD (2008) Shape control of colloidal metal nanocrystals. Small 4:310–325. doi:10.1002/smll.200701295

Toma A et al (2005) Monoclonal antibody A7-superparamagnetic iron oxide as contrast agent of MR imaging of rectal carcinoma. Br J Cancer 93:131–136. doi:10.1038/sj.bjc.6602668

Waldmann TA (2003) Immunotherapy: past, present and future. Nat Med 9:269–277. doi:10.1038/nm0303-269

Wang M et al (2009) Immunolabeling and NIR-excited fluorescent imaging of HeLa cells by using NaYF4:Yb,Er upconversion nanoparticles. ACS Nano 3:1580–1586. doi:10.1021/nn900491j

Weissleder R et al (1989) Superparamagnetic iron-oxide—pharmacokinetics and toxicity. Am J Roentgenol 152:167–173

Whitesides GM (2003) The 'right' size in nanobiotechnology. Nat Biotechnol 21:1161–1165

Xia T et al (2006) Comparison of the abilities of ambient and manufactured nanoparticles to induce cellular toxicity according to an oxidative stress paradigm. Nano Lett 6:1794–1807. doi:10.1021/nl061025k

Yang L et al (2009) Single chain epidermal growth factor receptor antibody conjugated nanoparticles for in vivo tumor targeting and imaging. Small 5:235–243. doi:10.1002/smll.200800714

Zhang LJ, Webster TJ (2009) Nanotechnology and nanomaterials: promises for improved tissue regeneration. Nano Today 4:66–80. doi:10.1016/j.nantod.2008.10.014

Zhou J et al (2010) Dual-modality in vivo imaging using rare-earth nanocrystals with near-infrared to near-infrared (NIR-to-NIR) upconversion luminescence and magnetic resonance properties. Biomaterials 31:3287–3295. doi:10.1016/j.biomaterials.2010.01.040

Zrazhevskiy P, Sena M, Gao XH (2010) Designing multifunctional quantum dots for bioimaging, detection, and drug delivery. Chem Soc Rev 39:4326–4354. doi:10.1039/b915139g

Chapter 2
Soft Matter Composites Interfacing with Biomolecules, Cells, and Tissues

Athanassia Athanassiou, Despina Fragouli, Ilker Bayer, Paolo Netti, Loris Rizzello, and Pier Paolo Pompa

2.1 Introduction

The parameters that affect and optimize the interactions at bio/non-biointerfaces are revised and analyzed in this chapter. We focus on soft polymeric materials starting with their critical properties that determine the viability of biological systems in contact with them. In particular, the right combination of surface chemistry, topography, and mechanical properties of the employed materials can generate the ideal interface for the target biological organism. We present the state of the art of the applications of such bio/soft matter composites interactions in tissue engineering for scaffolds and skin wound dressings.

Biocompatible, bioinert polymers are already used as implants in the human body in order to mimic the activity of a body part. The recent challenge though for the research in this field that will be discussed herein is to develop biodegradable scaffolds where specific cells can grow, adhere, proliferate, get vascularized, and eventually develop a tissue. The control of surface topography, chemistry, and mechanical properties in combination with appropriate nanofillers or biological growth factors present in the extracellular matrix can guarantee clinical success to future engineered scaffolds.

In the field of skin wound healing, active dressings that can provide the right conditions for optimized progress of the healing are gaining increasing space. We revise the most recent research efforts in the area, focusing on hydrogel type and electrospun nanofibrous dressings. These two types of materials, due to their

A. Athanassiou (✉) • D. Fragouli • I. Bayer
Central Research Laboratory, Istituto Italiano di Tecnologia, Genova, Italy
e-mail: athanassia.athanassiou@iit.it

P. Netti
Center for Advanced Biomaterials for Health Care, Istituto Italiano di Tecnologia, Napoli, Italy

L. Rizzello • P.P. Pompa
Center for Biomolecular Nanotechnologies, Istituto Italiano di Tecnologia, Lecce, Italy

R. Cingolani (ed.), *Bioinspired Approaches for Human-Centric Technologies*,
DOI 10.1007/978-3-319-04924-3_2, © Springer International Publishing Switzerland 2014

particular mechanical and topographic characteristics, have demonstrated a big potentiality as active wound dressings especially combined with silver or other antimicrobial agents and antibiotics but also extracellular matrix growth factors.

At the end of the chapter, we present a special focus on nanosilver, the most common antibacterial system used so far as filler in the soft composite materials developed for interactions with biological systems.

2.2 Materials' Properties That Determine Bio-interactions Critical for the Ideal Scaffold Design

Two-dimensional polymeric-based surfaces have been used extensively as prototype systems for the study of the growth of diverse cell cultures. These studies are of particular importance since they clarify the influence of the materials' parameters, such as chemistry and surface topography, to the viability of the cells.

The interaction of different artificial surfaces with biomaterials is of high research interest for their utilization in biomedical applications. In fact, bio-interfaces able to control the behavior of biomolecules or cells at various surfaces are promising tools for the investigation of the mechanisms taking place and are of particular interest for the development of medical devices, scaffolds, and other systems. The biointerface functionality is defined by specific physicochemical properties of the materials' surface including not only its mechanical properties and surface topography but also chemical composition, surface energy, and polarity, which together define the surface wettability.

In particular, the mechanical properties of a surface are of great importance on the cell survival, proliferation, adhesion, differentiation, and metabolism. Specifically, cells interact with a surface only if they are able to actively generate force and to transmit this force to the surroundings, sensing thus the passive properties of their environment (Schwarz and Safran 2013). This fact strongly depends on the type of the cells, and indeed, it has been shown that the differentiation of stem cells can be guided by the mechanical properties of the substrate (Fu et al. 2010; Engler et al. 2006); soft matrices can be neurogenic, stiffer matrices myogenic, and rigid matrices are proved to be osteogenic. Furthermore, the growth and movement of cells can be defined by the stiffness of the substrate. Particularly, various types of cells have the ability to migrate along gradients in stiffness of an underlying substrate and this rigidity-guided movement is called "durotaxis" (Lo et al. 2000). For this reason polymeric surfaces with controlled mechanical surface properties have been developed able to elucidate the effect of the mechanical properties on the cells behavior or differentiation, without altering the other critical properties such as surface chemistry and topography (Fu et al. 2010; Best et al. 2013; Palchesko et al. 2012). However, in most cases, it is very difficult to isolate and study exclusively such effect, since this property is often combined with other critical surface parameters (Schmidt et al. 2012; Genchi et al. 2013; Gaharwar et al. 2013).

Surface topography plays a basic role on the immobilization and activity of bioentities. To elucidate the role of surface topography in mediating cell-surface interactions, it is necessary to isolate it from all other parameters (e.g., surface chemistry). A recent study has shown that by modifying the nanotopography of a polymeric surface, the fibroblast cells attachment and spreading can be accurately controlled, and it is enhanced compared to the corresponding flat surfaces (Reynolds et al. 2013). However, the topography but also the chemical composition determine the surface wettability, a combined factor which plays a major role on the interaction with the biomaterials (Ciofani et al. 2013; Siow et al. 2006; Joy et al. 2011; Keselowsky et al. 2005). In fact, the wetting characteristics of a surface affect significantly the adsorption of proteins and the cells attachment and proliferation (Lourenço et al. 2012). Both highly hydrophilic and hydrophilic surfaces may inhibit such interactions, while surfaces with moderate wettability favor the adsorption of proteins, resulting in a positive cell response (Bacakova et al. 2011). However, all types of surface wettability can be useful for applications that deal with interactions with biomaterials, ranging from anti-biofouling materials for the fabrication of artificial blood vessels (Sun et al. 2011) to directed cells growth. In the latter case, various groups have been focused in the development of special surface architectures with controlled wettability (Zelzer et al. 2008; Oliveira et al. 2011; Ueda and Levkin 2013) for the directed cells growth on defined areas.

In particular, there has been a lot of effort for the formation of polymeric surfaces with special wetting properties ranging from superhydrophobic with ultrahigh or ultralow adhesion (Bayer et al. 2011) to superhydrophilic surfaces. This is obtained by modifying the surface roughness and/or the surface chemistry in the whole area or on specific zones using different techniques. A novel way to obtain such type of characteristics is the fabrication of smart polymeric surfaces where the wetting properties can change upon the application of an external stimulus. In most of the cases, such stimuli can be heat or light irradiation resulting thus to a localized effect. For example, surfaces with reversible wettability can be fabricated utilizing thermoresponsive or photoresponsive polymers, such as poly (isopropylacrylamides) (Sun and Qing 2011) or polymers doped with photochromic molecules (Athanassiou et al. 2006). Another way to obtain reversible surface wettability is the fabrication of nanocomposite films with polymers and titanium dioxide nanomaterials. For example, it has been recently reported the possibility to change the surface wettability of such nanocomposite surfaces from hydrophobic to hydrophilic upon UV laser light irradiation (Caputo et al. 2008), and this effect can be further enhanced by inducing a microroughness on the specific surfaces (Caputo et al. 2009). This is attributed to the unique effect of titanium dioxide to change reversibly its surface wetting properties due to oxygen vacancies formed upon UV irradiation resulting in the formation of a hydroxylated surface. The use of laser light for the tuning of the surface wettability of such materials offers the possibility to form localized patterned surfaces with controlled wetting gradients as already presented (Villafiorita Monteleone et al. 2010). An alternative method for the control of the surface chemistry and surface roughness can be also the spraying of nanomaterials of different dimensions on microrough surfaces by using masks with controlled shape, and such process results in the formation of superhydrophobic surfaces with controlled water adhesion, making thus possible the localized interactions with biomaterials on defined areas (Milionis et al. 2013, 2014).

Although surfaces serve as model systems or as biosensors, the actual scaffolds to be implanted in the body need to be three dimensional with an interconnected porous network, since they must resemble the structure and shape of the deficient organ part that is to be regenerated. Such scaffolds are required to provide to the transplanted cells the biological environment and the 3-D support that is needed until the regenerated tissue is formed, structurally stabilized, and efficiently vascularized.

The recent advances on the fabrication of natural or synthetic polymeric materials, in the form of foams or fibrous scaffolds, as candidates for tissue regeneration able to provide directional cell attachment and promotion are discussed herein. The polymer-based materials for the fabrication of such scaffolds should be nontoxic to cells, biocompatible and biodegradable, and should interact positively with the cells to promote cell adhesion, proliferation, migration, and differentiated cell function. Furthermore, it should be highly porous in order to provide sufficient space for cellular activity, and with appropriate mechanical properties. More specifically, microscale parameters such as pore density, size, and configuration can affect the cell proliferation and differentiation (Karageorgiou and Kaplan 2005; Ng et al. 2009; Pamula et al. 2008), and therefore current research is focused on the development of porous material scaffolds that integrate with biological molecules or cells and regenerate tissues. However, one of the main challenges is the engineering of materials that can match both the mechanical properties and the biological environment of the tissue.

Synthetic and natural polymers, such as poly(α-hydroxy acids), polycarbonates, poly(fumarate)s, poly(urethane)s, polyesters, and their copolymers in the first case and collagen, polysaccharides, silk, gelatin, fibrin, and their derivatives in the second case, have been utilized for the formation of foams or fibrous matrices, for tissue engineering, e.g., bone and cartilage. Synthetic polymers can be designed in order to present desired mechanical and chemical properties compatible for scaffolds, to have appropriate biodegradation time, and they can be broadly available and cost-effective. In contrary to the synthetic, natural polymers present the appropriate affinity, making thus possible the promotion of desirable cell responses. However, they present several disadvantages, such as the poor mechanical strength and the complexities in the purification and extraction from the natural sources (Ng et al. 2012; Place et al. 2009a). The type and the properties of the foams or fibrous polymeric scaffolds are strongly dependent on the nature of the polymer utilized and on the type of tissue regenerated, while in the recent years, the scaffolds incorporate both microporous structures and nanostructures in order to better simulate the in vivo microenvironment and to enhance the cellular functions. Therefore, it is often used the combination of different methods for the fabrication of nanofeatures on the scaffolds but also the use of nanoparticles together with the polymeric materials for their fabrication (Ng et al. 2012; Dvir et al. 2011). Electrospinning, phase separation, gas foaming, 3-D printing, stereolithography, particulate leaching techniques, etc., are used, and the surface of the resulting scaffolds is sufficiently modified for the enhanced cell adhesion and proliferation.

Electrospun fibrous polymeric scaffolds have a very high surface-to-volume ratio, while a wide range of porosity with microscale interconnected pores, shape, and dimensions can be selected depending on the polymer solutions and processing parameters. One of the advantages of the electrospun fibrous scaffolds is the ability to orient the fibers but also to precisely control the porosity rendering thus such method ideal for a controlled and optimized solution for each type of scaffold application such as in vascular, neural, bone, cartilage, and tendon/ligament scaffolds (Moffa et al. 2013; Polini et al. 2013; Lee et al. 2010; Wang et al. 2011a; Nandakumar et al. 2010; Choi et al. 2008). Gas foaming techniques utilize the formation of gas bubbles by a chemical reaction or the expansion of CO_2 in polymer viscous matrices (Kim et al. 2012; van der Pol et al. 2010). In thermally induced phase separation process, a homogeneous polymer solution turns into a multiphase system characterized by a polymer-rich and a polymer-poor phase, under certain temperature conditions. After removal of the solvent, the polymer-rich phase solidifies to form a matrix, while the rest becomes pores. If the temperature is low enough, the solid–liquid demixing occurs with a frozen solvent and the concentrated polymer phase. Depending on the type of polymer solution and the process parameters, various types of scaffolds are formed for specific applications (Wei and Ma 2008; Mandoli et al. 2010; Jack et al. 2009). Particulate leaching is an easy and straightforward method to generate a porous polymeric structure and deals with the mixing of a polymer or prepolymer viscous melt or solution with a granular template of desired shape and size such as sugar or salt. After the polymerization or the solidification of the polymer, the template is leached remaining with the porous polymeric structure. Such method can be used for the fabrication of foams structures (Pamula et al. 2009; Mou et al. 2013) or in combination with other methods (e.g., phase separation, electrospinning) in order to form scaffolds with multiscale porosity (Liu and Ma 2009; Wei and Ma 2009; Kim et al. 2008a; Guarino et al. 2008). On the other hand, rapid prototyping methods such as 3-D printing (Seyednejad et al. 2011, 2012) and stereolithography offer the opportunity to prepare structures with precise complex and reproducible geometries that can help in the growth of the implanted cells but also in the biodegradability of the scaffolds in an accurate and highly manageable way. The 3-D design can be done via specific computer softwares, and therefore it can be tuned and modified according to specific needs. In the case of stereolithography, lasers have been used to successfully produce microstructured biomaterials for tissue engineering scaffolds, and a suite of different laser techniques has been reported to produce structures with a range of microstructure resolutions (Beke et al. 2012, 2013; Sušec et al. 2013; Johnson et al. 2013).

2.3 Bioactivated Cell-Instructive Scaffolds

The next generation of scaffolds requires the encoding of complex arrays of biofunctional signals to control and guide cellular events and tissue remodeling. The concept of tissue and cell guidance is rapidly evolving as more information on the biological control of the extracellular microenvironment on cellular function and tissue morphogenesis becomes available. These findings have burst a novel concept in bioactive material design based on nanometric control of structural and functional features to recapitulate the spatiotemporal molecular regulatory program and the three-dimensional architecture of the native extracellular matrix. Micro- and nanostructured scaffolds able to sequester and deliver biomolecular moieties in a tightly spatial and temporal controlled manner have been proposed as highly effective in tissue repairing, in guiding functional angiogenesis, and in controlling stem cell differentiation. Although these materials are a first attempt to mimic the complex and dynamic microenvironment presented in vivo, an increased symbiosis among material engineering, micro- and nanotechnology, drug delivery, and cell and molecular biology is needed to fabricate biomaterials that encode the whole array of biosignals to guide and control developmental processes in tissue- and organ-specific differentiation and morphogenesis.

Scaffold design concept has been constantly evolving during the last two decades passing from the original notion of an inert temporary material permissive to cell and tissue growth to the modern concept of proactive cell-instructive material, able to control and guide tissue morphogenesis (Hacker and Mikos 2006) (Fig. 2.1).

Originally, scaffolds were envisaged as provisional constructs that could only provide geometrical guidance to cell and tissue growth. According to the modern concept, instead, the ideal scaffold should provide an active guidance to the whole process of tissue repairing by displaying a series of chemical, biochemical, and biophysical cues to elicit specific events at the cellular and tissue level. Spatio-temporal presentation of biological signals must be combined with microstructural and mechanical properties to provide a proper cell-instructive environment not only within the scaffolds but also at the interface with the native tissues. The typical approach is to reestablish the essential features of the extracellular matrix (EMC) environment in a natural or synthetic material. Along this line, purified ECM components or decellularized ECMs derived from animals have been widely used in tissue engineering. Decellularized ECM has been successfully used as a scaffold for soft tissue applications (Voytik-Harbin et al. 1998), and single purified ECM components, such as collagen, hyaluronic acid, and fibrin, have been combined to create controlled and standardized materials with structure similar to native ECM (Battista et al. 2005; Chan and Mooney 2008). Albeit biological tissue-derived materials have some advantages, such as biocompatibility and cell receptors recognition, synthetic materials are chemically programmable and reproducible; moreover, they display a high degree of control of their properties offering the possibility to tailor their performance on the specific application. In order to improve the

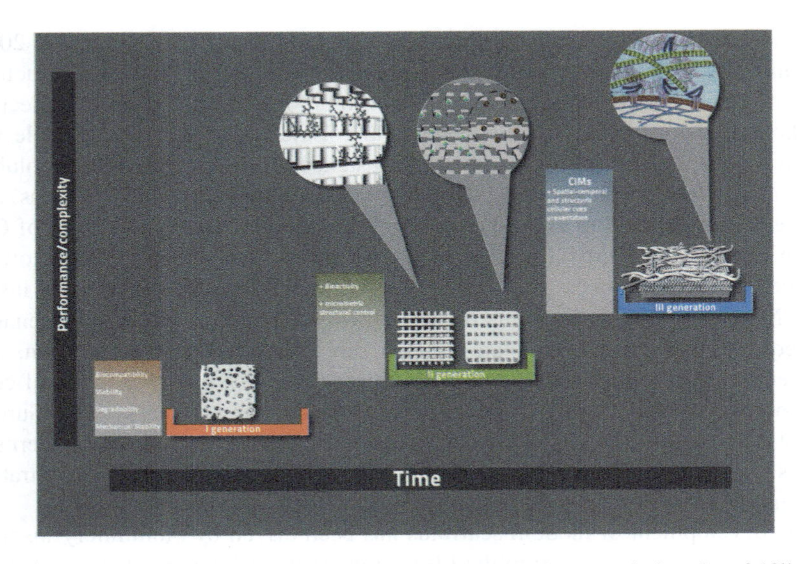

Fig. 2.1 Evolution of scaffold concept: first scaffold generation was designed to fulfill basic properties like biocompatibility, viability, mechanical stability, degradability, and porosity. They were conceived as an inert ancillary frame to temporarily replace the function of damaged tissue, while the cells seeded within its structure could deposit novel tissue that would progressively restore the original status. The appreciation of the central role of the microenvironment on tissue morphogenesis has stirred research direction along the design of a second generation of scaffolds that encode biological signals able to control and guide cell and tissue processes. Scaffolds of this generation were enriched with bioactive moieties, either physisorbed or chemically conjugated, that could be presented at cell surface to trigger specific events. However, to elicit specific events and correctly instruct a cell to perform a specific task, signals must be presented at the right time, at the right dose, and at the right site. Therefore, next scaffold generation should provide a tight control of presentation at nanometric scale of physical and biomolecular cues to recapitulate the spatiotemporal regulatory program and the three-dimensional architecture of the native extracellular matrix. This new generation of scaffolds should be able to provide the suitable instructive microenvironment for the cell to activate the correct morphogenic pathway

interaction with cells, biological active molecules have been incorporated within synthetic materials obtaining hybrid proactive materials to promote and control cell interaction and functions. The development of synthetic material designed to present a complex array of bioactive signals with a defined time and space program is at the frontier of biomaterials science for the realization of artificial replica of the extracellular matrix.

ECM is the natural medium in which cells grow, differentiate, and migrate and represents the gold standard material for tissue regeneration (Bosman and Stamenkovic 2003). The cell–ECM interaction is highly specific and reciprocal. Cells produce, organize, and eventually degrade the macromolecular components of the ECM, and, in turn, ECM sequesters and presents molecular signals that control and guide cell response. ECM is a dynamic environment in which several proliferation–adhesion–differentiation motifs are continuously generated, sequestered, and released often according to cellular stimuli (Katz and Streuli 2007; Fittkau et al. 2005; Stupack and Cheresh 2002). Moreover, solid-state, structural ECM molecules, such as heparin, act as reservoirs for secreted signaling molecules for their on-demand release (Rapraeger 2000; Wijelath et al. 2002; Taipale and KeskiOja 1997). Growth factors (GFs), for instance, are locally stored in insoluble/ latent forms through specific binding with glycosaminoglycans (e.g., heparins) and released upon demand to elicit their biological activity. The sequestration of GFs within the ECM in inert form is necessary for rapid signal transduction, allowing extracellular signal processing to take place in time frames similar to those inside cells. Moreover, spatial gradients of GFs play a major role in ECM maintenance and equilibrium because they are able to direct cell adhesion, migration, and differentiation deriving from given progenitor cells and organize patterns of cells into complex structures, such as vascular networks and the nervous system (Gurdon et al. 1994; Tanabe and Jessell 1997; Burgess et al. 2000). Thus, spatial patterns in tissues are dictated by both the architectural features of the ECM and concentration profiles/gradients of diffusible bioactive factors (Kong and Mooney 2007).

The development of modern scaffolds has been driven by biomimicry-inspired design to recapitulate in a simplified form the essential features of the molecular and structural microenvironment existing in the ECM. For instance, several micro- and nanofabrication strategies, including molecular and nanoparticulate self-assembly, micro and nanoprinting, electrospinning, and molecular and nano-templating (Hutmacher 2001; Sachlos and Czernuszka 2003; Teo et al. 2006; Guarino et al. 2007; Beniash et al. 2005; Place et al. 2009b; Mehta et al. 2012), have been used in an attempt to reproduce the spatial organization of the fibrillar structure of the ECM that provides essential guidance for cell organization, survival, and function (Sachlos and Czernuszka 2003; Guarino et al. 2007). Topographic and stereomorphological cellular cues can be provided by controlling fiber dimension and arrangement (Teo et al. 2006); chrono- and spatial-programmed presentation of bioactive moieties can be encoded by placing morphogenic factor-loaded degradable microparticles in predefined regions of the scaffold (Mehta et al. 2012; Luciani et al. 2008); finally, the exposition of matricellular cues can be controlled, even dynamically, by grafting integrin adhesive motifs (Causa et al. 2007) (Fig. 2.2).

The necessity to control the presentation of microenvironmental cues at cell level denotes the key shift from the concept of shape to cell guidance that accompanies modern scaffold design strategies. However, the attainment of tight control over space, time, and molecular arrangement of the cascade of signals required to control and guide the process of tissue or organ repair is, albeit theoretically achievable, practically and economically non-pursuable (Place et al. 2009b). The recapitulation of the complex molecular events occurring within the extracellular space during the process of tissue repair and regeneration should be reproduced in the most essential features using simplified strategies. For instance, within its fibrillar components, ECM has a vast range of integrin-binding motifs, each of them with a specific function and activity (Causa et al. 2007; Ventre et al. 2012). Most of these motifs have been identified and their corresponding short sequence

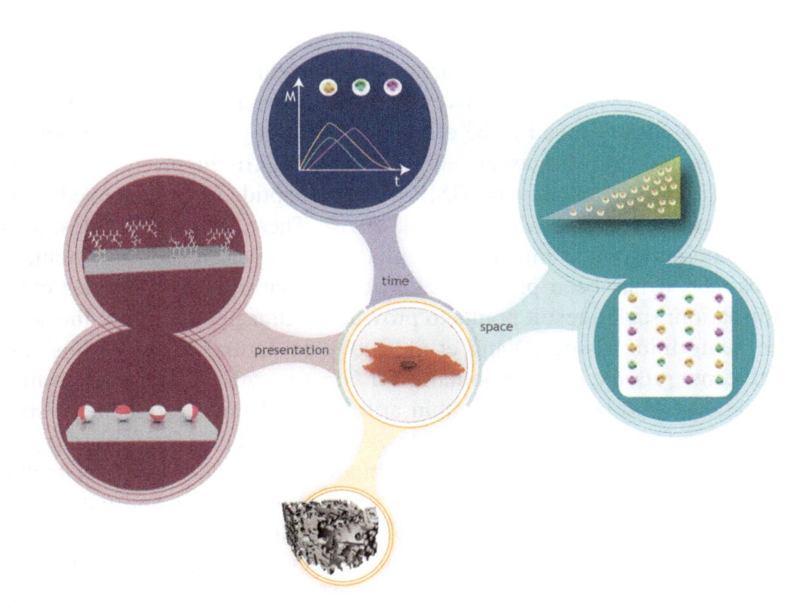

Fig. 2.2 Schematic of bioactivated scaffolds—next generation of scaffolds should control the presentation of bioactive signals in time, space and configuration/conformation. Molecular conformation must be suitable for cell interaction to elicit the desired response and can be tailored with the aid of molecular spacer. Time and space presentation of the signal must be arranged and accorded with specific profiles. The synchronization over time of a specific signal can be achieved by the use of engineered GFs-encapsulated microdepots (Biondi et al. 2008). Embedding microdepots releasing GFs at known release rates in a defined spatial distribution within the scaffold it is virtually possible to recreate any, even complex, molecular microenvironment (Sun et al. 2004; Whitesides et al. 2001). The combination of micropositioning systems and mathematical modeling describing the complex and multiple mechanisms governing the release kinetics from single microspheres within the scaffold can be of help in realizing scaffolds with highly controlled architecture by computer-aided scaffold design (CASD) (Sun et al. 2004; Hutmacher et al. 2004)

peptides synthetically reproduced (Ventre et al. 2012). The accessibility to an entire library of integrin-binding peptides makes it possible to reproduce the integrin-mediated cross talk realistically and in a simplified manner by inserting small molecular units within the scaffold instead of the whole fibrillar protein such as collagen, fibronectin, or laminin. However, the insertion of all possible matricellular cues mimicking peptides in a scaffold would certainly make a more realistic replica of the natural molecular niche for cells but would make scaffold production impractical and perhaps unnecessarily complex. Furthermore, since during any tissue repairing process GFs are continuously produced within the extracellular space and dynamically presented at cell surface, the use of these generally labile proteins within the scaffold requires sophisticated technologies to preserve their activity for a medium–long time period (Borselli et al. 2007). The use of peptides capable of eliciting comparable morphogenic activity allows a dramatic reduction in the level of scaffold complexity. Even if these peptides generally elicit cell response at a higher dose compared to their natural or recombinant counterparts, they provide a viable alternative in terms of cost and handling. QK peptide, for instance, has been proved to be effective in eliciting angiogenic response and has been already exploited as an alternative to VEGF in promoting scaffolds (Finetti et al. 2012). Analogously, BMP mimetic peptide already proved a potent osteogenic active molecule (Zouani et al. 2010). These small molecules, as their natural counterparts, often impart a potentiated biological response if bound to a solid substrate. It has been proved that materials with grafted peptides enhance tissue formation; such a result points to provide a better integration of the scaffold with the neoforming tissue (Wang et al. 2007). In natural ECM, GAGs (glycosaminoglycans) provide binding domains for GFs (growth factor), and this mechanism of action could be encoded within artificial ECM by introducing a specific binding domain for the mimicking peptides. Alginate and poly(acrylamide) gel, for instance, have been sulfated to enhance the binding affinity to some GFs, including VEGF, PDGF, and HGF, potentiating the angiogenic activity and extending the flexibility of the scaffold for growth factor presentation and preservation (Merkel et al. 2002; Rouet et al. 2005; Chaterji and Gemeinhart 2007). Furthermore, the modulation of binding affinity within the scaffolds structure provides a viable strategy to control stable gradients of GFs (Fig. 2.2) or their mimicking peptides, which are proved to be essential in controlling and guiding morphogenetic processes (Griffith and Swartz 2006).

In natural ECM, there is a continuous production of GFs that are sequestered within molecular recess and eventually used upon cell request. Sources of GFs or their mimicking peptides, at a specific location within a synthetic scaffold, can be provided with the use of micro- or nanoparticles loaded with bioactive moieties and programmed to deliver according to a specific profile (Fig. 2.2). Integration of GF-loaded microparticles engineered to release sequentially various GFs has been already discussed in the literature (Luciani et al. 2008; Richardson et al. 2001; Saltzman and Olbricht 2002). According to this approach, it is possible to control the spatial distribution and the gradients of bioactive agents at different locations within the scaffold (Luciani et al. 2008; Borselli et al. 2007; Chen et al. 2007). A more advanced method to manufacture microsphere-integrated scaffolds able to regulate GFs release kinetics both temporally and spatially may take advantage of micromanipulation-based techniques. Possible developments and advancement include the control over the presentation of relevant signals, not only within the physical domain of the scaffolds but also within the host surrounding tissues. Microdepot acting as a single point source may be micropositioned by 3-D printing and soft lithography to obtain highly regulated structures able to trigger the extent and possibly the architecture/structure of tissue formation (Sun et al. 2004; Whitesides et al. 2001). The combination of micropositioning systems and mathematical modeling describing the complex and multiple mechanisms governing the release kinetics from single microspheres within the scaffold can be of help in creating scaffolds with a highly controlled architecture using computer-aided scaffold design programs (CASD) (Whitesides et al. 2001; Hutmacher et al. 2004).

Over the past decades, the concept of scaffolds has been strongly redefined: from the original definition of a space-filling material to the most modern vision of programmable bioactive material, able to guide and control complex cellular processes. Thanks to a sapient integration of cellular and molecular biology combined with the advancement in material science and nanotechnology, future scaffolds can be envisaged as a simplified, yet effective, replica of the natural ECM—with the potentiality to make tissue engineering a real clinical success.

2.4 Introduction to Skin Wound Active Dressing Materials

The skin is the largest organ in the human body and the one interfacing with the external environment, keeping protected the rest of the body but also receiving sensory stimuli. It consists of three layers. The outermost layer is the bloodless epidermis and is bonded to the underlying dermis layer. In the dermis are included blood vessels, collagen and elastin fibers, glands, hair follicles, and nerves' endings. The innermost layer is the subcutis, an energy reservoir and impact protective layer, composed of mainly fat tissue. When the skin layers are damaged, an acute wound is formed. The treatment of acute wounds should involve first the cleaning, to reduce the risk of infection, and then the closure, where appropriate dressings are involved. The wound closure helps in the reduction of the infections risks, brings the separated tissues close together, and promotes the healing process. Such healing process goes through four phases: (1) hemostasis, (2) inflammation, (3) proliferation, and (4) maturation remodeling. As the healing progresses, the different phases often overlap, as schematically demonstrated in Fig. 2.3. When the healing of an acute wound does not go through the usual phases, failing to close in the expected time due to intrinsic or extrinsic causes, then a chronic wound can develop. In such wound, the septic infections are common, but resolving their origin can help in restarting the healing process.

The dressing of a skin wound has a crucial role in the healing process since it provides the right conditions that assure its optimized progress till the final closure. There are already numerous wound dressings in the market, each one tackling diverse types of wounds, acute or chronic. These dressings can be categorized according to their interactions with the wound: (1) passive dressings that just cover the wound (i.e., gauzes), (2) interactive dressings that promote the healing by being oxygen and water vapor permeable but not permeable to bacteria (i.e., transparent films, foams, gels), and (3) active dressings that deliver substances that contribute to the healing process (alginates, chitosan, hydrocolloids). Usually, the skin wound dressing types that are available in the market are traditional gauzes and tulles, transparent films, and foams that cannot absorb the exudates but are moisture permeable and dressings that upon contact with the wound exudates form a gel creating a moist environment (hydrocolloids, alginates, hydrofibers). Lately, the availability of active dressings containing silver or other antimicrobial agents or antibiotics is progressively increasing.

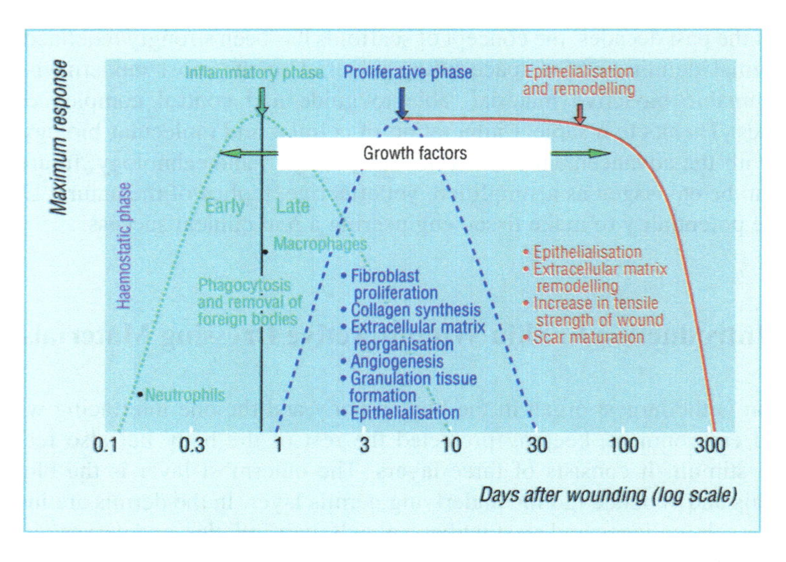

Fig. 2.3 The four overlapping phases of acute wound healing (Enoch et al. 2006)

The majority of the research efforts in this field are concentrated to hydrogel type and nanofibrous, especially electrospun, materials that have a big potentiality as active wound dressings, providing new possibilities for the wound-healing market.

2.5 Hydrogel Materials with Antibacterial Agents for Skin Regeneration

Hydrogels are hydrophilic polymers which can be swollen by water and have found biomedical applications for tissue engineering and drug delivery. For instance, alginate- and chitosan-based materials can uptake large amounts of water compared to their initial weight when in contact with moist media such as open tissue wounds. As a result, they gelatinize. During the formation of alginate- or chitosan-based gels, they exchange or loose ions and eventually can become structurally unstable. Hence, various methods have been developed to maintain structural longevity in hydrogels obtained from natural polymers (Malmsten 2011). Natural polymer-based hydrogels are generally classified into various categories depending on the preparation method, the charge, and the mechanical and structural characteristics. In this chapter, we will present the state of the art developed in recent years on hydrogels based on natural polymers and their various applications in the field of wound healing and treatment.

Hydrophilic and organic antimicrobial agents and drugs can be readily incorporated into sodium alginate- and chitosan-based polymers in aqueous solutions.

Sodium alginate solutions containing hydrophilic antibacterial agents can be turned into films or beads which will swell and gelatinize upon contact with, for instance, hydrated skin wounds. A recent work combined povidone–iodine (PVPI) and sodium alginate into antimicrobial calcium cross-linked films and beads which released PVPI in a controlled manner in moist media or in water (Liakos et al. 2013). PVPI is encapsulated in the films forming circular microdomains. Upon immersion into moist media such as bacteria- or fungi-laden agar or aqueous media or contaminated water, these films swell, gelatinize, and start releasing the antimicrobial agent (PVPI) slowly inhibiting the growth. The films also display antimicrobial and antifungal activity when exposed to agar media heavily populated by *E. coli* and *Candida albicans* fungi as seen in Fig. 2.4. This was achieved by natural gelation and swelling of alginate in such media. These alginate films can also encapsulate hydrophobic antimicrobial agents such as natural essential oils (EOs) (Liakos et al. 2014). The process differs from direct mixing in aqueous solution in that surfactant stabilized emulsions need to be prepared. Namely, elicriso italic, chamomile blue, cinnamon, lavender, tea tree, peppermint, eucalyptus, lemongrass, and lemon oils were encapsulated in the films as potential active substances. Glycerol was used to induce plasticity and surfactants were added to improve the dispersion of EOs in the sodium alginate matrix.

The topography, chemical composition, mechanical properties, and humidity resistance of the films were studied. Antimicrobial tests were conducted on films containing different percentages of EOs against *E. coli* bacteria and *Candida albicans* fungi (Liakos et al. 2014). Such diverse types of essential oil-fortified alginate films can find many applications mainly as disposable wound dressings but also in food packaging, medical device protection and disinfection, and indoor air quality improvement applications, to name a few. Not all essential oils encapsulated in alginic matrices present similar effects against inhibiting bacterial or fungal growth as exemplified in Fig. 2.5.

There has been much interest in forming 3-D hydrogel structures from natural polymers containing large amounts of water but being structurally stable and functional (antimicrobial and drug releasing). In order to enhance their mechanical robustness, researchers use physical or chemical cross-linking procedures to create three-dimensional (3-D) polymeric networks. The most common biopolymer hydrogels are obtained from alginic acid polymers, chitosan, gelatin, and β-cyclodextrin (enzymatically obtained from starch). Due to their high water content and soft, porous 3-D structure (see Fig. 2.6), they can easily simulate in vivo extracellular matrix (ECM) microenvironment in biomedical applications. Hydrogels can be applied externally or can be injectable and can carry cells or drugs into the body in a minimally invasive manner. Hydrogels have also been used for the creation of 3-D scaffolds for cell culture and transplantation and as carriers for local release of proteins and drugs (Lee et al. 2013; Fonseca et al. 2014).

Alginic acid-based natural polymers are linear polysaccharides with homopolymeric blocks of (1,4)-linked β-D-mannuronate and α-L-guluronate that are extracted from seaweed and shrimp shells (see Fig. 2.7). They are widely used in making various forms of biomedical materials. In general, alginate forms a hydrogel via

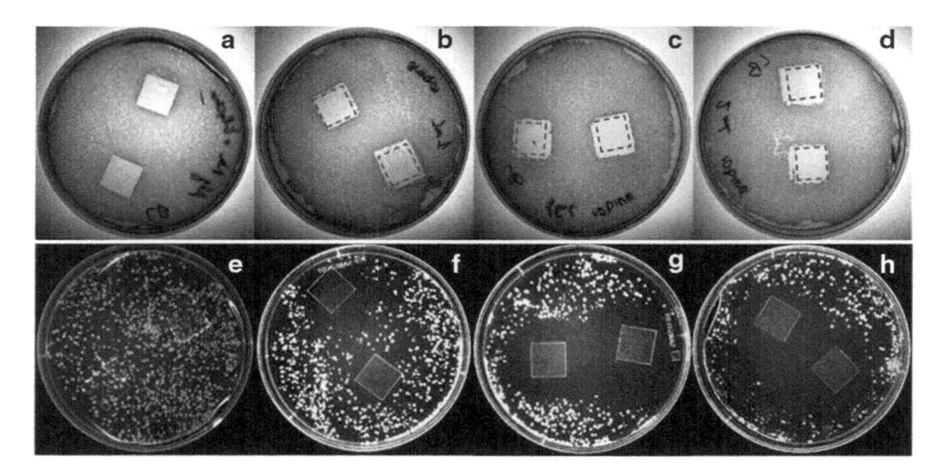

Fig. 2.4 Photographs of Petri dishes containing heavily populated *E. coli* bacteria after 48 h incubation in the presence of (**a**) 70 wt% NaAlg/30 wt% glycerol film (control film), (**b**) film 1, (**c**) film 2, and (**d**) film 3. The *red noncontinuous line* indicates the borders of the glass slide. Photographs of Petri dishes containing *C. albicans* after 48 h incubation in the presence of (**e**) 70 wt% NaAlg/30 wt% glycerol film, (**f**) film 1, (**g**) film 2, and (**h**) film 3. Film 1, film 2 and film 3 indicate increasing concentrations of PVPI (Liakos et al. 2013)

ionic interactions between carboxylic acids and divalent cations such as Ca^{2+}, Mg^{2+}, and Ba^{2+} as depicted in Fig. 2.8. Applications of alginate hydrogels range from injecting cells and drugs to wound dressings and dental implants due to their low toxicity, low cost, and gelling ability by the action of divalent cations.

There is still an active research interest in rendering alginate-based hydrogels more robust by controlling their mechanical and biophysical properties such as elastic modulus, swelling ratio, and degradation rate, although control over rapid ionic cross-linking and rapid loss of ions is still highly challenging. Therefore, intermolecular cross-linking methods such as conjugating various types of cross-linkers to the alginate backbone have been developed, but such reagents and reaction conditions for conjugation and cross-linking are typically toxic to encapsulated cells and can cause denaturation of growth factors or complications in wound treatment and healing.

The structure and mechanical behavior of gelatin gels have already been widely studied in the past (Wan et al. 2008; Van Vlierberghe et al. 2011; Mazzitelli et al. 2013). Gelatin normally dissolves in aqueous solutions at temperatures around body temperature where it exists as flexible single coils. On cooling down, transparent gels are formed, if the concentration is higher than the critical gelation concentration. These gels are formed by physical cross-links, also called "junction zones," originating from a partial transition to "ordered" triple-helical collagen-like sequences, separated by peptide residues in the "disordered" conformation. Because of its unique gelation and biomimetic properties, gelatin is interesting to use as a hydrogel for biomedical applications (Van Vlierberghe et al. 2011). There exist several methods to cross-link gelatin hydrogels. The disadvantage of most

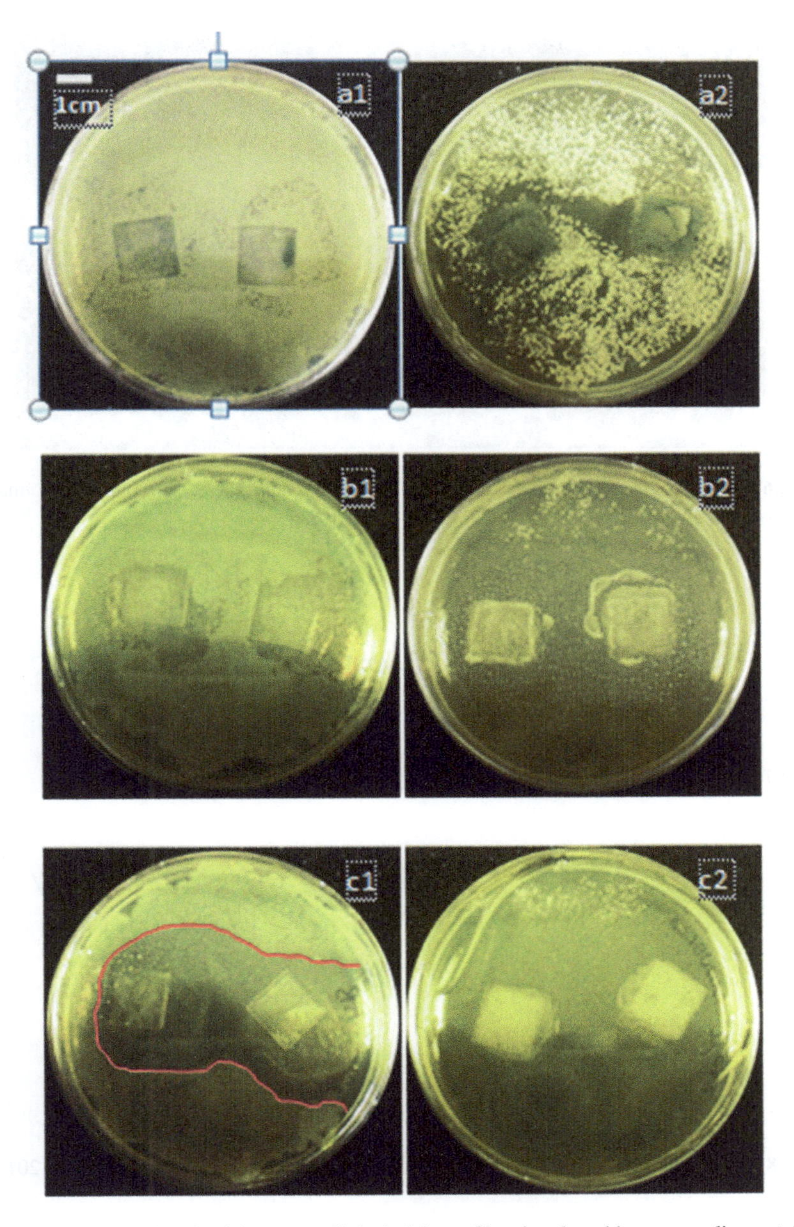

Fig. 2.5 EO-encapsulated calcium cross-linked alginate films incubated in agar media containing bacteria and fungi. (**a1**) Chamomile blue incubated with *E. coli* and (**a2**) chamomile blue incubated with *C. albicans*. (**b1**) Peppermint incubated with *E. coli*, (**b2**) peppermint with *C. albicans*, (**c1**) cinnamon incubated with *E. coli* (the *continuous red line* represents the inhibition zone to guide the eye), and (**c2**) cinnamon incubated with *C. albicans* (Liakos et al. 2014)

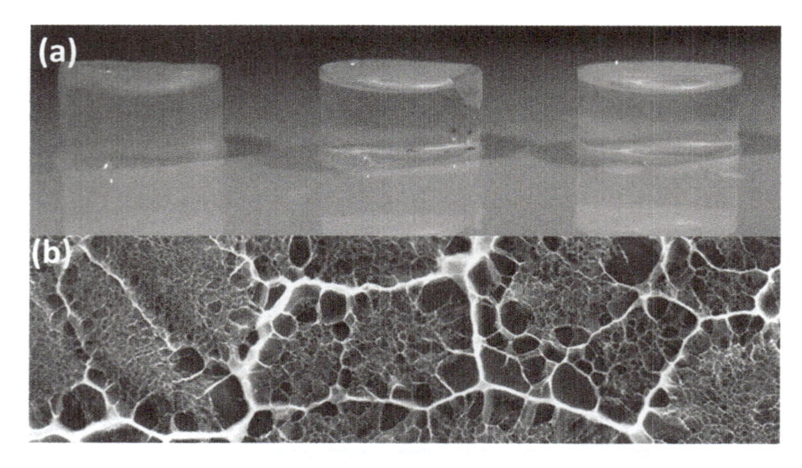

Fig. 2.6 (**a**) Photograph of alginate hydrogels. (**b**) Cryo-scanning electron microscopy image of alginate hydrogel (Lee et al. 2013)

Fig. 2.7 Chemical structure of alginic acid polymer

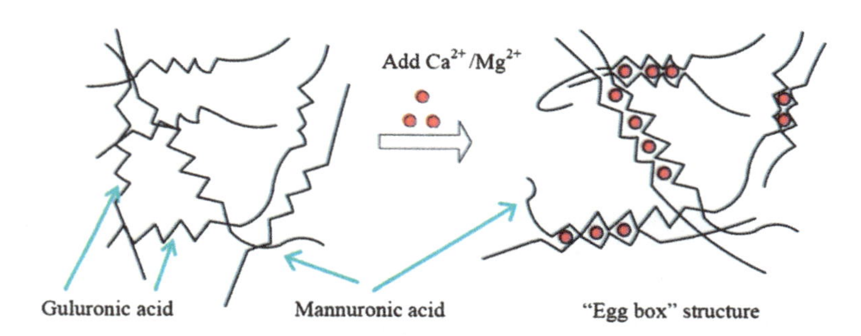

Fig. 2.8 Cross-linking of alginic acid with calcium or magnesium ions (Fonseca et al. 2014)

chemical cross-linking procedures is the fact that they are irreversible and can contain chemical traces that can hinder wound healing. Recent works demonstrated that cross-linking via disulfide bond formation by oxidation of thiolated compounds could offer a solution for this problem, since this process is reversible. Cleavage of the disulfide linkages via reducing agents (e.g., dithiothreitol) results in thiolated, soluble macromolecules. The mechanical properties of thiolated gelatin hydrogels as depicted in Fig. 2.9 depend on the contributions of both the physical

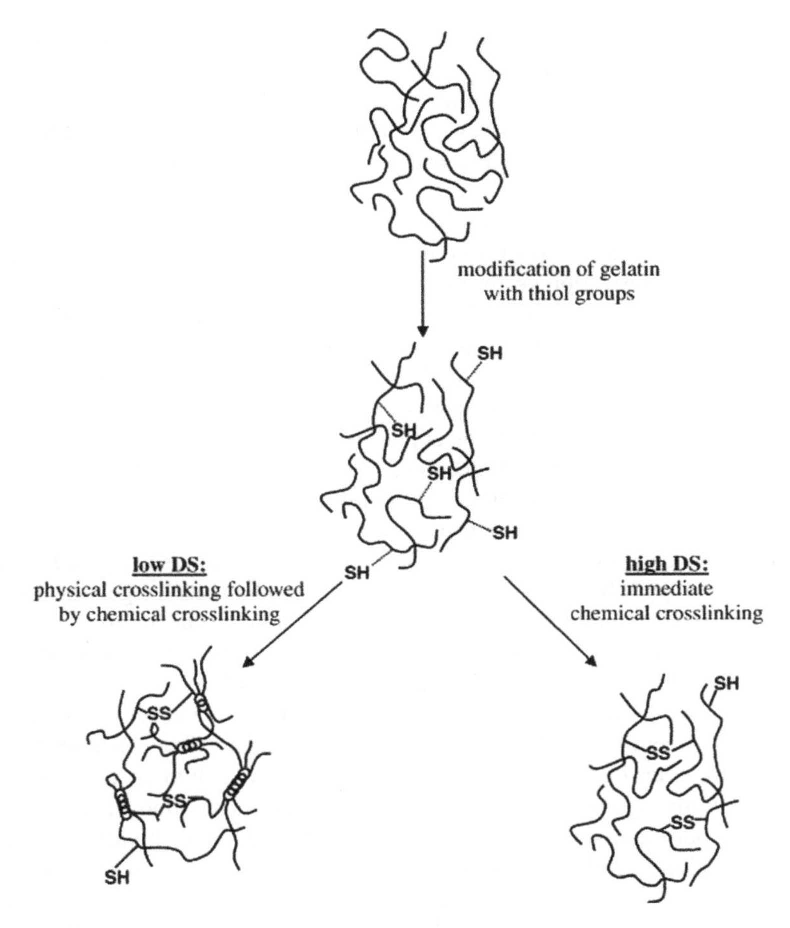

Fig. 2.9 Schematic representation of the influence of the synthesis route on the formation of the gelatin network (Wan et al. 2008)

cross-linking and the chemical cross-linking by disulfide formation. Above the sol–gel temperature, the gel strength only depends on the chemical network, due to the thermoreversibility of the physical entanglements. Common cross-linking agents are *N*-acetylhomocysteine thiolactone and Traut's reagent.

Moreover, recent works demonstrated fabrication of gelatin-based hydrogel patches (Mazzitelli et al. 2013). The effect of different preparation parameters were analyzed with respect to the rheological and pharmaceutical characteristics of hydrogel blend patches as transdermal delivery formulation. Mixtures of pectin and gelatin were employed for the production of patches, with adjustable properties, following a two-step gelation procedure. The first gelation, a thermal one, is trigged by the presence of gelatin, whereas, the second gelation, an ionic one, is due to the formation of the typical egg box structure of pectin. In particular, the patch structural properties were assessed by oscillation stress sweep measurements which provided information concerning their viscoelastic properties. In addition, different modalities for drug loading were analyzed with respect to drug homogeneous distribution; testosterone was employed as model drug for transdermal administration. Finally, the performances of the produced transdermal patches were studied, in terms of reproducibility and reliability, by determination of in vitro drug release profiles.

Transdermal patches are usually formulated to assure a sustained systemic drug release, from a few days up to a couple of weeks. In this respect, the accurate rheological characterization performed on patches with different formulations had the aim to select those presenting the best viscoelastic properties, allowing an easy administration (i.e., skin application) and duration of use. As further objective aimed to evaluate the drug product performance, specific tests for determining the drug release from the produced patches were performed. Determination of drug or metal ion (in the case of silver- or copper-based patches) release profiles from transdermal medicines, although does not represent a measure of bioavailability, gives important information on the drug release characteristics that have the potential to alter the biological performance of the drug in the dosage form. As an example to nanoparticle-laden hydrogels, silver nanocomposite hydrogels were recently developed by using acrylamide and biodegradable gelatin (Reddy et al. 2013). Silver nanoparticles were generated throughout the hydrogel networks using in situ method by incorporating Ag^{+} ions and the subsequent treatment with sodium borohydride as shown in Fig. 2.10. The effect of gelatin on the swelling studies was investigated. The hydrogel synthesized silver nanocomposites were also characterized. The biodegradable gelatin-based silver nanocomposite hydrogels were tested for antibacterial properties and exhibited a strong antibacterial activity against bacillus. These agents can easily find applications in wound and burn dressings. Moreover, cross-linked gelatin–chondroitin sulfate hydrogels exhibit excellent properties for the controlled release of small cationic antibacterial proteins into wounds (Kuijpers et al. 2000). Combining chondroitin sulfate with gelatin in a cross-linked gel increases the interaction between the cationic protein and the hydrogel, causing an increased loading capacity and an extended release time for wound treatment. As two different antibacterial proteins, recombinant thrombocidin, rTC-1, and lysozyme, were used resulting in similar release results, it is, hence, expected that such release systems can be used for a broad range of cationic antibacterial proteins without major adaptations. The effectiveness of these hydrogels in skin treatment was demonstrated on polyester films (Dacron) coated with a skin-like tissue as seen in Fig. 2.11. Finally, these hydrogels are biocompatible and degrade almost completely within several weeks of application, thus allowing tissue integration, which is advantageous for the healing characteristics of porous biomaterials, and may improve the long-term infection resistance of these materials.

Similar to alginic acid polymers, chitosan-based hydrogels have also received a great deal of attention due to their well-documented biocompatibility, low toxicity, and degradability by human enzymes and their natural antibacterial properties (Giri et al. 2012; Bhattarai et al. 2010; Fiejdasz et al. 2013). These and other properties

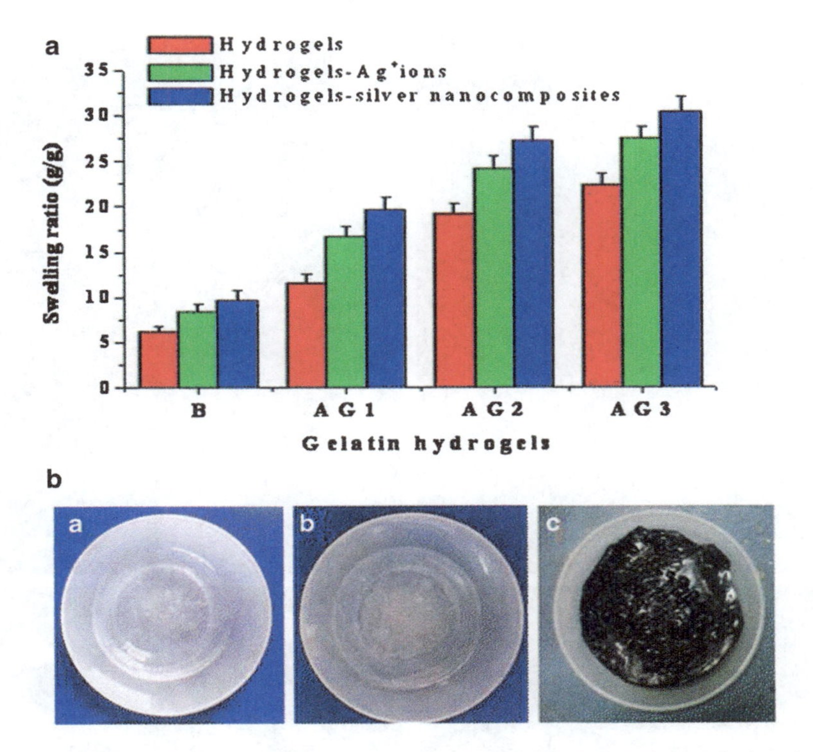

Fig. 2.10 (**a**, *upper panel*) swelling behavior of pure hydrogel, ions-loaded hydrogel, and nanohydrogels. (**b**, *lower panel*) (a) plain hydrogel. (b) Ag+ ions-loaded hydrogel. (c) Ag nanocomposite hydrogels (Reddy et al. 2013)

such as hydrophilicity, existence of functional amino groups, and a net cationic charge have made chitosan a suitable polymer for the intelligent delivery of macromolecular compounds, such as peptides, proteins, antigens, oligonucleotides, and genes. Chitosan hydrogels have been prepared with a variety of different shapes, geometries, and formulations that include liquid gels, powders, beads, films, tablets, capsules, microspheres, microparticles, sponges, nanofibrils, and inorganic composites. In each preparation, chitosan is either physically associated or chemically cross-linked to form the hydrogel. As a hydrogel, chitosan networks should satisfy the following: (1) interchain interactions must be strong enough to form semipermanent junction points in the network and (2) the network should promote the access and residence of water molecules within. Gels that meet these demands may be prepared by non-covalent strategies that rely on electrostatic, hydrophobic, and hydrogen bonding forces. Figure 2.12 shows the schematics of four major physical interactions (i.e., ionic, polyelectrolyte, interpolymer complex, and hydrophobic associations) that lead to the gelation of a chitosan solution (Bhattarai et al. 2010). Because the network formation by all of these interactions is purely physical, gel formation can be reversed. Due to cationic amino groups of

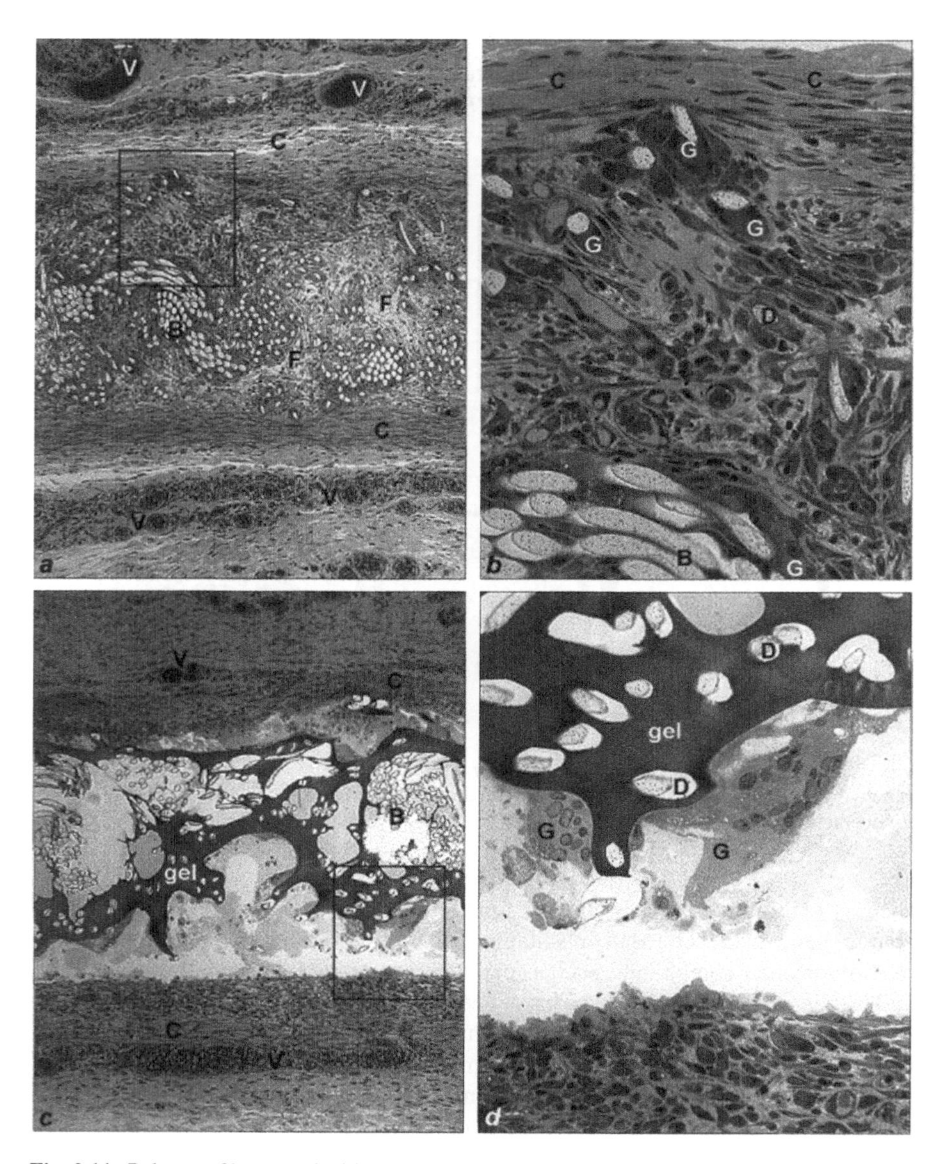

Fig. 2.11 Polyester film coated with soft tissue. Dacron-pt (**a**; 5×), Dacron-pt (**b**; 20×), Dacron-pt-gel-0.8 (**c**; 5×), and Dacron-pt-gel–ChS-0.8 (**d**; 20×) after 10 days of implantation [B = Dacron fiber bundles, V = blood vessels, F = fibrin, D = Dacron fiber, C = capsule, G = giant cell, gel = cross-linked gel (gelatin or gelatin–ChS)] (Kuijpers et al. 2000)

chitosan, ionic interactions can occur between chitosan and negatively charged molecules and anions. Ionic complexation of mixed charge systems can be formed between chitosan and small anionic molecules, such as sulfates, citrates, and phosphates or anions of metals like Pt (II), Pd (II), and Mo (VI). While

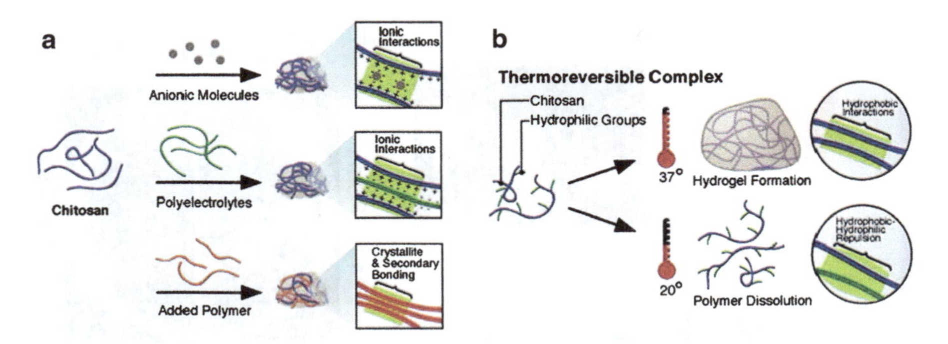

Fig. 2.12 Schematic representation of chitosan-based hydrogel networks derived from different physical associations: (**a**) networks of chitosan formed with ionic molecules, polyelectrolyte polymer, and neutral polymers; (**b**) thermoreversible networks of chitosan graft copolymer resulting semisolid gel at body temperature and liquid below room temperature (Bhattarai et al. 2010)

polyelectrolytes form electrostatic interactions with chitosan, they are different from the ions or ionic molecules used in ionic complexation in that they are larger molecules with a broad molecular weight range, such as polysaccharides, proteins, and synthetic polymers (Fig. 2.12). They are complexed without the use of organic precursors, catalysts, or reactive agents, alleviating the concern about safety in the body or cross-reactions with a therapeutic payload. In addition, because PECs consist of only chitosan and the polyelectrolyte, their complexation is straightforward and reversible.

Chitosan–alginate blend-based nanocomposite hydrogels containing sugars (see Fig. 2.13) were also shown to be highly effective in wound treatment (Travan et al. 2009). The role of chitosan is fundamental in the formation and stabilization of well-dispersed small silver nanoparticles, for instance. Reproducibility of size distribution together with a demonstrated stability of the nanoparticles over time can be achieved in chitosan-based polymer matrices. Moreover, the use of sugar-based additives adds a considerable appeal to the results obtained. The simultaneous presence of a sugar-based bioactive polymer for cell stimulation (Fig. 2.13) and of silver nanoparticles in the gel for antibacterial activity represents a major achievement in would treatment. Such approaches can bridge the gap between nanotechnology and glycobiology (Travan et al. 2009; Morais et al. 2013).

In open-wound treatment, there is the major risk of infection that presents serious consequences, which can compromise the recovery success. To prevent those infections, several approaches are used such as sterility protocols and antibiotics administration. However, these protocols are not always effective, and the antibiotic activity can even fail due to pathogenic resistance development. Therefore, recently, studies were made to ascertain the use of certain ions as antimicrobial agents, such as cerium (Ce), which has revealed antimicrobial properties against several microorganisms (Morais et al. 2013). This way, it can be incorporated in different biomaterials to grant them antimicrobial ability, contributing to a better

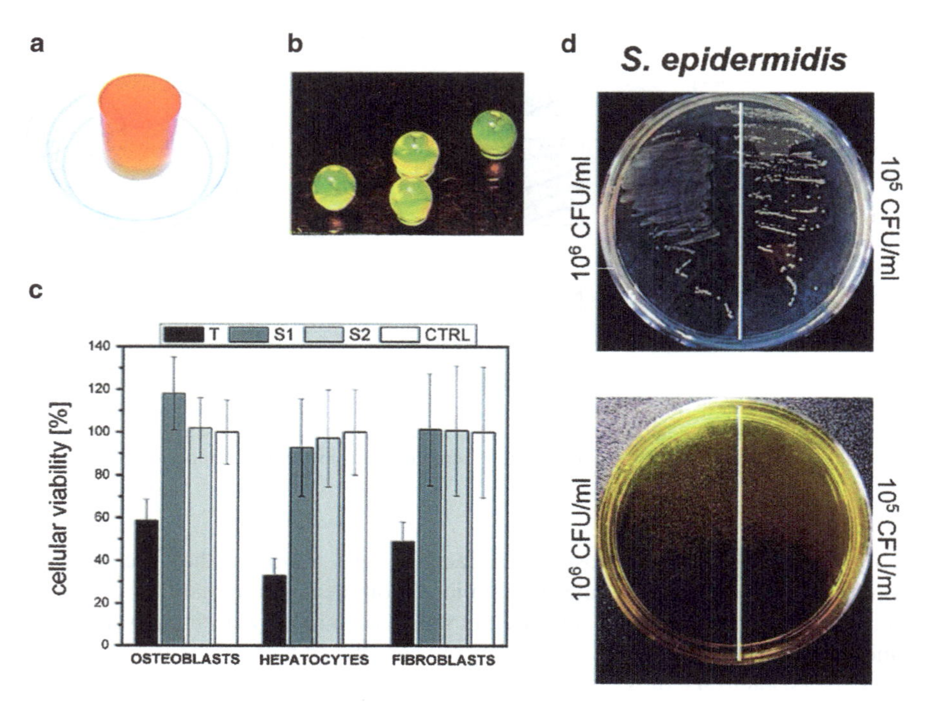

Fig. 2.13 (**a**) Mixed alginate – chitosan–sugar cylindrical hydrogel containing silver nanoparticles. (**b**) Alginate–silver microspheres. (**c**) Cytotoxicity analysis (MTT assay) on mouse fibroblast (NIH-3T3), human hepatocarcinoma (HepG2), and human osteosarcoma (MG63) cell lines of functional gel microspheres external solutions (S1 and S2, external solutions not diluted and 1:10 diluted, respectively; T, cytotoxicity positive control, cells treated with Triton 1 %; CTRL, cytotoxicity negative control, cells treated with 0.015 M NaCl solution). (**d**) Growth of *S. epidermidis* on 20 % Mueller – Hinton AC gel (*upper Petri dish*) and on 20 % Mueller – Hinton AC-nAg gel (*lower Petri dish*) (Travan et al. 2009)

wider spectrum wound sterilization and healing performance. A recent study evaluated the biological performance of hydrogels based on alginate, chitosan, and hyaluronic acid blends, which were found to enhance tissue generation. Furthermore, in order to obtain a hydrogel not only with a tissue generation enhancement ability but also with an antimicrobial ability to avoid infections, Ce(III) ions were incorporated in one of these hydrogels, and its biological performance was also studied and effectiveness of Ce(III) was demonstrated (Morais et al. 2013).

Fluorinated chitosan hydrogels were shown to be highly effective in wound treatment (Wijekoon et al. 2013). Recently, series of novel, biocompatible hydrogels able to repeatedly take up and deliver oxygen at beneficial levels have been developed by conjugating various perfluorocarbon (PFC) chains to methacrylamide chitosan via Schiff base nucleophilic substitution, followed by photopolymerization to form hydrogels. This new class of fluorinated and biologically derived chitosan materials can be formed into injectable or moldable photo-cross-linked hydrogels allowing controlling both the capacity and rate of oxygen delivery, providing beneficial oxygen levels for days in a wound (Wijekoon et al. 2013). Since these systems are capable of reloading oxygen more than once, they can be utilized for long periods of time potentially weeks for treatment and cell regeneration. Fibroblast cells were shown to respond favorably to such enhanced oxygen environments even without supplemental oxygen which should directly translate to accelerated wound healing in vivo.

Another material of choice for construction is cyclodextrins (CD) towards biopolymer hydrogels with antimicrobial properties (Glisoni et al. 2013). For instance, two types of hydrophilic networks with conjugated beta-cyclodextrin (β-CD) were recently developed with the aim of engineering useful platforms for the localized release of an antimicrobial 5,6-dimethoxy-1-indanone N4-allyl thiosemicarbazone (TSC) in the soft and moist tissue such as the eye and its potential application in ophthalmic diseases. Poly(2-hydroxyethyl methacrylate) soft contact lenses (SCLs) coated with β-CD, namely, pHEMA-co-β-CD, and superhydrophilic hydrogels (SHHs) of directly cross-linked hydroxypropyl-β-CD were synthesized and characterized regarding their structure (ATR/FT-IR), drug loading capacity, swelling, and in vitro release in artificial lacrimal fluid. Incorporation of TSC to the networks was carried out both during polymerization (DP method) and after synthesis (PP method). The first method led to similar drug loads in all the hydrogels, with minor drug loss during the washing steps to remove unreacted monomers, while the second method evidenced the influence of structural parameters on the loading efficiency (proportion of CD units, mesh size, swelling degree). Both systems provided a controlled TSC release for at least 2 weeks, TSC concentrations (up to 4000 μg/g dry hydrogel) being within an optimal therapeutic window for the antimicrobial ocular treatment. Microbiological tests against *P. aeruginosa* and *S. aureus* confirmed the ability of TSC-loaded pHEMA-co-β-CD network to inhibit bacterial growth as demonstrated in Fig. 2.14.

As we exemplified in this section, hydrogels are playing an increasing role in regenerative medicine and wound care owing to their growing functional sophistication. This is being fortified by advances in hydrogel synthesis, particularly through molecular and genetic engineering, which provide greater control of hydrogel structure and hence the emergence of hydrogels with new functionalities particularly existence of multifunctional aspects such as antimicrobial properties as well as cell proliferation and structural stability. In order to exploit and expand biomedical uses of hydrogels based on biopolymers, it is necessary to fully understand the relationship between hydrogel structure and function. This section is by no means a comprehensive review of such materials but aimed to highlight the key attributes of biopolymer hydrogels that modulate their function, with discussions and examples on the link between these attributes and hydrogel behavior, and identifying possible future applications to elucidate them.

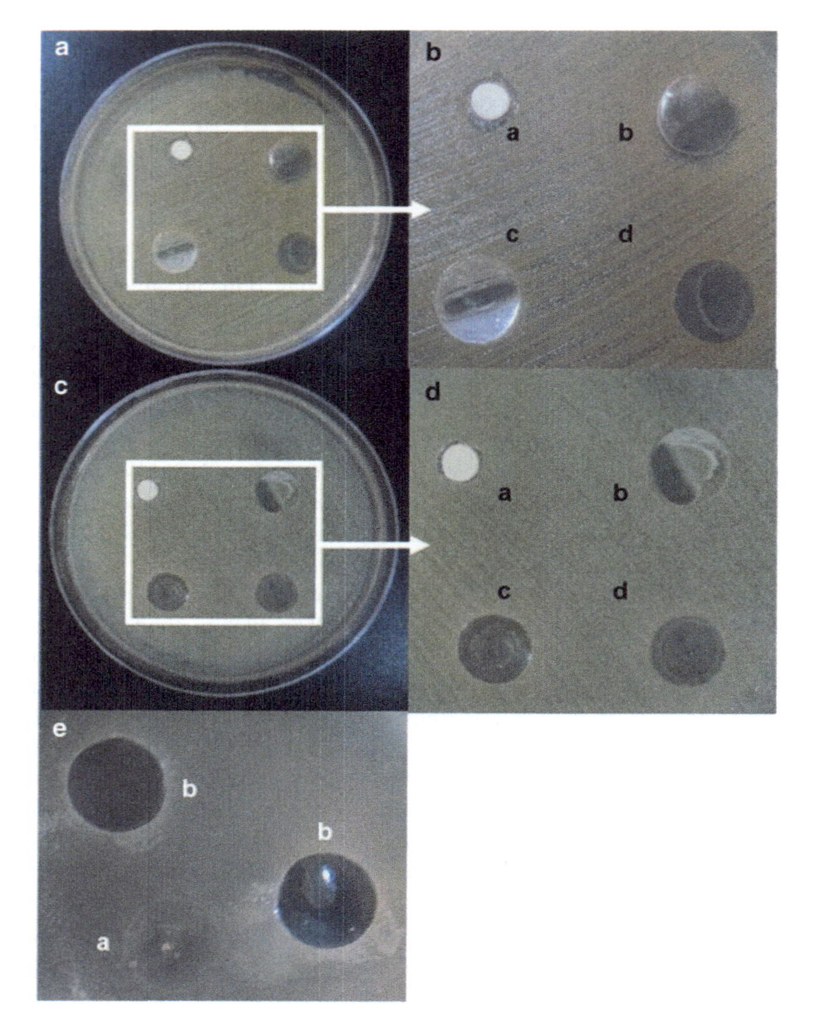

Fig. 2.14 Antibacterial activity in (**a**, **b**, and **e**) against *S. aureus* ATCC 6538 and (**c** and **d**) against *P. aeruginosa* ATCC 9027 cultures after 24 h. (a) Paper disk loaded with 200 μg of TSC (positive control), (b) SCL without TSC (negative control), (c) TSC-loaded SCL obtained by the PP method with stirring of 24 h and (d) TSC-loaded SCL obtained by the DP method. All the SCLs are pHEMA-co-β-CD with 10 % (w/v) of mono-MA-β-CD. (**b** and **d**) The magnification of (**a**) and (**c**), respectively. (**e**) Bacterial growth beneath the surface of (a) TSC-free and (b) TSC-loaded SCLs (Glisoni et al. 2013)

2.6 Fibrous Materials with Antibacterial and Tissue Regenerating Activity for Skin Wound Healing

The use of hydrogel materials described in Sect. 2.5 as wound dressings has some drawbacks, such as swelling and low active surface, that can be overcome using fibrous composite materials. These materials can be conventional fibrous dressings, such as woven cotton, properly modified to attain also antibacterial properties, or nonwoven synthetic or natural polymeric fibers made with conventional methods or by electrospinning for fibers of nanometric dimensions. Such fibers can incorporate various active nutrient or antibacterial and antimicrobial compounds that can aid the wound-healing process. In order to develop fibrous wound dressings, various methods such as dry spinning, wet spinning, spinning with viscose-type spinnerets, or even functionalization of textiles have been presented so far in the literature. In the majority of these approaches, natural polymers were used, like chitin, chitosan (Pillai et al. 2009; Notin et al. 2006), alginates (Qin 2008; Neibert et al. 2012), cellulose, silk fibroin, combination of those (Fan et al. 2005, 2006), or also their combination with synthetic polymers.

Over the last years, these techniques have been progressively replaced by electrospinning. Electrospinning is a highly versatile, effective, easily scalable, and low-cost technique to fabricate ultrathin fibers that cannot be produced with any other technique, with diameters in the submicron and nanometer range depending on the polymeric materials used and the processing conditions. Another advantage of electrospun nanofibrous wound dressing with respect to all the other dressing types is based to the fact that they can mimic the architecture of EMC due to the nanometer scale of the fibers' diameter and to their overall nanotopography. As reported above, wound healing is a complex and dynamic process of restoring cellular structures and tissue layers through interactions of cells, growth factor, and EMC (Calne 2011). The biological functionality of EMC has not yet being fully reproduced in wound dressing materials, possibly due to its complexity and multifunctionality. Indeed, the EMC is the main constituent of the dermal skin layer containing proteoglycans, collagen, hyaluronic acid, fibronectin, and elastin, all components essential for skin regeneration. A recent review on electrospun materials used for wound healing makes a very complete synopsis on the activity of the EMC components during the wound-healing process (Rieger et al. 2013). Nevertheless, although the complete biological activity of the EMC is not replicated, the use of specific polymers in combination with the particular topography of the electrospun mats can provide to the tissues the ideal environment to promote wound healing. By loading them with active principles present in the EMC, exactly like in the case of the bioactivated cell-instructive scaffolds described in Sect. 2.3, the tissue regeneration activity can be greatly assisted when such active dressings are put in the proximity of the wound. In tissue engineering, electrospun mats were proved ideal scaffolds for cells adhesion, growth, proliferation, and differentiation (Moffa et al. 2013; Polini et al. 2013). Here, we focus on the research efforts made in the field of active wound dressings.

In the electrospinning technique, a high electric field is applied in order to create fibers with a diameter ranging from a few nanometers to larger than 1 μm. A basic electrospinning apparatus consists of a syringe filled with the target polymer solution, a syringe pump, a high voltage supply, and a collector. The metallic needle of the syringe serves as electrode to induce electrical charges within the solution, under the influence of a strong electrostatic field. When the charge repulsion overcomes the surface tension of the polymeric solution, a charged polymeric jet is formed and is accelerated towards the collector. During the flight of the jet, the solvent evaporates and polymeric nanofibers are collected.

The electrospun fiber mats have high surface area, much higher than films of hydrogel materials or even that other fibrous dressing made in conventional ways. In this way, that can assure optimized exude absorption, moisture permeation, and gas transport (Zhang et al. 2005). On the top, this technique is highly versatile in terms of used materials. Indeed, electrospun fibers can be made of natural or synthetic polymers or different combinations of both. Finally, the electrospun mats can attain different functionalities by tuning the different polymer concentrations and by incorporating in the nanofibers different drugs, active biological molecules, antibacterial agents, etc.

2.7 Electrospun Mats Without Active Agents

Natural polymers, such as polysaccharides and proteins are the most common electrospun materials used for treatment of skin wounds due to their inherent properties that assist the process of healing. In the majority of the cases, they are used in combination with synthetic polymers due to their intrinsic low processability (e.g., poor solubility and high surface tension) (Lee et al. 2009) but also in order to enhance the mechanical properties and tune the morphological features of the produced mats. In particular, the polysaccharide chitosan has demonstrated intrinsic hemostatic and antibacterial properties, and for this reason many research works have been focused on its electrospinning. Since it cannot be electrospun alone, it is used in combination with other polymers. For example, an electrospun matrix of chitosan, collagen, and polyethylene oxide was fabricated followed by further cross-linking using glutaraldehyde vapor. Animal studies showed increased wound-healing rate using this matrix as wound dressing compared to gauzes and commercial collagen sponges (Chen et al. 2008). Also the electrospun combination of chitosan and silk fibroin has demonstrated good antibacterial activity and biocompatibility using murine fibroblasts. Although only in vitro tests were performed, the results suggest that such composite nanofibrous membranes can be used in wound healing (Cai et al. 2010). A successful combination of electrospun nanofibers includes chitosan, hydroxybenzotriazole, and polyvinyl alcohol blend. This underwent cytotoxicity tests and was found nontoxic to human fibroblast cells, suggesting its suitability as wound dressing material (Charernsriwilaiwat et al. 2010). A natural polysaccharide that has shown great potentiality for the regeneration of tissues is the alginate, but few works have been done on its electrospinning since it easily forms fibers using the wet spinning technique of sodium alginate in a calcium salt aqueous solution. Uniform electrospun nanofibers were obtained by a blend of a cell adhesive peptide modified alginate, unmodified alginate, and PEO and demonstrated good human dermal fibroblast cells adhesion (Jeong et al. 2010). Another study has better demonstrated the potentiality of blended PVA-sodium alginate electrospun nanofibrous mats as wound dressings by in vivo experiments. The healing performances of wounds using the prepared electrospun dressings were compared with commercially available dressings with promising results (Üstündağ et al. 2010). A polysaccharide that is the main component of the natural extracellular matrix in connective tissues is the hyaluronic acid and as such is expected to play an important role in the wound-healing process. Indeed, electrospun mats of hyaluronic acid compared in a preclinical study with five commercial gauzes and antibiotic dressings showed increased performances in the healing of wounds (Uppal et al. 2011). Among the natural protein polymers that have been electrospun for wound dressing applications, collagen is possibly the most popular since it is an important extracellular matrix component that promotes wound healing. Electrospun membranes of polylactide–polyglycolide/collagen were found to be very effective as wound-healing accelerators of open wounds in rats especially in the early-stage healing (Liu et al. 2010a). The effects of polycaprolactone/collagen electrospun nanofibers in aligned and random arrangements on phenotypic expression of human adipose stromal cells in vitro were studied recently. The cells demonstrated higher synthesis capacity for critical extracellular matrix molecules in the aligned nanofibers, demonstrating the potentiality of the latter for accelerated wound repair (Xiaoling and Wang 2012). Electrospun nanofibrous membranes of modified polycaprolactone–collagen were found suitable for the attachment and proliferation of fibroblast, suggesting the potential to be used for the treatment of skin defects and burn wounds (Venugopal et al. 2006). Finally, electrospun silk has been evaluated in terms of conformational and biocompatible characteristics related to wound dressings. Six distinct electrospun silk material groups in the hydrated state exhibited absorption, water vapor transmission, oxygen permeation, and enzymatic biodegradation, essential characteristics for dressings of wounds. In the dry state, three of the electrospun silk materials were found to be the best potential candidates for wound dressings (Wharram et al. 2010). Another protein, the gelatin has been electrospun with poly(vinyl alcohol) starting from their aqueous solutions. The produced nanofibers fibers were subsequently cross-linked with glutaraldehyde vapor and heat treated. Due to the cytocompatibility of the mats, proved through test in vitro with fibroblasts, they were suggested as potential wound dressings (Yang et al. 2011). Blends of low-molecular-weight fish scale collagen peptides and chito-oligosaccharide with polyvinyl alcohol were electrospun to form nanofibrous membranes. The membranes showed good antibacterial activity especially against gram-positive *Staphylococcus aureus* and a bit less against gram-negative Escherichia coli, indicating that the membranes released intracellular materials, particularly with *S. aureus*. The electrospun membranes showed also good biocompatibility using in vitro measurements with human skin fibroblasts. The authors claimed that low-molecular-weight fish scale collagen peptides are superior to mammalian collagen for wound repairing (Wang et al. 2011b). Finally, electrospun fibrinogen nanofibers were proposed as wound dressing, since fibrinogen is a protein present in the blood plasma with important role in wound healing (Wnek et al. 2003).

2.8 Electrospun Mats Loaded with Active Agents

In the skin wound healing, active agents are considered substances that intervene in the course of one or more phases of the process facilitating its finalization. A variety of electrospun mats loaded with active agents have been proposed for topical antimicrobial, drug, antibiotic, or bioactive molecules delivery.

Loading in the course of electrospinning Silk–PEO electrospun mats containing epidermal growth factor were fabricated, from a common solution, for the promotion of wound-healing processes. The incorporated epidermal growth factor was slowly released (25 % release in 170 h). Using a human three-dimensional model, the authors demonstrated that the biofunctionalized silk mats, when used as dressings, aid the healing of wounds by increasing the time of wound closure by the epidermal tongue by 90 %. On the top, the mats were preserving their structural integrity during the healing time (Schneider et al. 2009). Among the wound dressing fibrous materials, the ones that contain silver nanoparticles for antibacterial activity are quite popular. In a work on gelatin nanofibers, silver nanoparticles were formed in situ in the gelatin solution starting from their $AgNO_3$ precursor at least 12 h after the preparation of the solution, with the amount of nanoparticles increasing with increasing time. Electrospinning of the nanoparticles-containing solutions lead to nanocomposite fibers that were further cross-linked with moist glutaraldehyde vapor to improve their stability in an aqueous medium. The fibrous mats showed good antibacterial activity with decreasing strength against *Pseudomonas aeruginosa*, followed by *Staphylococcus aureus*, *Escherichia coli*, and methicillin-resistant *S. aureus* (Rujitanaroj et al. 2008). In another work, silver nanoparticles were synthesized in situ in the spinning formic acid solution of chitosan or *N*-carboxyethyl chitosan and PEO. The nanoparticles were uniformly dispersed in the nanofibers, and 15 % wt. of them was decorating the fibers' surface. The composite electrospun mats were proposed for antibacterial wound dressing materials (Penchev et al. 2009). Instead of silver, also TiO_2 nanoparticles have been used as antibacterial fillers. Indeed, in situ generated TiO_2 in electrospun polyurethane fibers was efficient against *Ps. aeruginosa* and *S. aureus*. The membranes also showed water vapor transmission and immediate adherence to L929 cells, all properties essential for wound dressing applications (Yan et al. 2011). In other research works, plant extracts have been used as fillers in electrospun nanofibers either to promote cell proliferation or to induce an antibacterial activity to the developed dressings. In particular, cellulose acetate fiber mats containing either asiaticoside (from the plant *Centella asiatica*) or curcumin (from the plant *Curcuma longa* L.) were successfully prepared. Normal human dermal fibroblasts were attached and proliferate better on the electrospun mats when asiaticoside was included, whereas the presence of curcumin imparted their antioxidant activity (Suwantong et al. 2010). Moreover, the crude bark extract of the plant *Tecomella undulate* was loaded in PCL/PVP electrospun fibers that were found to inhibit the growth of *P. aeruginosa*, *S. aureus*, and *E. coli* (Suganya et al. 2011). Lysozyme, an enzyme found in abundance in egg white and a natural form of protection from gram-positive pathogens, was used as an additive in electrospun mats of chitosan–ethylenediaminetetraacetic acid and polyvinyl alcohol. The rate of wound healing of the composite mats was found to be accelerated compared to gauze controls, in experiments performed in vivo using male Wistar rats, indicating that lysozyme-loaded nanofibers have a potential for wound healing (Charernsriwilaiwat et al. 2012). Furthermore antibiotics were successfully electrospun in combination with the right polymers. In particular, electrospun nanofibrous membranes of PEG–PLA incorporating the hydrophilic antibiotic drug, tetracycline hydrochloride, were found to preserve the bioactivity. The antibiotic was released over 6 days and was found to be effective in inhibiting growth of *S. aureus*. Such a local sustained delivery of antibiotics makes these membranes promising as wound dressings for ulcers caused by diabetes or other diseases (Xu et al. 2010). Finally, the group of Xiaohong Li has used emulsion electrospinning to embed fibroblast growth factor into ultrafine poly(ethylene glycol)-based fibers with a core–sheath structure to promote the wound-healing process. In vivo tests in the dorsal area of diabetic rats showed that the gradual growth factor release increased the wound recovery rate with improved vascularization, enhanced collagen deposition and maturation, complete re-epithelialization, and formation of skin appendages. The authors suggest the use of such electrospun fibrous mats to accelerate the healing of diabetic skin ulcers (Yang et al. 2012).

In few cases of electrospun mats developed for wound dressings, the active agents are loaded to the fibers after the mats preparation, a method that has given also promising results. As an example, we mention silk fibroin mats that were prepared by electrospinning and subsequently coated with silver nanoparticles. The composite mats were fabricated as prototypic wound dressings and demonstrated good antimicrobial properties against *Staphylococcus aureus* and *Pseudomonas aeruginosa* (Uttayarat et al. 2012). Another example of postproduction functionalization is the loading of a cationic drug neomycin onto the cationic exchange nanofibers of poly(styrene sulfonic acid-co-maleic acid) and polyvinyl alcohol. Prior to loading, the fibers were subjected to thermal cross-linking to produce ion exchange nanofiber mats. In vivo, wound-healing tests performed in Wistar rats revealed that the functionalized mats decreased the acute wound size during the first week after tissue damage better than gauze and blank nanofiber mats. On the top, neomycin-loaded nanofiber mats demonstrated satisfactory antibacterial activity against both gram-positive and gram-negative bacteria (Nitanan et al. 2013).

2.9 Multicomponent Electrospun Mats

The ideal wound dressing materials should follow the different phases of the wound-healing process by providing to the wound the right substances at the right time in order to optimize the wound-healing processes and times. A few works have demonstrated the use of multicomponent electrospun mats, for a simultaneous or a stepwise release of the active agents in specific stages of the wound-healing process. In particular, composite electrospun mats of poly(lactic-co-glycolic acid) with mesoporous silica nanoparticles were used for the co-encapsulation and prolonged simultaneous release of the hydrophilic model drug rhodamine B and the hydrophobic model drug fluorescein. The codrug delivery system can be very useful for wound dressings that require combined therapy of several kinds of drugs (Song et al. 2012a). Further work of the group on the same system showed that the release of the two drugs can be monitored separately. Most of the fluorescein was released rapidly during the 324 h of the trial, but the rhodamine B showed a sustained release behavior (Song et al. 2012b).

Multicomponent systems can be also considered all the core–shell electrospun fibers. Especially for wound dressing applications, the use of electrospun membranes that consist of core–shell fibers is gaining increasing interest. To prepare such fibers using electrospinning, two different polymers can be separately delivered to the inner and outer channel of a coaxial-tube spinneret. Different active agents can be loaded to the core and to the shell of the fibers in order to obtain their sustainable delivery to the wound. Wang et al. used poly(DL-lactic acid) and poly (3-hydroxybutyrate), two biodegradable polymers, for the production of core–shell nanofibers with the possibility to swap the material for the core and the shell. Using poly(3-hydroxybutyrate) as the shell, the loaded dimethyloxalylglycine drug could be released in a controllable manner. Whereas the single component fibers showed an immediate release, the core–shell fibers showed two-stage release kinetics when the drug was embedded in the core. The amount released in the first stage was 25 % within 60 h, independent from the shell thickness. In the second stage, the release rate was controlled by the thickness of the shell and was linear (Wang et al. 2010). Another very recent work demonstrated the use of core–shell nanofibers of gelatin and poly(L-lactic acid)-co-poly-(ε-caprolactone) to encapsulate multiple epidermal induction factors such as the epidermal growth factor, insulin, hydrocortisone, and retinoic acid. When the same fibers were blend spun, an initial 44.9 % burst release of the active agents was observed during the first 15 days, whereas no burst release was detected from the core–shell nanofibers. Moreover, the proliferation and differentiation to epidermal lineages of stem cells on the core–shell nanofibers were higher with respect to the blended fibers (Jin et al. 2013). In a similar way, the antibiotic gentamicin was encapsulated in coaxial fibers containing a skin of PLA and a core of collagen using electrospinning in order to provide to wounds a strong and time-controllable antibacterial release (Torres-Giner et al. 2012).

2.10 A Special Focus on Antibacterial Silver Nanoparticles

Infectious diseases by human pathogens have been considered one of the first causes of mortality and disability since the last century. The discovery and global commercialization of antibiotics in the second half of the twentieth century was a milestone of modern medicine. However, together with the development of effective antibacterial drugs, the issue of antimicrobial resistance is also raising concerns worldwide, due to an almost indiscriminate abuse in the last decades (Powers 2004; Spellberg 2008; Spellberg et al. 2008; Morens et al. 2010). Bacteria, in fact, may rapidly evolve specific molecular determinants able to interact with the drug in an unpredictable way, leading to its inactivation, degradation, or expulsion (Andersson and Hughes 2010; Schwaber et al. 2004; Levy and Marshall 2004). As a consequence, several active molecules discovered in the last decades are now rather inadequate also for the treatment of pathologies commonly considered as weakly hazardous. Thus, new effective solutions are required through innovative, multidisciplinary approaches, which should include the design and development of new antibacterial compounds meeting the requirements of low cost of production, specificity, and long-term efficacy (to avoid the significant limitation of bacterial resistance to classical drugs). In this regard, nanotechnology may provide some previously unexplored methods and techniques to develop innovative antimicrobial drugs and devices. In particular, silver-based nanomaterials in the form of colloidal nanoparticles (AgNPs) are emerging as promising candidates for the next generation of systemic drugs, thanks to broad-spectrum efficacy and their intrinsic ability to reach even very peripheral body districts and to cross biological barriers. On the other side, nanoengineered silver-based nanocomposites are increasingly explored for the realization of safe intracorporeal implants to avoid the formation of localized infections.

Although silver has been considered a “poisoning metal” for microorganisms since antiquities (Liau et al. 1997; Klasen 2000a, b), the current advancement of nanotechnology is enabling the realization of different types of AgNPs and silver nanocomposites with high controlled and tuned physicochemical characteristics at nanoscale level (e.g., in terms of size, shape, and surface chemistry) (Dahl et al. 2007). Herein, we aim to provide to the readers the most recent knowledge about the use of AgNPs as antimicrobial agent, a topic that is increasingly attracting great interest, as also confirmed by the annual worldwide production of nanosilver of more than 300 tons (Nowack et al. 2011; Kumar et al. 2008). In particular, we review the biocidal effects of AgNPs, with a special focus on both the advantages and open issues rising in this topic and on the molecular mechanisms of nanosilver action. In addition, we discuss the limits and drawbacks in the methods exploited for the antibacterial tests, providing useful guidelines for the design of efficient antibacterial nanosystems. Although there is a huge and increasing number of studies available on this subject (Eckhardt et al. 2013; Chernousova and Epple 2013; Hajipour et al. 2012; Lemire et al. 2013), it should be considered that literature data are rather contrasting (especially regarding the role played by the physicochemical properties of NPs and the actual dose), mainly because of the general lack of standardized nanomaterials and assays employed for characterizing the biocidal effects.

The effect of the physicochemical properties of AgNPs (e.g., size, shape, and surface chemistry) on their antimicrobial activity is discussed next. Concerning the size, smaller AgNPs demonstrate a stronger bactericidal activity compared to bigger particles. For instance, Choi and collaborator demonstrated that AgNPs in the range of 5–20 nm are more effective compared to bigger NPs, to AgCl (in the form of colloids), and to free Ag^+ ions (from a silver salt) (Choi and Hu 2008). In this case, the toxicity effects have been related to production of reactive oxygen species (ROS) combined to strong membrane damage. This was later confirmed by Sondi et al. (Sondi and Salopek-Sondi 2004). The strong efficiency of small AgNPs was also demonstrated by other works, who reported that AgNPs with a diameter of c.a. 10 nm have a stronger tendency to bind the membrane of gram-negative bacteria, as compared to bigger nanoparticles, thus leading to a more pronounced damage (Morones et al. 2005). The authors also stated that the release of Ag^+ ions from the particles surface represents a major contribution to the overall bactericidal effects.

Apart from size, also surface charge has been demonstrated to have an important role. In particular, positively charged AgNPs were found to elicit a strong activity against microorganisms, while negatively charged particles were less toxic (El Badawy et al. 2011). This behavior was explained in terms of electrostatic interactions between the negative membrane of bacteria and the positive charge covering the surface of particles. In particular, the electrostatic interactions may increase the dose of silver in the close proximity of microorganisms.

With respect to the AgNPs shape, truncated triangular silver nanoplates, with a (111) lattice plane, were observed to elicit a strong antibacterial activity, compared to both rod- and spherical-shaped AgNPs and to Ag^+. However, despite these experimental data highlighted a direct correlation between the NPs shape and the biological outcomes, a crucial role was again ascribed to the NPs surface charge, since truncated silver nanoplates had a positive charge (Pal et al. 2007). The above studies concluded that the toxicity mechanisms may be related to both AgNPs and Ag^+ ions released from their surfaces, though not providing a definite conclusion. Only recently, an elegant work solved this problem, demonstrating that the bactericidal effects are mainly due to the silver ions (Xiu et al. 2012). The authors fabricated AgNPs of ~5 and ~11 nm and stored them under anaerobic conditions, where the release of Ag^+ is completely prevented (Liu et al. 2010b; Liu and Hurt 2010). Interestingly, the viability assays on *E. coli* showed that AgNPs have no detectable effects under anaerobic conditions (in which there is no Ag^+ release), also using NPs concentrations higher than the minimum lethal concentration (MLC). On the other side, incubation of *E. coli* and AgNPs under aerobic conditions showed significant toxicity. It is thus evident that the physicochemical characteristics of AgNPs do not play a crucial role in determining the toxicity, rather than are important in terms of influencing the rate of Ag^+ release from the nanoparticle surfaces. For instance, the specific surface area (per mass unit) is higher in smaller AgNPs, thus allowing a higher rate of silver ion release. There are several other works that explored the bactericidal effects of AgNPs (Smetana et al. 2008; Panacek et al. 2006, 2009; Vertelov et al. 2008; Kim et al. 2008b, 2009; Navarro et al. 2008). However, it should be considered that there is a general level of data disagreement, especially regarding the final dose of AgNPs required for eliciting a strong bactericidal effect, the preferential molecular targets of NPs, and the real molecular mechanisms underlying toxicity.

The most acknowledged theory regarding the bactericidal effect of silver indicates a mechanism of direct membrane damage, due to chemical interaction between Ag^+ and bacterial membrane proteins. In particular, Ag^+ is a soft cation and, according to the hard–soft acid–base theory (HSAB) of Pearson, it may strongly bind soft ligand, such as the sulfur groups of proteins. In addition, other coordination complexes have been proposed between Ag^+ and all the different amino acids, in which the binding affinity was theoretically and experimentally calculated (Nomiya et al. 2000; Jover et al. 2008, 2009; Kasuga et al. 2012). As a consequence of the interaction event, bacterial membrane may undergo a general loss of function, especially regarding the impairment of the respiratory chain, followed by dissipation of proton motive force and ATP production, and increased permeability which does not allow the membrane to compensate the external osmotic pressure (Eckhardt et al. 2013; Dibrov et al. 2002). The decrease in ATP level, combined with membrane loss of activity, may then generate further metabolic concerns, especially for crucial enzyme-dependent metabolic pathways. Additionally, another possible mechanism of membrane damage-related toxicity includes the formation of breaks or pits (Li et al. 2011; Mirzajani et al. 2011). In particular, silver ions have been proposed to destroy the $\beta - 1 \rightarrow 4$ glycosidic bonds connecting the main building blocks of the peptidoglycan, namely, the *N*-acetylglucosamine and *N*-acetylmuramic acid, which are consequently released into the media (Mirzajani et al. 2011). In this scenario, positively charged AgNPs situated in close proximity to the cell membrane may be also subjected to a strong pH decrease (down to values of 3, due to the bacterial proton motive force) that, in turn, might promote localized Ag^+ release, which further increases the NPs toxicity.

Following membrane damage/poration, external Ag^+ and even AgNPs (although this latter occurrence has not been clearly demonstrated) may gain direct access to the cytosol, where silver ions may induce further damage. Upon reaching the cytosol, Ag^+ ions may interact with a number of important enzymes, unfolding them and decreasing, for instance, the enzymatic activity of the respiratory chain dehydrogenase (Li et al. 2011). Moreover, Ag^+ ions can interfere with the enzymes by replacing their native metal cation from the binding site (e.g., in the case of metalloproteins). Silver ions may also strongly bind DNA, with a preferential binding site to guanine N7 and adenine N7 (Arakawa et al. 2001). This may lead, in turn, to inaccurate DNA condensation, as well as errors in DNA replication and transcriptions, that may cause random mutations.

All these considerations assume that Ag^+ directly induces a specific damage, due to physical/chemical interaction events. On the other side, silver ions may also lead to indirect damages by means of reactive oxygen species (ROS) production. In this respect, singlet oxygen, hydrogen peroxide, superoxide radical anion, and hydroxyl radical are known to target lipids, DNA, RNA, and proteins, causing severe effects, including malfunction of membranes, proteins, and DNA replication machinery (Cabiscol et al. 2000). The issue of Ag^+ -related ROS production remains, however, quite controversial, as some research works addressed strong correlation (Choi and Hu 2008; Inoue et al. 2002; Hwang et al. 2008), while other experimental data displayed no significant trends (Sintubin et al. 2011; Xiu et al. 2011). This is likely due to the ability of microorganisms to resist oxidative stress by adopting several molecular strategies, which include direct immediate detoxification carried out by enzymes (i.e., catalase, superoxide dismutase, and peroxidase) (Fang 2004) and a long-term detoxification controlled by a transcriptional expression of several proteins (including OxyR, SoxRS, and PerR). These strategies enable bacteria a high survival probability against ROS-related stress.

However, it should be considered that a detailed and universal description of the antibacterial mechanisms of AgNPs is still not available, also due to general lack of standardized materials and protocols to be employed for the assays. In particular, the synthesis of high-quality AgNPs, in terms of narrow size and shape distribution, remained a challenge for several years, and only in the recent years some good results were achieved (Burda et al. 2005; Wennemers 2012; Liang et al. 2010; Belser et al. 2009; Upert et al. 2012). A typical reaction is governed, in fact, by different thermodynamic factors. Capturing the distinct stages of a controlled atomic nucleation around few atoms represented a serious challenge, which has been only solved recently. However, most of the data available to date about the bactericidal properties of AgNPs have been obtained with particles having almost uncontrolled physicochemical properties or particles that were not characterized. Together with the absence of an analytical approach for particles characterization and testing, this hindered the possibility to have a confident explanation of the various phenomena. In this respect, an important point is that AgNPs should be characterized by means of different techniques (e.g., dynamic light scattering, UV-visible spectroscopy, transmission electron, and/or scanning electron microscopy), both in aqueous medium and after incubation in the bacterial culture medium. The specific components of the media may, in fact, interact with the particle surface (e.g., forming a protein corona), significantly changing their original physicochemical properties and, consequently, also the observed biological outcomes (Walczyk et al. 2010; Monopoli et al. 2011a, b). In particular, the colloidal stability of AgNPs in biological growth media is an important parameter to keep under control: NPs may form aggregates/agglomerates and precipitates, consequently compromising the effective dose of silver and, also, the NPs efficacy. Furthermore, also the medium proteins and salts may bind free Ag^+ (released from the AgNPs surface), reducing the overall final dose available.

Another point is the kinetic of silver oxidation that may be strongly affected by the specific medium used. In this latter case, a correct procedure includes the use of different methods for quantifying, in situ, the Ag^+ release from the NPs surface. For instance, the inductively coupled plasma spectrometry-based techniques (i.e.,

ICP-OES and ICP-MS, which are rather sensitive but require physical separation of Ag^+ from AgNPs) and UV–Vis analyses (having the advantage of correlating the decrease of AgNPs surface plasmon absorption band with NPs dissolution, even in complex media) (Zook et al. 2011) can be both useful to address the Ag^+ release.

From the above considerations, the same batch of AgNPs may behave in a completely different way when tested in different media or at different aging. Finally, most of the available commercial kits used to address the viability of bacteria, upon AgNPs treatment, are based on the use of fluorescent/colorimetric probes. In this latter case, the probe itself may directly interact with the NPs, providing false-positive or false-negative results, and AgNPs may directly interfere with the optical readout of some assays (such as in the case of bacterial viability assays). It is thus evident that a standardized method to study the interactions of NPs with bacteria is still far to be accomplished, and that future efforts should be strongly focused in such direction.

As a final point, we would like to drive the reader's attention to some of the advantages and disadvantages of the use of AgNPs or Ag^+ for fabricating effective antibacterial devices. In particular, while a classical laboratory test in solution will indicate that silver salts are significantly more effective than AgNPs, these latter represent a "pool" of Ag^+ ions that can be finely engineered/functionalized with specific targeting molecules, in order to reach a specific body compartment. Moreover, NPs possess an intrinsic Trojan horse effect, which enable them to cross biological membranes and barriers (for instance, allowing an abundant cellular uptake). In this respect, NPs are ideal candidates for defeating intracellular pathogen-related infections, where microorganisms proliferate within host cells, hiding from both standard antibiotics and host immune system. In addition, AgNPs may offer the characteristic of localized and controlled long-term release, since they can be finely engineered in order to control the kinetics of Ag^+ oxidation from their surface. This topic is of crucial importance in applications such as chronic infections, medical devices, and wound healing. Nevertheless, AgNPs are not probably the best choice for the treatment of acute infections, since an immediate release of Ag^+ is not feasible at physiologic conditions. On the other side, silver ions may be ideal candidates for fast defeating a bacterial colony, due to the high immediate dose accessible (though silver ions are not able to cross biological membranes and have a poor targeting efficiency). Moreover, unlike the laboratory model experiments (usually carried out in solution), for in vivo assays, NPs typically lead to higher effective dose as compared to silver ions.

The data available on the bactericidal effects of AgNPs represent a good chance, for pharmaceutical companies, to develop a new category of antibiotic compounds. However, several issues should be considered. First, the capability of finely controlling the Ag^+ release from the particles surface is a fundamental topic to be addressed, especially regarding the possibility of long-term release. Second, research tests should be based on standardized assays, reference materials, and specific SOPs (standard operating procedures, e.g., for NPS characterization and dispersion). Third, the indiscriminate use of AgNPs may lead to several worrying effects, including the possibility of enhancing the bacterial silver resistance. In this respect, it has been demonstrated that some particular strains of *E. coli* and *Salmonella* spp. already possess a peculiar operon, named *sil*, encoding for different proteins responsible for silver resistance (Gupta et al. 1998, 1999, 2001). In particular, the *sil* gene cluster codifies for periplasmic silver-binding proteins and molecular efflux pumps, which work in cooperation for expelling Ag^+ ions from the cytoplasm (or even the periplasmic space) to the extracellular space. Finally, the uncontrolled environmental release of silver (in the form of bulk, Ag^+, and AgNPs) is increasing the chance of exposure to humans (with unpredictable toxicity consequences), as well as it represents a serious risk from an ecological viewpoint, a topic that will be discussed with more details in the following paragraph.

2.10.1 Implications for the Environment and Human Risk Exposure

The environmental release of silver, in all its forms (i.e., ions, nanoparticles, and clusters), is constantly rising, and it is actually quantified to be c.a. 20 tons per year (Gottschalk et al. 2009). Hence, several research efforts aimed to understand the potential ecological consequences of silver release, in terms of investigating the toxic effects to the different organisms populating specific ecosystems. Also in this case, there is a significant data disagreement, since several works labeled nanosilver as a potential polluting agent, while other data considered it as negligible and not dangerous (Hansen and Baun 2012; Grieger et al. 2012; Blaser et al. 2008; Musee et al. 2011; Nowack et al. 2012). For instance, the release of silver in the soil has been proved to induce a dramatic decrease in the reproduction potential of the nematode *Caenorhabditis elegans* as a consequence of increased oxidative stress (Roh et al. 2009). Other environmental model organisms, such as the green alga *Chlamydomonas reinhardtii* or *Danio rerio*, displayed toxicity effects upon AgNPs treatments (Navarro et al. 2008; Asharani et al. 2008), suggesting that nanosilver is a potential pollutant. However, it should be highlighted that the ecotoxicology assays are usually performed by means of model experiments (i.e., in laboratory), which are not similar to real conditions. Here, in fact, the physicochemical characteristics of silver are quite unpredictable, in terms of particles size, shape, and agglomeration state. Hence, understanding the real effects of nanosilver on a specific fauna could represent, most probably, an extremely difficult challenge, due to the high and complex variables characterizing the system.

The rise in environmental presence of AgNPs is also increasing the possibility of human risk exposure. For this reason, many studies focused on exploring the potential adverse effects of nanosilver on eukaryotes (nanotoxicity assessment) (Christensen et al. 2010; Ahamed et al. 2010). Inhalation of vapors, aerosols, or particulates and oral or skin adsorption are the major routes of entry of silver compounds into the body. Upon inhalation, AgNPs may deposit in the respiratory tract, causing damage through direct contact with tissues. Then, they can reach the bloodstream and diffuse throughout all the central and peripheral body districts, causing extensive toxicity to different organs (Sue et al. 2001; Wadhera and Fung 2005; Takenaka et al. 2001). Several data indicate that AgNPs may be the cause of DNA damage and apoptosis in fibroblasts and liver cells and lead to cell death and oxidative stress in human skin carcinoma and fibrosarcoma cells (Arora et al. 2008, 2012). Also for eukaryotic cell lines, some molecular mechanisms of AgNPs action have been proposed and include increased LDH outflow, misregulation of GSH-related detoxification, reduced mitochondrial function, apoptosis, DNA fragmentation, ROS generation, and metallothionein sequestration (Arora et al. 2008; Hussain et al. 2005, 2006; Braydich-Stolle et al. 2005; Hsin et al. 2008; Ahamed et al. 2008; Park et al. 2010). It should be mentioned, as in the case of the low reproducibility of AgNPs bactericidal assays, that the data on eukaryotic toxicity are not conclusive, due to similar limitations of the lack of NP reference materials and standardized protocols for the tests, which hindered to achieve a correct risk assessment of AgNPs.

References

Ahamed M, Karns M, Goodson M, Rowe J, Hussain SM, Schlager JJ, Hong Y (2008) DNA damage response to different surface chemistry of silver nanoparticles in mammalian cells. Toxicol Appl Pharmacol 233(3):404–410

Ahamed M, Alsalhi MS, Siddiqui MK (2010) Silver nanoparticle applications and human health. Clin Chim Acta 411(23–24):1841–1848

Andersson DI, Hughes D (2010) Antibiotic resistance and its cost: is it possible to reverse resistance? Nat Rev Microbiol 8(4):260–271

Arakawa H, Neault JF, Tajmir-Riahi HA (2001) Silver(I) complexes with DNA and RNA studied by Fourier transform infrared spectroscopy and capillary electrophoresis. Biophys J 81(3): 1580–1587

Arora S, Jain J, Rajwade JM, Paknikar KM (2008) Cellular responses induced by silver nanoparticles: in vitro studies. Toxicol Lett 179(2):93–100

Arora S, Rajwade JM, Paknikar KM (2012) Nanotoxicology and in vitro studies: the need of the hour. Toxicol Appl Pharmacol 258(2):151–165

Asharani PV, Lian Wu Y, Gong Z, Valiyaveettil S (2008) Toxicity of silver nanoparticles in zebrafish models. Nanotechnology 19(25):255102

Athanassiou A, Lygeraki MI, Pisignano D, Lakiotaki K, Varda M, Mele E, Fotakis C, Cingolani R, Anastasiadis SH (2006) Photocontrolled variations in the wetting capability of photochromic polymers enhanced by surface nanostructuring. Langmuir 22:2329

Bacakova L, Filova E, Parizek M, Ruml T, Svorcik V (2011) Modulation of cell adhesion, proliferation and differentiation on materials designed for body implants. Biotechnol Adv 29:739

Battista S, Guarnieri D, Borselli C, Zeppetelli S, Borzacchiello A, Mayol L, Gerbasio D, Keene DR, Ambrosio L, Netti PA (2005) The effect of matrix composition of 3D constructs on embryonic stem cell differentiation. Biomaterials 26:6194

Bayer IS, Fragouli D, Martorana PJ, Martiradonna L, Cingolani R, Athanassiou A (2011) Solvent resistant superhydrophobic films from self-emulsifying carnauba wax–alcohol emulsions. Soft Matter 7:7939

Beke S, Anjum F, Tsushima H, Ceseracciu L, Chieregatti E, Diaspro A, Athanassiou A, Brandi F (2012) Towards excimer-laser-based stereolithography: a rapid process to fabricate rigid biodegradable photopolymer scaffolds. J R Soc Interface 9:3017

Beke S, Anjum F, Ceseracciu L, Romano I, Athanassiou A, Diaspro A, Brandi F (2013) Rapid fabrication of rigid biodegradable scaffolds by excimer laser mask projection technique: a comparison between 248 and 308 nm. Laser Phys 23:035602

Belser K, Vig Slenters T, Pfumbidzai C, Upert G, Mirolo L, Fromm KM, Wennemers H (2009) Silver nanoparticle formation in different sizes induced by peptides identified within split-and-mix libraries. Angew Chem Int Ed Engl 48(20):3661–3664

Beniash E, Hartgerink JD, Storrie H, Stendahl JC, Stupp SI (2005) Self-assembling peptide amphiphile nanofiber matrices for cell entrapment. Acta Biomater 1(4):387–397

Best JP, Javed S, Richardson JJ, Cho KL, Kamphuis MMJ, Caruso F (2013) Stiffness-mediated adhesion of cervical cancer cells to soft hydrogel films. Soft Matter 9:4580

Bhattarai N, Gunn J, Zhang M (2010) Chitosanbased hydrogels for controlled, localized drug delivery. Adv Drug Deliv Rev 62(1):83–99

Biondi M, Ungaro F, Quaglia F, Netti PA (2008) Controlled drug delivery in tissue engineering. Adv Drug Deliv Rev 60(2):229–242

Blaser SA, Scheringer M, Macleod M, Hungerbuhler K (2008) Estimation of cumulative aquatic exposure and risk due to silver: contribution of nano-functionalized plastics and textiles. Sci Total Environ 390(2–3):396–409

Borselli C, Oliviero O, Battista S, Ambrosio L, Netti PA (2007) Induction of directional sprouting angiogenesis by matrix gradients. J Biomed Mater Res A 80A(2):297–305

Bosman FT, Stamenkovic I (2003) Functional structure and composition of the extracellular matrix. J Pathol 200(4):423–428

Braydich-Stolle L, Hussain S, Schlager JJ, Hofmann MC (2005) In vitro cytotoxicity of nanoparticles in mammalian germline stem cells. Toxicol Sci 88(2):412–419

Burda C, Chen X, Narayanan R, El-Sayed MA (2005) Chemistry and properties of nanocrystals of different shapes. Chem Rev 105(4):1025–1102

Burgess BT, Myles JL, Dickinson RB (2000) Quantitative analysis of adhesion-mediated cell migration in three-dimensional gels of RGD-grafted collagen. Ann Biomed Eng 28(1): 110–118

Cabiscol E, Tamarit J, Ros J (2000) Oxidative stress in bacteria and protein damage by reactive oxygen species. Int Microbiol 3(1):3–8

Cai Z-X, Mo X-M, Zhang K-H, Fan L-P, Yin A-L, He C-L, Wang H-S (2010) Fabrication of chitosan/silk fibroin composite nanofibers for wound-dressing applications. Int J Mol Sci 11: 3529–3539

Calne S (2011) Acellular matrices for the treatment of wounds. Wounds International, London

Caputo G, Nobile C, Kipp T, Blasi L, Grillo V, Carlino E, Manna L, Cingolani R, Cozzoli PD, Athanassiou A (2008) Reversible wettability changes in colloidal TiO2 nanorod thin-film coatings under selective UV laser irradiation. J Phys Chem C 112:701

Caputo G, Cortese B, Nobile C, Salerno M, Cingolani R, Gigli G, Cozzoli PD, Athanassiou A (2009) Reversibly light-switchable wettability of hybrid organic/inorganic surfaces with dual - micro-/nanoscale roughness. Adv Funct Mater 19:1149

Causa F, Netti PA, Ambrosio L (2007) A multi-functional scaffold for tissue regeneration: the need to engineer a tissue analogue. Biomaterials 28(34):5093–5099

Chan G, Mooney DJ (2008) New materials for tissue engineering: towards greater control over the biological response. Trends Biotechnol 26:382–392

Charernsriwilaiwat N, Opanasopit P, Rojanarata T, Ngawhirunpat T, Supaphol P (2010) Preparation and characterization of chitosan -hydroxybenzotriazole/polyvinyl alcohol blend nanofibers by the electrospinning technique. Carbohydr Polym 81:675–680

Charernsriwilaiwat N, Opanasopit P, Rojanarata T, Ngawhirunpat T (2012) Lysozyme-loaded, electrospun chitosan-based nanofiber mats for wound healing. Int J Pharm 427(2):379–384

Chaterji S, Gemeinhart RA (2007) Enhanced osteoblast-like cell adhesion and proliferation using sulfonate-bearing polymeric scaffolds. J Biomed Mater Res A 83A(4):990–998
Chen RR, Silva EA, Yuen WW, Mooney DJ (2007) Spatio-temporal VEGF and PDGF delivery patterns blood vessel formation and maturation. Pharm Res 24(2):258–264
Chen J-P, Chang G-Y, Chen J-K (2008) Electrospun collagen/chitosan nanofibrous membrane as wound dressing. Colloids Surf A Physicochem Eng Asp 313–314:183–188
Chernousova S, Epple M (2013) Silver as antibacterial agent: ion, nanoparticle, and metal. Angew Chem Int Ed 52(6):1636–1653
Choi O, Hu Z (2008) Size dependent and reactive oxygen species related nanosilver toxicity to nitrifying bacteria. Environ Sci Technol 42(12):4583–4588
Choi JS, Lee SJ, Christ GJ, Atala A, Yoo JJ (2008) The influence of electrospun aligned poly (ε-caprolactone)/collagen nanofiber meshes on the formation of self-aligned skeletal muscle myotubes. Biomaterials 29:2899
Christensen FM, Johnston HJ, Stone V, Aitken RJ, Hankin S, Peters S, Aschberger K (2010) Nano-silver—feasibility and challenges for human health risk assessment based on open literature. Nanotoxicology 4(3):284–295
Ciofani G, Genchi GG, Liakos I, Athanassiou A, Mattoli V, Bandiera A (2013) Human recombinant elastin-like protein coatings for muscle cell proliferation and differentiation. Acta Biomater 9:5111
Dahl JA, Maddux BL, Hutchison JE (2007) Toward greener nanosynthesis. Chem Rev 107(6): 2228–2269
Dibrov P, Dzioba J, Gosink KK, Hase CC (2002) Chemiosmotic mechanism of antimicrobial activity of Ag(+) in Vibrio cholerae. Antimicrob Agents Chemother 46(8):2668–2670
Dvir T, Timko BP, Kohane DS, Langer R (2011) Nanotechnological strategies for engineering complex tissues. Nat Nanotechnol 6:13
Eckhardt S, Brunetto PS, Gagnon J, Priebe M, Giese B, Fromm KM (2013) Nanobio silver: its interactions with peptides and bacteria, and its uses in medicine. Chem Rev 113(7):4708–4754
El Badawy AM, Silva RG, Morris B, Scheckel KG, Suidan MT, Tolaymat TM (2011) Surface charge-dependent toxicity of silver nanoparticles. Environ Sci Technol 45(1):283–287
Engler A, Sen S, Sweeney H, Discher D (2006) Matrix elasticity directs stem cell lineage specification. Cell 126:677
Enoch S, Grey JE, Harding KG (2006) ABC of wound healing: recent advances and emerging treatments. BMJ 332:962
Fan L, Yumin D, Zhang B, Yang J, Cai J, Zhang L, Zhou J (2005) Preparation and properties of alginate/water-soluble chitin blend fibers. J Macromol Sci A Pure Appl Chem 42(6):723–732
Fan L, Du Y, Zhang B, Yang J, Zhou J, Kennedy JF (2006) Preparation and properties of alginate/ carboxymethyl chitosan blend fibers. Carbohydr Polym 65(4):447–452
Fang FC (2004) Antimicrobial reactive oxygen and nitrogen species: concepts and controversies. Nat Rev Microbiol 2(10):820–832
Fiejdasz S, Szczubiałka K, Lewandowska-Łańcucka J, Osyczka AM, Nowakowska M (2013) Biopolymer-based hydrogels as injectable materials for tissue repair scaffolds. Biomed Mater 8:035013
Finetti F, Basile A, Capasso D, Di Gaetano S, Di Stasi R, Pascale M, Turco CM, Ziche M, Morbidelli L, D'Andrea LD (2012) Functional and pharmacological characterization of a VEGF mimetic peptide on reparative angiogenesis. Biochem Pharmacol 84(3):303–311
Fittkau MH, Zilla P, Bezuidenhout D, Lutolf MP, Human P, Hubbell JA, Davies N (2005) The selective modulation of endothelial cell mobility on RGD peptide containing surfaces by YIGSR peptides. Biomaterials 26(2):167–174
Fonseca KB, Gomes DB, Lee K, Santos SG, Sousa AF, Silva EA, Mooney DJ, Granja PL, Barrias CC (2014) Injectable MMP-sensitive alginate hydrogels as hMSC delivery systems. Biomacromolecules 15:380–390
Fu J, Wang Y-K, Yang MT, Desai RA, Yu X, Liu Z, Chen CS (2010) Mechanical regulation of cell function with geometrically modulated elastomeric substrates. Nat Methods 7:733

Gaharwar AK, Rivera C, Wu C-J, Chan BK, Schmidt G (2013) Photocrosslinked nanocomposite hydrogels from PEG and silica nanospheres: structural, mechanical and cell adhesion characteristics. Mater Sci Eng C 33:1800
Genchi GG, Ciofani G, Liakos I, Ricotti L, Ceseracciu L, Athanassiou A, Mazzolai B, Menciassi A, Mattoli V (2013) Bio/non-bio interfaces: a straightforward method for obtaining long term PDMS/muscle cell biohybrid constructs. Colloids Surf B: Biointerfaces 105:144
Giri TK, Thakur A, Alexander A, Ajazuddin, Badwaik H, Tripathi DK (2012) Modified chitosan hydrogels as drug delivery and tissue engineering systems: present status and applications. Acta Pharm Sin B 2(5):439–449
Glisoni RJ, García-Fernández MJ, Pino M, Gutkind G, Moglioni AG, Alvarez-Lorenzo C, Concheiro A, Sosnik A (2013) β-Cyclodextrin hydrogels for the ocular release of antibacterial thiosemicarbazones. Carbohydr Polym 93(2):449–457
Gottschalk F, Sonderer T, Scholz RW, Nowack B (2009) Modeled environmental concentrations of engineered nanomaterials (TiO(2), ZnO, Ag, CNT, Fullerenes) for different regions. Environ Sci Technol 43(24):9216–9222
Grieger KD, Linkov I, Hansen SF, Baun A (2012) Environmental risk analysis for nanomaterials: review and evaluation of frameworks. Nanotoxicology 6(2):196–212
Griffith LG, Swartz MA (2006) Capturing complex 3D tissue physiology in vitro. Nat Rev Mol Cell Biol 7(3):211–224
Guarino V, Causa F, Ambrosio L (2007) Bioactive scaffolds for bone and ligament tissue. Expert Rev Med Devices 4(3):405–418
Guarino V, Causa F, Taddei P, di Foggia M, Ciapetti G, Martini D, Fagnano C, Baldini N, Ambrosio L (2008) Polylactic acid fibre-reinforced polycaprolactone scaffolds for bone tissue engineering. Biomaterials 29:3662
Gupta A, Maynes M, Silver S (1998) Effects of halides on plasmid-mediated silver resistance in Escherichia coli. Appl Environ Microbiol 64(12):5042–5045
Gupta A, Matsui K, Lo JF, Silver S (1999) Molecular basis for resistance to silver cations in Salmonella. Nat Med 5(2):183–188
Gupta A, Phung LT, Taylor DE, Silver S (2001) Diversity of silver resistance genes in IncH incompatibility group plasmids. Microbiology 147(Pt 12):3393–3402
Gurdon JB et al (1994) Activin signaling and response to a morphogen gradient. Nature 371 (6497):487–492
Hacker MC, Mikos AG (2006) Trends in tissue engineering research. Tissue Eng 12:2049
Hajipour MJ, Fromm KM, Ashkarran AA, de Aberasturi DJ, de Larramendi IR, Rojo T, Serpooshan V, Parak WJ, Mahmoudi M (2012) Antibacterial properties of nanoparticles. Trends Biotechnol 30(10):499–511
Hansen SF, Baun A (2012) When enough is enough. Nat Nanotechnol 7(7):409–411
Hsin YH, Chen CF, Huang S, Shih TS, Lai PS, Chueh PJ (2008) The apoptotic effect of nanosilver is mediated by a ROS- and JNK-dependent mechanism involving the mitochondrial pathway in NIH3T3 cells. Toxicol Lett 179(3):130–139
Hussain SM, Hess KL, Gearhart JM, Geiss KT, Schlager JJ (2005) In vitro toxicity of nanoparticles in BRL 3A rat liver cells. Toxicol In Vitro 19(7):975–983
Hussain SM, Javorina AK, Schrand AM, Duhart HM, Ali SF, Schlager JJ (2006) The interaction of manganese nanoparticles with PC-12 cells induces dopamine depletion. Toxicol Sci 92(2): 456–463
Hutmacher DW (2001) Scaffold design and fabrication technologies for engineering tissues—state of the art and future perspectives. J Biomater Sci Polym Ed 12(1):107–124
Hutmacher DW, Sittinger M, Risbud MV (2004) Scaffold-based tissue engineering: rationale for computer-aided design and solid free-form fabrication systems. Trends Biotechnol 22(7): 354–362
Hwang ET, Lee JH, Chae YJ, Kim YS, Kim BC, Sang BI, Gu MB (2008) Analysis of the toxic mode of action of silver nanoparticles using stress-specific bioluminescent bacteria. Small 4 (6):746–750

Inoue Y, Hoshino M, Takahashi H, Noguchi T, Murata T, Kanzaki Y, Hamashima H, Sasatsu M (2002) Bactericidal activity of Ag-zeolite mediated by reactive oxygen species under aerated conditions. J Inorg Biochem 92(1):37–42
Jack KS, Velayudhan S, Luckman P, Trau M, Grøndahl L, Cooper-White J (2009) The fabrication and characterization of biodegradable HA/PHBV nanoparticle–polymer composite scaffolds. Acta Biomater 5:2657
Jeong SI, Krebs MD, Bonino CA, Khan SA, Alsberg E (2010) Electrospun alginate nanofibers with controlled cell adhesion for tissue engineering. Macromol Biosci 10:934–943
Jin G, Prabhakaranb MP, Kaib D, Ramakrishnaa S (2013) Controlled release of multiple epidermal induction factors through core–shell nanofibers for skin regeneration. Eur J Pharm Biopharm 85(3):689–698
Johnson DW, Sherborne C, Didsbury MP, Pateman C, Cameron NR, Claeyssens F (2013) Macrostructuring of emulsion-templated porous polymers by 3D laser patterning. Adv Mater 25:3178
Jover J, Bosque R, Sales J (2008) A comparison of the binding affinity of the common amino acids with different metal cations. Dalton Trans 45:6441–6453
Jover J, Bosque R, Sales J (2009) Quantitative structure-property relationship estimation of cation binding affinity of the common amino acids. J Phys Chem A 113(15):3703–3708
Joy A, Cohen DM, Luk A, Anim-Danso E, Chen C, Kohn J (2011) Control of surface chemistry, substrate stiffness, and cell function in a novel terpolymer methacrylate library. Langmuir 27: 1891
Karageorgiou V, Kaplan D (2005) Porosity of 3D biomaterial scaffolds and osteogenesis. Biomaterials 26:5474
Kasuga NC, Yoshikawa R, Sakai Y, Nomiya K (2012) Syntheses, structures, and antimicrobial activities of remarkably light-stable and water-soluble silver complexes with amino acid derivatives, silver(I) N-acetylmethioninates. Inorg Chem 51(3):1640–1647
Katz E, Streuli CH (2007) The extracellular matrix as an adhesion checkpoint for mammary epithelial function. Int J Biochem Cell Biol 39(4):715–726
Keselowsky BG, Collard DM, Garcia AJ (2005) Integrin binding specificity regulates biomaterial surface chemistry effects on cell differentiation. Proc Natl Acad Sci USA 102:5953
Kim TG, Chung HJ, Park TG (2008a) Macroporous and nanofibrous hyaluronic acid/collagen hybrid scaffold fabricated by concurrent electrospinning and deposition/leaching of salt particles. Acta Biomater 4:1611
Kim KJ, Sung WS, Moon SK, Choi JS, Kim JG, Lee DG (2008b) Antifungal effect of silver nanoparticles on dermatophytes. J Microbiol Biotechnol 18(8):1482–1484
Kim KJ, Sung WS, Suh BK, Moon SK, Choi JS, Kim JG, Lee DG (2009) Antifungal activity and mode of action of silver nano-particles on Candida albicans. Biometals 22(2):235–242
Kim HJ, Park IK, Kim JH, Cho CS, Kim MS (2012) Gas foaming fabrication of porous biphasic calcium phosphate for bone regeneration. Tissue Eng Regen Med 9:63
Klasen HJ (2000a) A historical review of the use of silver in the treatment of burns. II. Renewed interest for silver. Burns 26(2):131–138
Klasen HJ (2000b) Historical review of the use of silver in the treatment of burns. I. Early uses. Burns 26(2):117–130
Kong HJ, Mooney DJ (2007) Microenvironmental regulation of biomacromolecular therapies. Nat Rev Drug Discov 6(6):455–463
Kuijpers AJ, van Wachem PB, van Luyn MJA, Brouwer LA, Engbers GHM, Krijgsveld J, Zaat SAJ, Dankert J, Feijen J (2000) In vitro and in vivo evaluation of gelatin-chondroitin sulphate hydrogels for controlled release of antibacterial proteins. Biomaterials 21(17):1763–1772
Kumar A, Vemula PK, Ajayan PM, John G (2008) Silver-nanoparticle-embedded antimicrobial paints based on vegetable oil. Nat Mater 7(3):236–241
Lee KY, Jeong L, Kang YO, Lee SJ, Park WH (2009) Electrospinning of polysaccharides for regenerative medicine. Adv Drug Deliv Rev 61(12):1020–1032

Lee E-J, Teng S-H, Jang T-S, Wang P, Yook S-W, Kim H-E, Koh Y-H (2010) Nanostructured poly (e-caprolactone)–silica xerogel fibrous membrane for guided bone regeneration. Acta Biomater 6:3557

Lee C, Shin J, Lee JS, Byun E, Ryu JH, Um SH, Kim DI, Lee H, Cho S-W (2013) Bioinspired, calcium-free alginate hydrogels with tunable physical and mechanical properties and improved biocompatibility. Biomacromolecules 14(6):2004–2013

Lemire JA, Harrison JJ, Turner RJ (2013) Antimicrobial activity of metals: mechanisms, molecular targets and applications. Nat Rev Microbiol 11(6):371–384

Levy SB, Marshall B (2004) Antibacterial resistance worldwide: causes, challenges and responses. Nat Med 10(12 Suppl):S122–S129

Li WR, Xie XB, Shi QS, Duan SS, Ouyang YS, Chen YB (2011) Antibacterial effect of silver nanoparticles on Staphylococcus aureus. Biometals 24(1):135–141

Liakos I, Rizzello L, Bayer IS, Pompa PP, Cingolani R, Athanassiou A (2013) Controlled antiseptic release by alginate polymer films and beads. Carbohydr Polym 92(1):176–183

Liakos I, Rizzello L, Scurr DJ, Pompa PP, Bayer IS, Athanassiou A (2014) All-natural composite wound dressing films of essential oils encapsulated in sodium alginate with antimicrobial properties. Int J Pharm 463(2):137–145

Liang HY, Wang WZ, Huang YZ, Zhang SP, Wei H, Xu HX (2010) Controlled Synthesis of Uniform Silver Nanospheres. J Phys Chem C 114(16):7427–7431

Liau SY, Read DC, Pugh WJ, Furr JR, Russell AD (1997) Interaction of silver nitrate with readily identifiable groups: relationship to the antibacterial action of silver ions. Lett Appl Microbiol 25(4):279–283

Liu J, Hurt RH (2010) Ion release kinetics and particle persistence in aqueous nano-silver colloids. Environ Sci Technol 44(6):2169–2175

Liu X, Ma PX (2009) Phase separation, pore structure, and properties of nanofibrous gelatin scaffolds. Biomaterials 30:4094

Liu S-J, Kau Y-C, Chou C-Y, Chen J-K, Wu R-C, Yeh W-L (2010a) Electrospun PLGA/collagen nanofibrous membrane as early-stage wound dressing. J Membr Sci 355:53–59

Liu J, Sonshine DA, Shervani S, Hurt RH (2010b) Controlled release of biologically active silver from nanosilver surfaces. ACS Nano 4(11):6903–6913

Lo CM, Wang HB, Dembo M, Wang YL (2000) Cell movement is guided by the rigidity of the substrate. Biophys J 79(1):144

Lourenço BN, Marchioli G, Song W, Reis RL, van Blitterswijk CA, Karperien M, van Apeldoorn A, Mano JF (2012) Wettability influences cell behavior on superhydrophobic surfaces with different topographies. Biointerphases 7:46

Luciani A, Coccoli V, Orsi S, Ambrosio L, Netti PA (2008) PCL microspheres based functional scaffolds by bottom-up approach with predefined microstructural properties and release profiles. Biomaterials 29(36):4800–4807

Malmsten M (2011) Antimicrobial and antiviral hydrogel. Soft Matter 7:8725–8736. doi:10.1039/C1SM05809F

Mandoli C, Mecheri B, Forte G, Pagliari F, Pagliari S, Carotenuto F, Fiaccavento R, Rinaldi A, Di Nardo P, Licoccia S, Traversa E (2010) Thick soft tissue reconstruction on highly perfusive biodegradable scaffolds. Macromol Biosci 10:127

Mazzitelli S, Pagano C, Giusepponi D, Nastruzzi C, Perioli L (2013) Hydrogel blends with adjustable properties as patches for transdermal delivery. Int J Pharm 454(1):47–57

Mehta M, Schmidt-Bleek K, Duda GN, Mooney DJ (2012) Biomaterial delivery of morphogens to mimic the natural healing cascade in bone. Adv Drug Deliv Rev 64:1257–1276

Merkel TC, Freeman BD, Spontak RJ, He Z, Pinnau I, Meakin P, Hill AJ (2002) Ultrapermeable, reverse-selective nanocomposite membranes. Science 296(5567):519–522

Milionis A, Martiradonna L, Anyfantis GC, Cozzoli PD, Bayer IS, Fragouli D, Athanassiou A (2013) Control of the water adhesion on hydrophobic micropillars by spray coating technique. Colloid Polym Sci 291:401

Milionis A, Fragouli D, Martiradonna L, Anyfantis GC, Cozzoli PD, Bayer IS, Athanassiou A (2014) Spatially controlled surface energy traps on superhydrophobic surfaces. ACS Appl Mater Interfaces 6:1036–1043

Mirzajani F, Ghassempour A, Aliahmadi A, Esmaeili MA (2011) Antibacterial effect of silver nanoparticles on Staphylococcus aureus. Res Microbiol 162(5):542–549

Moffa M, Polini A, Sciancalepore AG, Persano L, Mele E, Passione LG, Potente G, Pisignano D (2013) Microvascular endothelial cell spreading and proliferation on nanofibrous scaffolds by polymer blends with enhanced wettability. Soft Matter 9:5529

Monopoli MP, Walczyk D, Campbell A, Elia G, Lynch I, Bombelli FB, Dawson KA (2011a) Physical-chemical aspects of protein corona: relevance to in vitro and in vivo biological impacts of nanoparticles. J Am Chem Soc 133(8):2525–2534

Monopoli MP, Bombelli FB, Dawson KA (2011b) Nanobiotechnology: nanoparticle coronas take shape. Nat Nanotechnol 6(1):11–12

Morais DS, Rodrigues MA, Lopes MA, Coelho MJ, Maurício AC, Gomes R, Amorim I, Ferraz MP, Santos JD, Botelho CM (2013) Biological evaluation of alginate-based hydrogels, with antimicrobial features by Ce(III) incorporation, as vehicles for a bone substitute. J Mater Sci Mater Med 24(9):2145–2155

Morens DM, Folkers GK, Fauci AS (2010) The challenge of emerging and re-emerging infectious diseases (vol 430, pg 242, 2004). Nature 463(7277):122

Morones JR, Elechiguerra JL, Camacho A, Holt K, Kouri JB, Ramirez JT, Yacaman MJ (2005) The bactericidal effect of silver nanoparticles. Nanotechnology 16(10):2346–2353

Mou Z-L, Duan L-M, Qi X-N, Zhang Z-Q (2013) Preparation of silk fibroin/collagen/hydroxyapatite composite scaffold by particulate leaching method. Mater Lett 105:189

Musee N, Thwala M, Nota N (2011) The antibacterial effects of engineered nanomaterials: implications for wastewater treatment plants. J Environ Monit 13(5):1164–1183

Nandakumar A, Fernandes H, de Boer J, Moroni L, Habibovic P, van Blitterswijk CA (2010) Fabrication of bioactive composite scaffolds by electrospinning for bone regeneration. Macromol Biosci 10:1365

Navarro E, Piccapietra F, Wagner B, Marconi F, Kaegi R, Odzak N, Sigg L, Behra R (2008) Toxicity of silver nanoparticles to Chlamydomonas reinhardtii. Environ Sci Technol 42(23): 8959–8964

Neibert K, Gopishetty V, Grigoryev A, Tokarev I, Al-Hajaj N, Vorstenbosch J, Philip A, Minko S, Maysinger D (2012) Wound-healing with mechanically robust and biodegradable hydrogel fibers loaded with silver nanoparticles. Adv Healthc Mater 1(5):621–630

Ng R, Zhang X, Liu N, Yang ST (2009) Modifications of nonwoven polyethylene terephthalate fibrous matrices via NaOH hydrolysis: effects on pore size, fiber diameter, cell seeding and proliferation. Process Biochem 44:992

Ng R, Zang R, Yang KK, Liu N, Yang S-T (2012) Three-dimensional fibrous scaffolds with microstructures and nanotextures for tissue engineering. RCS Adv 2:10110

Nitanan T, Akkaramongkolporn P, Rojanarata T, Ngawhirunpat T, Opanasopit P (2013) Neomycin-loaded poly(styrene sulfonic acid-co-maleic acid) (PSSA-MA)/polyvinyl alcohol (PVA) ion exchange nanofibers for wound dressing materials. Int J Pharm 448(1):71–78

Nomiya K, Takahashi S, Noguchi R, Nemoto S, Takayama T, Oda M (2000) Synthesis and characterization of water-soluble silver(I) complexes with L-histidine (H2his) and (S)-(-)-2-pyrrolidone-5-carboxylic acid (H2pyrrld) showing a wide spectrum of effective antibacterial and antifungal activities. Crystal structures of chiral helical polymers [Ag(Hhis)]n and ([Ag (Hpyrrld)]2)n in the solid state. Inorg Chem 39(15):3301–3311

Notin L, Viton C, Lucas J-M, Domard A (2006) Pseudo-dry-spinning of chitosan. Acta Biomater 2:297–311

Nowack B, Krug HF, Height M (2011) 120 years of nanosilver history: implications for policy makers. Environ Sci Technol 45(4):1177–1183

Nowack B, Ranville JF, Diamond S, Gallego-Urrea JA, Metcalfe C, Rose J, Horne N, Koelmans AA, Klaine SJ (2012) Potential scenarios for nanomaterial release and subsequent alteration in the environment. Environ Toxicol Chem 31(1):50–59
Oliveira SM, Song W, Alves NM, Mano JF (2011) Chemical modification of bioinspired superhydrophobic polystyrene surfaces to control cell attachment/proliferation. Soft Matter 7:8932
Pal S, Tak YK, Song JM (2007) Does the antibacterial activity of silver nanoparticles depend on the shape of the nanoparticle? A study of the Gram-negative bacterium Escherichia coli. Appl Environ Microbiol 73(6):1712–1720
Palchesko RN, Zhang L, Sun Y, Feinberg AW (2012) Development of polydimethylsiloxane substrates with tunable elastic modulus to study cell mechanobiology in muscle and nerve. PLoS ONE 7:e51499
Pamula E, Bacakova L, Filova E, Buczynska J, Dobrzynski P, Noskova L, Grausova L (2008) The influence of pore size on colonization of poly(L-lactide-glycolide) scaffolds with human osteoblast-like MG 63 cells in vitro. J Mater Sci Mater Med 19:425
Pamula E, Filová E, Bacáková L, Lisá V, Adamczyk D (2009) Resorbable polymeric scaffolds for bone tissue engineering. J Biomed Mater Res A 89A:432
Panacek A, Kvitek L, Prucek R, Kolar M, Vecerova R, Pizurova N, Sharma VK, Nevecna T, Zboril R (2006) Silver colloid nanoparticles: synthesis, characterization, and their antibacterial activity. J Phys Chem B 110(33):16248–16253
Panacek A, Kolar M, Vecerova R, Prucek R, Soukupova J, Krystof V, Hamal P, Zboril R, Kvitek L (2009) Antifungal activity of silver nanoparticles against Candida spp. Biomaterials 30(31): 6333–6340
Park EJ, Yi J, Kim Y, Choi K, Park K (2010) Silver nanoparticles induce cytotoxicity by a Trojan-horse type mechanism. Toxicol In Vitro 24(3):872–878
Penchev H, Paneva D, Manolova N, Rashkov I (2009) Electrospun Hybrid nanofibers based on chitosan or N-carboxyethylchitosan and silver nanoparticles. Macromol Biosci 9:884–894
Pillai CKS, Paul W, Sharma CP (2009) Chitin and chitosan polymers: chemistry, solubility and fiber formation. Prog Polym Sci 34(7):641–678
Place ES, George JH, Williams CK, Stevens MM (2009a) Synthetic polymer scaffolds for tissue engineering. Chem Soc Rev 38:1139
Place ES, Evans ND, Stevens MM (2009b) Complexity in biomaterials for tissue engineering. Nat Mater 8(6):457–470
Polini A, Scaglione S, Quarto R, Pisignano D (2013) Composite electrospun nanofibers for influencing stem cell fate. Methods Mol Biol 1058:25–40
Powers JH (2004) Antimicrobial drug development—the past, the present, and the future. Clin Microbiol Infect 10:23–31
Qin Y (2008) The gel swelling properties of alginate fibers and their applications in wound management. Polym Adv Technol 19:6–14
Rapraeger AC (2000) Syndecan-regulated receptor signaling. J Cell Biol 149(5):995–997
Reddy PR, Varaprasad K, Sadiku R, Ramam K, Reddy GVS, Raju KM, Reddy N (2013) Development of gelatin based inorganic nanocomposite hydrogels for inactivation of bacteria. J Inorg Organomet Polym Mater 23(5):1054–1060
Reynolds NP, Styan KE, Easton CD, Li Y, Waddington L, Lara C, Forsythe JS, Mezzenga R, Hartley PG, Muir BW (2013) Nanotopographic surfaces with defined surface chemistries from amyloid fibril networks can control cell attachment. Biomacromolecules 14:2305
Richardson TP, Peters MC, Ennett AB, Mooney DJ (2001) Polymeric system for dual growth factor delivery. Nat Biotechnol 19(11):1029–1034
Rieger KA, Birch NP, Schiffman JD (2013) Designing electrospun nanofiber mats to promote wound healing—a review. J Mater Chem B 1:4531–4541
Roh JY, Sim SJ, Yi J, Park K, Chung KH, Ryu DY, Choi J (2009) Ecotoxicity of silver nanoparticles on the soil nematode Caenorhabditis elegans using functional ecotoxicogenomics. Environ Sci Technol 43(10):3933–3940

Rouet V, Hamma-Kourbali Y, Petit E, Panagopoulou P, Katsoris P, Barritault D, Caruelle JP, Courty J (2005) A synthetic glycosaminoglycan mimetic binds vascular endothelial growth factor and modulates angiogenesis. J Biol Chem 280(38):32792–32800
Rujitanaroj P-o, Pimpha N, Supaphol P (2008) Wound-dressing materials with antibacterial activity from electrospun gelatin fiber mats containing silver nanoparticles. Polymer 49: 4723–4732
Sachlos E, Czernuszka JT (2003) Making tissue engineering scaffolds work. Review: the application of solid freeform fabrication technology to the production of tissue engineering scaffolds. Eur Cell Mater 5:29–39, discussion 39–40
Saltzman WM, Olbricht WL (2002) Building drug delivery into tissue engineering. Nat Rev Drug Discov 1(3):177–186
Schmidt S, Madaboosi N, Uhlig K, Köhler D, Skirtach A, Duschl C, Möhwald H, Volodkin DV (2012) Control of cell adhesion by mechanical reinforcement of soft polyelectrolyte films with nanoparticles. Langmuir 28:7249
Schneider A, Wang XY, Kaplan DL, Garlick JA, Eglesa C (2009) Biofunctionalized electrospun silk mats as a topical bioactive dressing for accelerated wound healing. Acta Biomater 5(7): 2570–2578
Schwaber MJ, De-Medina T, Carmeli Y (2004) Epidemiological interpretation of antibiotic resistance studies - what are we missing? Nat Rev Microbiol 2(12):979–983
Schwarz US, Safran SA (2013) Physics of adherent cells. Rev Mod Phys 85:1327
Seyednejad H, Gawlitta D, Dhert WJA, van Nostrum CF, Vermonden T, Hennink WE (2011) Preparation and characterization of a three-dimensional printed scaffold based on a functionalized polyester for bone tissue engineering applications. Acta Biomater 7:1999
Seyednejad H, Gawlitta D, Kuiper RV, de Bruin A, van Nostrum CF, Vermonden T, Dhert WJA, Hennink WE (2012) In vivo biocompatibility and biodegradation of 3D-printed porous scaffolds based on a hydroxyl-functionalized poly(ε-caprolactone). Biomaterials 33:4309
Sintubin L, De Gusseme B, Van der Meeren P, Pycke BF, Verstraete W, Boon N (2011) The antibacterial activity of biogenic silver and its mode of action. Appl Microbiol Biotechnol 91(1):153–162
Siow KS, Britcher L, Kumar S, Griesser HJ (2006) Plasma methods for the generation of chemically reactive surfaces for biomolecule immobilization and cell colonization—a review. Plasma Process Polym 3:392
Smetana AB, Klabunde KJ, Marchin GR, Sorensen CM (2008) Biocidal activity of nanocrystalline silver powders and particles. Langmuir 24(14):7457–7464
Sondi I, Salopek-Sondi B (2004) Silver nanoparticles as antimicrobial agent: a case study on E. coli as a model for Gram-negative bacteria. J Colloid Interface Sci 275(1):177–182
Song B, Wu C, Chang J (2012a) Controllable delivery of hydrophilic and hydrophobic drugs from electrospun poly(lactic-co-glycolic acid)/mesoporous silica nanoparticles composite mats. J Biomed Mater Res B Appl Biomater 100(8):2178–2186
Song B, Wu C, Chang J (2012b) Dual drug release from electrospun poly(lactic-co-glycolic acid)/ mesoporous silica nanoparticles composite mats with distinct release profiles. Acta Biomater 8 (5):1901–1907
Spellberg B (2008) Dr. William H. Stewart: mistaken or maligned? Clin Infect Dis 47(2):294
Spellberg B, Guidos R, Gilbert D, Bradley J, Boucher HW, Scheld WM, Bartlett JG, Edwards J, Amer IDS (2008) The epidemic of antibiotic-resistant infections: a call to action for the medical community from the Infectious Diseases Society of America. Clin Infect Dis 46(2): 155–164
Stupack DG, Cheresh DA (2002) ECM remodeling regulates angiogenesis: endothelial integrins look for new ligands. Sci STKE 2002(119):e7
Sue YM, Lee JY, Wang MC, Lin TK, Sung JM, Huang JJ (2001) Generalized argyria in two chronic hemodialysis patients. Am J Kidney Dis 37(5):1048–1051

Suganya S, Senthil Ram T, Lakshmi BS, Giridev VR (2011) Herbal drug incorporated antibacterial nanofibrous mat fabricated by electrospinning: an excellent matrix for wound dressings. J Appl Polym Sci 121(5):2893–2899
Sun T, Qing G (2011) Biomimetic smart interface materials for biological applications. Adv Mater 23:H57
Sun W, Darling A, Starly B, Nam J (2004) Computer-aided tissue engineering: overview, scope and challenges. Biotechnol Appl Biochem 39:29–47
Sun T, Qing G, Su B, Jiang L (2011) Functional biointerface materials inspired from nature. Chem Soc Rev 40:2909
Sušec M, Ligon SC, Stampfl J, Liska R, Krajnc P (2013) Hierarchically porous materials from layer-by-layer photopolymerization of high internal phase emulsions. Macromol Rapid Commun 34:938
Suwantong O, Ruktanonchai U, Supaphol P (2010) In vitro biological evaluation of electrospun cellulose acetate fiber mats containing asiaticoside or curcumin. J Biomed Mater Res A 94(4): 1216–1225
Taipale J, KeskiOja J (1997) Growth factors in the extracellular matrix. FASEB J 11(1):51–59
Takenaka S, Karg E, Roth C, Schulz H, Ziesenis A, Heinzmann U, Schramel P, Heyder J (2001) Pulmonary and systemic distribution of inhaled ultrafine silver particles in rats. Environ Health Perspect 109(Suppl 4):547–551
Tanabe Y, Jessell TM (1997) Diversity and pattern in the developing spinal cord (vol 274, pg 1115, 1996). Science 276(5309):21
Teo W-E, He W, Ramakrishna S (2006) Electrospun scaffold tailored for tissue-specific extracellular matrix. Biotechnol J 1(9):918–929
Torres-Giner S, Martinez-Abad A, Gimeno-Alcañiz JV, Ocio MJ, Lagaron JM (2012) Controlled delivery of gentamicin antibiotic from bioactive electrospun polylactide-based ultrathin fibers. Adv Eng Mater 14:B112–B122
Travan A, Pelillo C, Donati I, Marsich E, Benincasa M, Scarpa T, Semeraro S, Turco G, Gennaro R, Paoletti S (2009) Non-cytotoxic silver nanoparticle-polysaccharide nanocomposites with antimicrobial activity. Biomacromolecules 10(6):1429–1435
Ueda E, Levkin PA (2013) Emerging applications of superhydrophilic-superhydrophobic micropatterns. Adv Mater 25:1234
Upert G, Bouillere F, Wennemers H (2012) Oligoprolines as scaffolds for the formation of silver nanoparticles in defined sizes: correlating molecular and nanoscopic dimensions. Angew Chem Int Ed Engl 51(17):4231–4234
Uppal R, Ramaswamy GN, Arnold C, Goodband R, Wang Y (2011) Hyaluronic acid nanofiber wound dressing-production, characterization, and in vivo behavior. J Biomed Mater Res B Appl Biomater 97(1):20–29
Üstündağ GC, Karaca E, Özbek S, ÇavuşoǦlu I (2010) In vivo evaluation of electrospun poly (vinyl alcohol)/sodium alginate nanofibrous mat as wound dressing. Tekstil ve Konfeksiyon 20:290–298
Uttayarat P, Jetawattana S, Suwanmala P, Eamsiri J, Tangthong T, Pongpat S (2012) Antimicrobial electrospun silk fibroin mats with silver nanoparticles for wound dressing application. Fiber Polym 13:999–1006
van der Pol U, Mathieu L, Zeiter S, Bourban P-E, Zambelli P-Y, Pearce SG, Bouré LP, Pioletti DP (2010) Augmentation of bone defect healing using a new biocomposite scaffold: an in vivo study in sheep. Acta Biomater 6:3755
Van Vlierberghe S, Schacht E, Dubruel E (2011) Reversible gelatin-based hydrogels: finetuning of material properties. Eur Polym J 47(5):1039–1047
Ventre M, Causa F, Netti PA (2012) Determinants of cell-material crosstalk at the interface: towards engineering of cell instructive materials. J R Soc Interface 9(74):2017–2032
Venugopal JR, Zhang Y, Ramakrishna S (2006) In vitro culture of human dermal fibroblasts on electrospun polycaprolactone collagen nanofibrous membrane. Artif Organs 30(6):440–446

Vertelov GK, Krutyakov YA, Efremenkova OV, Olenin AY, Lisichkin GV (2008) A versatile synthesis of highly bactericidal Myramistin(R) stabilized silver nanoparticles. Nanotechnology 19(35):355707

Villafiorita Monteleone F, Caputo G, Canale C, Cozzoli PD, Cingolani R, Fragouli D, Athanassiou A (2010) Light-controlled directional liquid drop movement on TiO2 nanorods-based nanocomposite photopatterns. Langmuir 26:18557

Voytik-Harbin SL, Brightman AO, Waisner BZ, Robinson JP, Lamar CH (1998) Small intestinal submucosa: a tissue-derived extracellular matrix that promotes tissue-specific growth and differentiation of cells in vitro. Tissue Eng 4:157

Wadhera A, Fung M (2005) Systemic argyria associated with ingestion of colloidal silver. Dermatol Online J 11(1):12

Walczyk D, Bombelli FB, Monopoli MP, Lynch I, Dawson KA (2010) What the cell "sees" in bionanoscience. J Am Chem Soc 132(16):5761–5768

Wan LQ, Jiang J, Arnold DE, Guo XE, Lu HH, Mow VC (2008) Mow, Calcium concentration effects on the mechanical and biochemical properties of Chondrocyte-Alginate constructs. Cell Mol Bioeng 1(1):93–102

Wang DA, Varghese S, Sharma B, Strehin I, Fermanian S, Gorham J, Fairbrother DH, Cascio B, Elisseeff JH (2007) Multifunctional chondroitin sulphate for cartilage tissue-biomaterial integration. Nat Mater 6(5):385–392

Wang C, Yan K-W, Lin Y-D, Hsieh PCH (2010) Biodegradable core/shell fibers by coaxial electrospinning: processing, fiber characterization, and its application in sustained drug release. Macromolecules 43(15):6389–6397

Wang S, Zhang Y, Wang H, Dong Z (2011a) Preparation, characterization and biocompatibility of electrospinning heparin-modified silk fibroin nanofibers. Int J Biol Macromol 48:345

Wang Y, Zhang CL, Zhang Q, Li P (2011b) Composite electrospun nanomembranes of fish scale collagen peptides/chito-oligosaccharides: antibacterial properties and potential for wound dressing. Int J Nanomedicine 6:667–676

Wei G, Ma PX (2008) Nanostructured biomaterials for regeneration. Adv Funct Mater 18:3568

Wei G, Ma PX (2009) Partially nanofibrous architecture of 3D tissue engineering scaffolds. Biomaterials 30:6426

Wennemers H (2012) Peptides as asymmetric catalysts and templates for the controlled formation of Ag nanoparticles. J Pept Sci 18(7):437–441

Wharram SE, Zhang X, Kaplan DL, McCarthy SP (2010) Electrospun silk material systems for wound healing. Macromol Biosci 10(3):246–257

Whitesides GM, Ostuni E, Takayama S, Jiang X, Ingber DE (2001) Soft lithography in biology and biochemistry. Annu Rev Biomed Eng 3:335–373

Wijekoon A, Fountas-Davis N, Leipzig ND (2013) Fluorinated methacrylamide chitosan hydrogel systems as adaptable oxygen carriers for wound healing. Acta Biomater 9(3):5653–5664

Wijelath ES, Murray J, Rahman S, Patel Y, Ishida A, Strand K, Aziz S, Cardona C, Hammond WP, Savidge GF, Rafii S, Sobel M (2002) Novel vascular endothelial growth factor binding domains of fibronectin enhance vascular endothelial growth factor biological activity. Circ Res 91(1):25–31

Wnek GE, Carr ME, Simpson DG, Bowlin GL (2003) Electrospinning of nanofiber fibrinogen structures. Nano Lett 3(2):213–216

Xiaoling F, Wang H (2012) Spatial arrangement of polycaprolactone/collagen nanofiber scaffolds regulates the wound healing related behaviors of human adipose stromal cells. Tissue Eng Part A 18(5–6):631–642

Xiu ZM, Ma J, Alvarez PJ (2011) Differential effect of common ligands and molecular oxygen on antimicrobial activity of silver nanoparticles versus silver ions. Environ Sci Technol 45(20): 9003–9008

Xiu ZM, Zhang QB, Puppala HL, Colvin VL, Alvarez PJ (2012) Negligible particle-specific antibacterial activity of silver nanoparticles. Nano Lett 12(8):4271–4275

Xu X, Zhong W, Zhou S, Trajtman A, Alfa M (2010) Electrospun PEG-PLA nanofibrous membrane for sustained release of hydrophilic antibiotics. J Appl Polym Sci 118(1):588–595
Yan L, Si S, Chen Y, Yuan T, Fan H, Yao Y, Zhang Q (2011) Electrospun in-situ hybrid polyurethane/nano-TiO2 as wound dressings. Fiber Polym 12(2):207–213
Yang C, Wu X, Zhao Y, Xu L, Wei S (2011) Nanofibrous scaffold prepared by electrospinning of poly(vinyl alcohol)/gelatin aqueous solutions. J Appl Polym Sci 121(5):3047–3055
Yang Y, Xia T, Chen F, Wei W, Liu C, He S, Li X (2012) Electrospun fibers with plasmid bFGF polyplex loadings promote skin wound healing in diabetic rats. Mol Pharm 9(1):48–58
Zelzer M, Majani R, Bradley JW, Rose FRAJ, Davies MC, Alexander MR (2008) Investigation of cell–surface interactions using chemical gradients formed from plasma polymers. Biomaterials 29:172
Zhang Y, Lim CT, Ramakrishna S, Huang Z-M (2005) Recent development of polymer nanofibers for biomedical and biotechnological applications. J Mater Sci Mater Med 16:933–946
Zook JM, Long SE, Cleveland D, Geronimo CL, MacCuspie RI (2011) Measuring silver nanoparticle dissolution in complex biological and environmental matrices using UV-visible absorbance. Anal Bioanal Chem 401(6):1993–2002
Zouani OF, Chollet C, Guillotin B, Durrieu MC (2010) Differentiation of pre-osteoblast cells on poly(ethylene terephthalate) grafted with RGD and/or BMPs mimetic peptides. Biomaterials 31(32):8245–8253

Chapter 3
Biosensing Detection

Guglielmo Lanzani, Maria Rosa Antognazza, Massimo De Vittorio, Simona Petroni, and Francesco Rizzi

3.1 Introduction

Human perception of the environment relies on senses for transducing light, inertial, mechanical, and biochemical stimuli in electrical signals through a great variety of receptors: photoreceptors for sight, mechanoreceptors for touch and hearing, and chemoreceptors for taste and smell, in addition to thermoreceptors for temperature and nocioreceptors for pain/damage sensing. Artificial and biomimetic approaches to mimic these sensorial systems for prosthetic and robotic applications require new-concept and frontier technologies.

Here we report on recent advances on bioelectronics technologies, based on organic semiconductors, for interfacing living systems and for artificial retinas, and on MEMS biomimetic approaches to produce and probe mechanoreceptors for touch and hearing senses.

3.2 The Emerging Field of Organic Bioelectronics

Since the 1970s, organic semiconductors, in the form of molecular crystals, small molecules, or conjugated polymers, have been the key players of a revolution in electronics and optoelectronics. The joint effort in materials chemistry, fundamental research, and device engineering led to the demonstration and in some cases the commercialization of a new generation of plastic devices, including light-emitting diodes, transistors, and photovoltaic cells. As compared to inorganic

G. Lanzani (✉) • M.R. Antognazza
Center for Nanoscience and Technology, Istituto Italiano di Tecnologia, Milan, Italy
e-mail: guglielmo.lanzani@iit.it

M. De Vittorio • S. Petroni • F. Rizzi
Center for Biomolecular Nanotechnology, Istituto Italiano di Tecnologia, Lecce, Italy

R. Cingolani (ed.), *Bioinspired Approaches for Human-Centric Technologies*,
DOI 10.1007/978-3-319-04924-3_3,

semiconductors, organic materials offer attractive characteristics in terms of mechanical properties, possibility of chemical engineering, and interaction with visible light. Importantly, the technology required for processing materials and realizing devices is relatively cheap and easy, and it fits well with transparent, bendable, rollable, and lightweight plastic substrates. The counterbalance to be paid back is reduced electronic mobility and poor environmental stability. Major efforts are currently focusing on improving performances of solar cells and transistors, which are expected to represent the next applications to be delivered on the market.

At the same time, the research community is now experiencing a "second birth" of organic electronics, approaching the last, unexplored frontier: the interaction with a living system, in the attempt to realize new-concept, organic-based human-machine interfaces. The mixed term "organic bioelectronics" was used for the first time in 2007 by Berggren and Richter-Dahlfors in a seminal review (Berggren and Richter-Dahlfors 2007), by referring to the application of organic electronics in the broad field of life sciences. Historically, the key milestone of conducting and semiconducting polymers for biomedical applications stands in their use as active, functional materials, opposed to the adoption as standard passive components for coatings. Since then, the field has been growing at a surprisingly fast rate, as documented by the increasing number of publications, the number of funded projects in the field, and the organization of focused symposia at international conferences.

The strong interest manifested by the community stems from the peculiar properties of organic semiconductors: polymers are able to offer innovative, valuable solutions where traditional technologies, based on silicon or other inorganic semiconductors, fail. Besides the possibility of adopting cheaper and more versatile processing technologies, specifically suited to the in vivo applications, organic semiconductors, and more specifically conjugated polymers, show superior biocompatibility and adaptability to work at the interface with living tissues. At the macroscopic level, the soft surface of polymer thin films represents an ideal substrate to grow cells for in vitro studies as well as for in vivo interfacing even with extremely delicate tissues, such as the retina, the central and peripheral neural tissue, the intestinal and kidney epithelium, etc. At a submicroscopic level, the polymers' softness finds an explanation in their peculiar conjugated structure, constituted by alternating single and double carbon bonds, which is indeed very similar to the structure found in many biological molecules (the retinal molecule, for instance). Moreover, conducting and semiconducting polymers offer the unique capability of mixed electronic conduction and ionic conduction, thus opening a new interconnection perspective with living matter.

All mentioned properties make this class of materials extremely attracting for applications in biomedical engineering, neuro-technology, and life sciences. In few years, many devices have been demonstrated, able to work both in vitro and in vivo. In some cases, their performances outperform those reported so far by adopting standard, inorganic technologies and have already reached the necessary development for preclinical and clinical application. In the following, we will present some notable (even though not exhaustive) examples of in vitro and in vivo applications.

Different strategies are being pursued, based on different concepts and device architectures. Most of reported devices are intended for cellular electric activity elicitation and/or recording; in particular, we divide them in three classes: conductive organic bioelectrodes, organic electrochemical transistors, and organic field-effect transistors. In addition, we report emerging techniques for optical stimulation of cell activity, relying on the use of hybrid bio-opto-interfaces, sensitive to visible light. The organic-based cell photoactivation represents a completely new tool in the neuroscience field and is especially promising for the realization of an all-organic artificial retinal prosthesis.

3.3 Conductive Organic Bioelectrodes

Traditionally, metals and inorganic semiconductors such as gold, iridium, platinum, iridium/platinum alloys, and silicon have been used in bionic devices, especially for neural probes and sensors (Guimard et al. 2007; Moulton et al. 2012). Platinum for instance has been widely adopted in cochlear implant electrodes as well as for deep brain stimulation electrodes and artificial visual systems; in the last 50 years, most of brain function studies have been conducted by using tungsten electrodes. Current limits of bioelectrodes are mainly constituted by their rigidity and sharpness, which damage the tissue during insertion and exert chronic stress on the surrounding environment; their limited biocompatibility, leading to inflammatory reactions, encapsulation, rejection, or break; and the poor biostability and transparency. The ideal bioelectrode should satisfy two requirements (Muskovich and Bettinger 2012); first, it would be necessary to lower as much as possible the impedance of the contact: a neural probe should maximize neural signals, minimize noise, and maintain high capacitance, and this implies an intimate connection between the electrode and the biological tissue. Second, it is necessary to find biocompatible coatings, in order to avoid glial responses and rapid degradation of the electrodes in the harsh biological environment. The use of semiconducting polymers as coatings of single electrodes or multielectrode arrays dates back to the 1970s: indeed, they proved to successfully meet both requirements. Organic semiconductors are able to improve the mechanical contact, to decrease the mechanical mismatch at the interface with tissue, and they do have beneficial effects on the lifetime of the implant, by offering enhanced biocompatibility (Khodagholy et al. 2011a; Hassler et al. 2011). An additional, important advantage is the possibility of functionalization with biomolecules that stimulate the neuronal outgrowth and minimize the immune response. Among the huge class of carbon-based materials, recent trends involve use of carbon nanotubes, carbon fibers, and graphene. These materials have demonstrated their usefulness in a number of applications, and for this specific topic, we remind the reader to more specialized reviews (Bareket-Keren and Hanein 2013; Kotov et al. 2009).

Here we restrict our attention to semiconducting polymers, adopted in the latest years not just as coatings but for the realization of the whole electrode structure, in an all-organic biomedical device fashion. The most employed materials are polyanilines (PANI), polypyrroles (PPy), and polythiophenes (Guimard et al. 2007; Muskovich and Bettinger 2012). A fundamental requirement limiting the use of polymers for prolonged in vitro operation or in vivo conditions is that they must retain conductivity under physiological conditions (pH = 7 in aqueous media): this is verified in PPy but not in PANI, which has therefore limited its application in bioelectrodes; conversely, PPy has been extensively used for the electrical stimulation of neuronal lines, in neural probes, and in bio-actuators (George et al. 2005). Unfortunately, PPy is subjected to irreversible oxidation. Compared to PPy and PANI, polythiophenes offer the advantage of superior electrical properties, easier biochemical functionalization, better processability, and improved electrochemical stability under physiological conditions. These features have determined an increasing interest for this material. Biocompatibility has been widely demonstrated in a number of cells, such as PC12, fibroblasts, endothelial cells, neuroblastoma cells, and cortical neural cell lines as well as living neurons. PEDOT:PSS in particular is a heavily doped p-type organic semiconductor, in which holes on the PEDOT chains (the semiconductor) are compensated by sulfonate anions on the PSS (the dopant). Thanks to its optimal properties of conductivity, chemical and electrical long-term stability, relatively low interfacial impedance, and processability easiness, PEDOT:PSS have emerged as the "golden material" for neural interfaces applications, and it is currently in process for FDA approval.

The first demonstration of inherent PEDOT cytocompatibility was reported by Martin and co-workers: they were able to develop integrated systems made between the polymer and living cells, by means of in situ polymerization. They reported an integrated neuro-electrode interface with neuroblastoma cells characterized by impedance values one order of magnitude lower than PEDOT films prepared ex vitro; the same group demonstrated polymerization of a PEDOT network around living neuronal cells (Richardson-Burns et al. 2007a) and finally throughout living brain tissue (Richardson-Burns et al. 2007b). The reduced impedance of the contact prompted use of PEDOT:PSS for the fabrication of single electrodes as well as microelectrode arrays (MEAs).

In 2011 Malliaras and co-workers (Yang et al. 2011) realized PEDOT:PSS microelectrodes used as sensitive sensors for the detection of individual transmitter release events from single cells. In other words, they were able to fabricate a "semiartificial synapsis" in which individual exocytosis event is electrochemically detected by the polymer microelectrode. The possibility of using conducting polymers for such an application relies on three constraints: (1) they must have adequate temporal resolution; (2) they must be patterned to single cell dimensions; and (3) they must be carefully insulated to reduce background noise and to resolve the small currents associated with detection of individual release events. It was demonstrated that the PEDOT:PSS microelectrode, properly covered by a fluoropolymer and insulated by a photoresist, matches all these requirements, with a detection capability in the same range of standard recording devices based on carbon fibers electrodes.

Polymer-based MEAs have been extensively reviewed by Blau in 2011. The same author recently demonstrated (Blau et al. 2010) the realization of a bendable, non-cytotoxic, and biostable PEDOT:PSS array composed of 60 electrodes. Its recording performances were investigated in a number of possible applications, including cardiac activity from acute in vitro preparations from embryonic hearts, neural activity in mouse retinal whole mounts and in vitro dissociated cortico-hippocampal co-cultures, and sensory-driven synaptic activity from in vivo neo-cortical tissue.

Given the promising performances of PEDOT:PSS electrodes, there has been recently a strong effort for the development of conformable arrays specifically targeted to in vivo applications. Implantable electrodes (traditionally used for deep brain stimulation in epilepsy and Parkinson's disease studies) consist in invasive, high-density arrays of metal electrodes. In many cases (for instance, in visual prosthesis), it is necessary to develop surface electrodes, able to conform to the curvilinear shapes of organs, still to form high-quality electrical contacts. Malliaras and co-workers reported on the fabrication of a PEDOT:PSS 32 electrodes array, of a total thickness of 4 μm, which could be successfully employed in electrocorticography (Khodagholy et al. 2011a). Interestingly, the polymer-based device was able to record the electrophysiological activity with high accuracy, outperforming plain gold electrodes of similar geometry.

This important result will certainly open the way to other proof-of-concept devices, which possibly will speed up adoption of organic conductors and semi-conductors in neuroscience and biotechnologies. Considering that (1) use of electrodes is certainly the most assessed way to establish biotic-abiotic interfaces, that (2) organic semiconductors in combination with inorganic conductors have been widely characterized in the past decades, and that (3) nowadays the actual possibility of progress in neuroscience and medicine strongly relies on finding new materials and new available technologies, organic-based bioelectrodes will most probably represent the first field where polymers can find a practical use at the clinical level. Potential applications in neurosurgery have been indeed recently highlighted in an interesting perspective by Von Holst (2013), including epilepsy, dysfunctions of central and peripheral nerves, traumatic brain injuries, and intracranial tumors.

3.4 Organic Electrochemical Transistors

Besides electrodes intended for stimulation and recording, use of transistors is emerged as a useful tool to extract the small electric potentials generated by cell cultures and tissue slices, providing a better signal-to-noise ratio due to local amplification by the transistor circuitry. However, use of inorganic transistors for in vivo recordings has been hitherto severely hampered by their poor biocompatibility: even in the most recent works reporting integration of silicon FETs into in vivo probes, the transistors themselves served as a mean for addressing hundreds of electrodes, but they did not serve as direct sensing elements, requiring instead

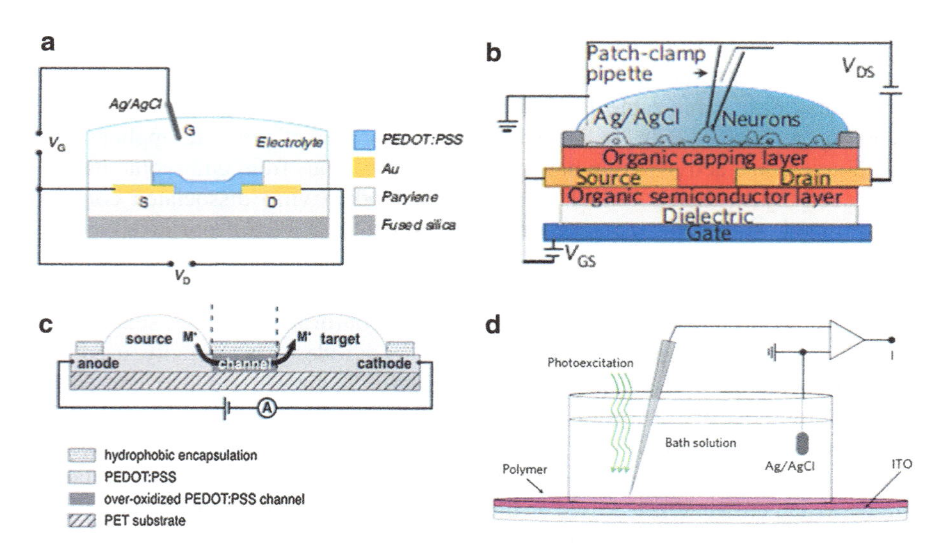

Fig. 3.1 Schematic diagram of (**a**) organic electrochemical transistor [reproduced with permission from Khodagholy et al. (2013b)], (**b**) organic field-effect transistor [reproduced with permission from Benfenati et al. (2013)], (**c**) organic electronic ion pump [reproduced with permission from Larsson et al. (2013)], and (**d**) biopolymer interface for cell photostimulation [reproduced with permission from Ghezzi et al. (2013)]

careful encapsulation to avoid inflammatory reactions. Organic electronics is emerging as a valuable alternative, not only for electrical activity recording but even for stimulation. Two kinds of architectures have been reported: the organic electrochemical transistor (OECT) and the organic field-effect transistor (OFET), schematically sketched in Fig. 3.1.

Unlike standard FET structures, where the active material is separated by the electrolyte through an insulating layer, in an OECT device the organic polymer is in direct contact with the electrolyte (White et al. 1984), the latter being a constitutive part of the device. Basically, the OECT device acts as a transconductance amplifier that converts a voltage modulation at the gate to a modulation of the drain current. The election material for the realization of OECT devices is nowadays PEDOT:PSS, thanks to its superior conductivity and cytocompatibility. In OECT structures the unique ability of organic electronic materials to conduct both electronic and ionic carriers is capitalized, serving thus as the ideal platform in integrated bioelectronic systems. More in detail, in PEDOT:PSS blends, PEDOT provides electronic conductivity, while PSS provides both electronic and cationic conductivity.

The transconductance of mechanically flexible PEDOT:PSS-based OECTs has been recently reported (Khodagholy et al. 2013a) in the mS range, a value which is two orders of magnitude larger than that planar silicon-based FETs. The reported values remain fairly constant from DC up to a frequency of the order of 1 kHz, a value determined by the process of ion transport between the electrolyte and the channel.

OECTs have raised interest in the community first of all as biosensors (Lin and Yan 2012; Lin et al. 2010), being employed, for instance, in DNA (Yan et al. 2009), enzymes (Zhu et al. 2004), and cell attachment sensing (Bolin et al. 2009). More recently, R. Owens and co-workers (Jimison et al. 2012) have demonstrated that it is possible to use an OECT structure in order to detect, in situ, minute disruptions in barrier tissue functions. In particular, they reported unprecedented temporal resolution and sensitivity in measuring variations of paracellular ionic fluxes induced by toxic compounds. New applications of organic semiconductors in toxicology, drug development, and disease diagnostics are therefore expected in the next future.

The possibility to realize OECT arrays able to direct interfacing with liquid electrolytes by lithographic processes was first demonstrated in 2011 (Khodagholy et al. 2011b). The transistors operated at low voltages and showed a response time in the order of 100 μs, thus compatible with biological processes recording. Highly conformable OECT arrays based on PEDOT:PSS were then used in vivo, in electrocorticography experiments for recording epileptiform discharges (Khodagholy et al. 2013b). Impressively, flexible transistor arrays were positively compared with surface electrodes, showing superior signal-to-noise ratios, and even with conventional penetrating electrodes. The observed differences rely on the key difference between the transistor arrays and the electrode arrays: in fact, the OECT locally amplifies the signal; conversely, in conventional electrode recordings the signal can be preamplified only outside the head of the animal, thus amplifying the noise generated by leads and interconnections as well.

Another interesting device capable of in vivo operation has been reported by Berggren and his collaborators (Larsson et al. 2013). Called the organic electronic ion pump (OEIP), it is essentially a variation on theme of the OECT principle (Fig. 3.1c). In the OEIP device structure, two PEDOT:PSS electrodes are patterned on a plastic substrate and are connected by a channel. The channel is made by overoxidized PEDOT:PSS, and, while electronically it is an insulator, it preserves the capability of conducting ions. The source electrolyte contains the positive ions to be delivered into the target electrolyte; oxidation of the source electrode (anode) forces ions to enter the anode itself from the source electrolyte. Since the channel is electronically insulating but allows ionic conductivity, ions will be pumped toward the cathode and finally delivered to the target electrolyte. Since ionic charges transported through the channel are fully or partially compensated by electronic charges flowing between the two electrodes, the current measured in the external circuit is directly proportional to the delivery rate of cations in the target electrolyte. It is important to note that, at variance with systems based on electrical stimulation, in the OEIP electrical signals are translated to delivery of specific chemical messengers, allowing to specifically target only the neurons expressing the cognate receptors. Interestingly, it is possible to exploit the OEIP concept not only for transporting metal ions but even for delivery of biomolecules, relevant for neuronal cell signaling. Some notable examples reported in in vitro studies include acetylcholine, aspartate, GABA, and glutamate (Isaksson et al. 2007). OEIPs were also realized in flexible geometries, suitable for surgical implantation. The controlled delivery of neurotransmitters was then assessed in the cochlear system of guinea pigs, thus demonstrating the practical possibility to modulate sensory functions in a very specific and quantitative way (Simon et al. 2009).

All in all, reported devices fully demonstrate that the technology is mature enough to compete with standard in vivo recording and stimulation tools, offering at the same time enhanced biocompatibility and unprecedented functionalities.

3.5 Organic Field-Effect Transistors

Organic field-effect transistor (OFET) architectures have been widely exploited for the realization and demonstration of biosensors in the latest years. Many possible applications have been reported, including pH, glucose, cholesterol, and enzyme sensing. Importantly, it is possible to operate some of these devices at very low voltages (in the liquid-gated configuration, for instance, or by using high capacitive gate dielectric materials), avoiding thus harmful electrochemical degradation and reducing the heat released to the surrounding: in one word, making them compatible with unavoidable biological constraints (Cramer et al. 2013a). Recent trends in OFET research are also leading to massive demonstration and development of bendable and rollable devices (Sekitani et al. 2010; Schwartz et al. 2013); moreover, at variance with inorganic semiconductors, low processing temperatures required by organic technology and availability of several printing technologies, such as screen printing and ink-jet printing, offer important perspectives in terms of devices' area scalability. Transparency and high thermal stability are two other important properties for some biomedical applications. For instance, it has been recently reported a flexible OFET based on a high-mobility organic semiconductor, operating at low voltages (2 V), is able to sustain high-temperature sterilization, required by medical applications (Kuribara et al. 2012).

All together, these characteristics justify the increasing interest toward possible applications in the biomedical field, aiming at in vivo operation.

The idea of using organic transistors for stimulating excitable cells activity dates back to 2008, when Stieglitz and co-workers (Feili et al. 2008) used pentacene transistors with silicon oxide as dielectric to stimulate a frog sciatic nerve and succeeded in recording cell responses. This first proved that OFETs could be used for matrix addressing in biomedical applications, even though in this case an externally applied potential of at least −35 V was required. Interestingly, the authors proposed a possible use of the same array for neural prosthetics devices and in particular for epiretinal stimulation.

Very recently, two works have been reported on the interaction between organic thin-film transistors and in vitro cells, capable of working at very low voltages.

Biscarini et al. (Cramer et al. 2013b) have demonstrated that a liquid-gated pentacene transistor is able both to stimulate and record the extracellular activity of stem murine cells cultured on top of the active polymer layer. The OFET response was monitored during the different phases of the neuronal differentiation process, and only when stem cells were differentiated into neurons, it was possible to measure electrical signals in the current following the stimulation.

Muccini et al. (Benfenati et al. 2013) demonstrated that a transparent organic transistor based on an n-type organic semiconductor, namely, *N*, *N*′-ditridecylperylene-3,4,9,10-tetracarboxylic diimide (P13), is able to provide both stimulation and recording of dorsal root ganglion primary neurons. Thanks to the improved, efficient coupling between the semiconductor and the neuronal cells, peculiar of the organic technology, it was possible to obtain a very good signal-to-noise ratio, exceeding by 16 times that of standard microelectrode array systems, without inducing any electroporation effect in the cell membrane. The good properties shown by the transistor in multicell activity recording and stimulation prompted the authors to be optimistic for the use of the device even in single cell recording.

3.6 Biopolymer Interfaces for Cell Photostimulation

In all abovementioned applications, electrical and/or ionic conductivity of organic semiconductors was exploited. Surprisingly, their most appealing properties, namely, the absorption and emission of light in the visible spectrum, which determined the flourish of organic optoelectronics with a plethora of devices (light-emitting diodes, organic photodetectors, organic photovoltaic cells, light-emitting transistors, light-emitting electrochemical cells), were not at all investigated in bioorganic interfaces until very recently. Indeed, only in 2011, organic semiconductors, working in a photodetector-like configuration, have been proposed as photoactive materials for optical excitation of neural networks. The use of organic photodetectors in medical and biological applications raises an important issue in the design of bioorganic interfaces, since the liquid electrolyte challenges the survival of organic device optoelectronic performances (capability of generating, transporting, and extracting charges), and degradation of the metal electrode is greatly accelerated in a liquid environment. A solution to the latter problem is the realization of devices in which the metal electrode is substituted by aqueous saline solutions.

In these examples, the device structure comprises an anodic contact (usually ITO) covered by the organic photosensitive layer and a saline electrolyte. It is clear that the complex polymer-liquid interface plays a key role in this specific case, and a number of studies aiming at characterizing such an interface have been reported (Cramer et al. 2009; Eisenthal 1996; Svennersten et al. 2011). Several conjugated polymers have been demonstrated to work as active layers in direct contact with liquid electrolytes (Gautam et al. 2011; Antognazza et al. 2009; Lanzarini et al. 2012; Gautam et al. 2010). Reported materials include regioregular poly (3-hexylthiophene-2,5-diyl) (rr-P3HT); poly-[*N*-90-heptadecanyl-2,7-carbazole-alt-5,5-(40,70-di-2-thienyl-20,10,30-benzothiadiazole) (PCDTBT); P3OT, poly (9,9-dioctylfluorene-co-benzothiadiazole) (F8BT); MEH-PPV; poly[2-methoxy-5-

(3′,7′-dimethyloctyloxy)-1,4-phenylene vinylene] (MDMO-PPV); and poly [2,6-(4,4-bis-(2-ethylhexyl)-4Hcyclopenta[2,1-b;3,4-b′]-dithiophene)-alt-4,7-(2,1,3-benzothiadiazole)] (PCPDTBT), as photoactive polymers, and poly {[N,N0-bis(2 octyldodecyl)naphthalene-1,4,5,8-bis-(dicarboximide)-2,6-diyl]-alt-5,50-(2,20-bithiophene)} (N2200) and PCBM as electron acceptors. Various electrolytes can be used for the saline solution, such as sodium iodide, sodium and potassium chloride, and sodium bromide. For direct interfacing to living cells, sodium chloride is the most interesting case, since it represents the most abundant component of the biological extracellular fluids and of any cell culture medium. Indeed, the same device configuration shows the generation of a photocurrent in the presence of common culturing and buffering media such as Dulbecco-modified minimum essential medium or buffered Krebs-Ringer's solutions. The main difference between hybrid and conventional OPDs is related to the interface phenomena between the polymer film and the electrolyte: in the hybrid device the conductance type changes from mainly electronic to ionic; in the solid-state cell, the mechanism is that of a standard Schottky barrier photodiode. The equilibrium condition at the interface is qualitatively similar: chemical potential (Fermi level) is equalized by charge transport across the interface. Yet the microscopic setting is dramatically different. In the solid device, charge carrier migration leads to space charge separation across the interface generating local electric fields that cause band bending. In the hybrid system, ion adsorption at the surface competes with charge transfer, also mediated by chemical reactions. A dipole layer forms at the surface, while a diffused ion layer spreads in the solution (i.e., Helmholtz layer). In general, hybrid photodetectors offer the opportunity to directly investigate the semiconducting polymer/electrolyte interface phenomena that appear of interest for multiple applications, such as photoelectrochemical cells, electrolyte-gated field-effect transistors, electrochemical transistors, tandem photovoltaic cells, and dye-sensitized solar cells. More specifically, they have a noticeable potential in the field of neuromorphic engineering for the development of artificial neural systems, whose design principles are based on those of biological nervous systems, as well as in bioinspired light-harvesting systems.

Lanzani and co-workers recently demonstrated that an organic photovoltaic blend (namely, P3HT:PCBM), coated on a transparent ITO conducting layer, is able to elicit electrical activity in primary neurons grown on top of it, upon stimulation in the visible range (Ghezzi et al. 2011). The reliability and reproducibility in the generation of neuron action potentials for pulsed illumination were excellent. Moreover, the opto-cell stimulation paradigm showed good spatial and temporal properties. It was also found that the same transduction process of light pulses into neuronal electrical activity is obtained by using a neat P3HT film deposited on ITO (Ghezzi et al. 2013). This observation indicates that the functioning of such a hybrid interface is different from that of conventional organic photovoltaic devices and that faradaic currents, injected in the cleft between the device and the neuron, are most probably not relevant here. Indeed, a large body of experimental evidence suggests the presence of a capacitive coupling between the organic layer and the neuron grown on top of it. It was also reported that the working principle of cell photoactivation is not limited to primary neuronal networks. The possibility to modulate in a controlled way the whole-cell conductance in primary rat astrocytes by means of optical stimulation, properly mediated by the active polymer film, has been recently demonstrated in Benfenati et al. (2014).

The present approach is exquisitely general in its working principles, and it represents a new tool for neural active interfacing, as a simpler alternative to the existing and widely used neuron optogenetic photostimulation techniques able to avoid potentially hazardous gene transfer protocols. The photostimulation is not specific for selected neuronal populations, as is the case for genetically encoded approaches, but the optical stimulation of neurons could be micrometrically shaped to stimulate selected neuronal populations owing to the high spatial selectivity of the photostimulation interface, and could lead to the development of new artificial optoelectronic neurointerfaces based on biocompatible organic materials.

The phenomenon of cell stimulation by polymer photoexcitation seems naturally fitting into artificial vision application. In particular, the high spatial and temporal resolution of the photoexcitation, together with the good biocompatibility properties demonstrated for the organic semiconductors, opens the way to the realization of a polymer-based artificial visual prosthesis. The goal here is to restore photosensitivity in retinas whose natural photoreceptors are damaged or lost. In 2013 Benfenati et al. reported that a polymer-based bioorganic interface is capable of restoring light sensitivity in blind retinas (Ghezzi et al. 2013). Acutely dissected blind retinas from albino rats were placed on P3HT-coated Glass:ITO substrates with the external layers in contact with the polymer. A 10 ms light pulse (4 μW/mm^2) was able to stimulate intense activity (detected by extracellular recordings in the ganglion cell layer), at levels indistinguishable from those of control retinas of normal rats, while no significant activity could be recorded in blinded retinas placed on Glass:ITO only substrates. The analysis of the temporal and pharmacological characteristics of the excitation proved that ganglion cell spiking was mediated by the activation of the external cell layer in contact with the polymer. Dose–response measurements (Fig. 3.2) revealed threshold intensity for photostimulation of about 0.3 μW/mm^2, closely matching the range of retinal irradiance during outdoor activity (0.1–10 μW/mm^2).

The reported results demonstrate that organic semiconductors can be a valid alternative to the more traditional devices used for retinal implants, mostly based on inorganic semiconductors and/or metallic electrodes (Zrenner 2012). The most successful retinal prostheses, namely, the epiretinal Argus device (Second Sight Medical Products) (Humayun et al. 2012) and the sub-retinal device Alpha (Retina Implant AG) (Zrenner et al. 2011), have obtained promising results and are currently under clinical testing. However, metal/silicon artificial devices still have to face and solve major common problems: need of power supply, scarce biocompatibility, low compliance, complexity of the fabrication process, electrode number, size and geometry, high impedance levels, resistive currents, and pronounced heat production, which is very detrimental to the retinal tissue. All these reasons have strongly limited the success of these metal-/silicon-based prostheses. Although the coupling mechanism between neural cells and the semiconducting

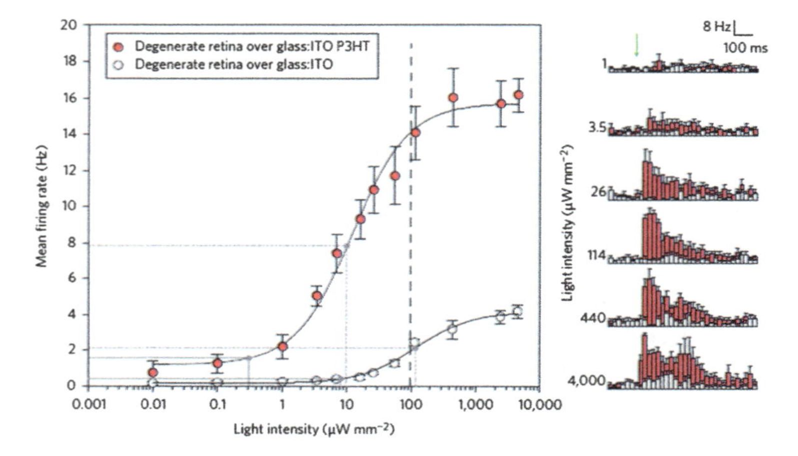

Fig. 3.2 A P3HT layer is able to induce neuronal firing and to restore light sensitivity in explanted blind retinas. Dose–response analysis of the mean (± s.e.m.) firing rate versus light intensity performed in degenerate retinas over P3HT-coated Glass:ITO (*red dots*) or Glass:ITO alone (*open dots*) shows sensitivity to irradiances compatible with physiological levels of illumination [reproduced with permission from Ghezzi et al. (2013)]

polymer is still only partially understood, its potential impact is clear-cut. The advantages offered by organic semiconductors are manifold and rely on material softness, reduced invasiveness, very low toxicity, and enhanced biocompatibility, no need for external biasing, very limited and spatially confined heat production, and reduced oxidation/reduction reactions at the interfaces, as a consequence of the capacitive-like coupling between the artificial and the natural tissue. Another major advantage is the spatial confinement of the stimulation, which could in principle improve the limited resolution of traditional implants. There are however many open issues, regarding in particular the long-term stability of the polymeric material, the tolerability over prolonged time in vivo, and the optimization of the device response, which represent an exciting challenge for material scientists, chemists, and physicist community, working at the forefront of biomedical technology.

3.7 Perspectives of Bioelectronic Interfaces

The several examples of organic-based devices for biomedical and neuroscience applications briefly summarized here above give a clear idea of the huge potential offered by conjugated materials. Reported performances in some cases already outmatch the ones of traditional inorganic devices, despite the fact that the field is still in its infancy. There is indeed a lot of room for discovering new possible applications, improving existing performances, and inventing new devices. Organic transistors, for instance, would greatly benefit from adopting new-generation, stable, and high-mobility n-type materials, recently reported in the literature, thus allowing the realization of ambipolar devices. Organic light-emitting diodes and light-emitting transistors represent fully unexplored opportunities in biotic-abiotic interfaces: they could however offer interesting opportunities, for instance, in the field of optogenetics. Concerning biopolymer interfaces for cell photoactivation, devices exploiting the capacitive charging, which leads to cell activity elicitation, would greatly benefit from adopting materials with high dielectric constant and coupling with properly engineered oxide layers. Finally, also electrochemical devices, which are now essentially based only on PEDOT:PSS, could be tremendously improved by development and careful chemical engineering of new materials.

On top of all, the many available processing techniques (such as ink-jet printing, soft lithography, screen printing, laser writing, and micromachining, just to cite some) hold the promise of realizing devices specifically targeted to different needs of various applications.

However, many issues remain to be addressed: long-term functioning, biostability, and full, long-term biocompatibility still wait for detailed analysis.

The path to full exploitation of organic bioelectronics will certainly go through a clear and detailed understanding of the biotic-abiotic interface phenomena; the complexity of the living tissue represents an obstacle that must and can be overtaken, since this is really crucial for the development and improvement of therapeutic applications and in vivo operation.

3.8 Flexible Piezoelectric/Flexoelectric MEMS for Bioinspired Sensors

Another challenge of bioinspired technologies is the realization of flexible materials to transduce a mechanical pressure/shear (stress) into a current, which are the basis for the realization of biomimetic tactile sensors and hearing sensors. In this section we discuss piezoelectric MEMS technologies developed for tactile sensing on flexible and compliant substrates. Based on a piezoelectric thin film of aluminum nitride (AlN) integrated on polymer, this technology exploits extensively the piezoelectric properties of the AlN, along with a 3D dome-shaped architecture, which leads to a strong flexoelectric behavior. In the next section we will deal with hearing and flow sensors to be used for the artificial ear or for proximity sensors.

The sense of touch allows one to detect and measure physical static or dynamic stimuli applied to the skin, and it constitutes an essential mean of knowledge and perception of the environment for humans, mammalians, and robots. In the human skin, the role of the detection of external stimuli on touch is provided by a great number of sensorial receptors, distributed with variable density and with different roles: mechanoreceptors to sense forces and pressure/vibration, thermoreceptors for temperature, and nocioreceptors for pain/damage.

The skin provides support and protection from the surrounding environment, and, by virtue of its compliance, it adapts to the touching object, transmitting its deformation to the mechanoreceptors underneath. In response, spikes of action potentials are generated and sent to the central nervous system, which processes and encodes the received signal.

The several thousands of mechanoreceptors in the human skin can be distinguished by their receptive field and rates of adaptation. Pacinian, Meissner, and Ruffini corpuscles and Merkel disks, each with a different role, can feel static and dynamic stimuli, normal and shear forces.

Mimicking the physiology and operation of these bio-mechanoreceptors is a challenging but necessary task, in order to realize artificial skins and to provide robots a real sense of touch. Texture, roughness, shape, slipperiness, and compliance of materials and surfaces would then be parameters accessible to the robotic intelligence, enabling higher levels of awareness of the environment and safe interaction in unstructured surroundings.

The compliance and adaptation of the flexible structure as in the human skin and the exploitation of piezoelectricity and flexoelectricity make it possible to emulate two mechanoreceptors at the same time: Merkel disks and Pacinian corpuscles. The sensor can therefore detect different types of forces: pressure as Merkel disks do in slow adapting mode, exploiting the flexoelectric effect, and vibrations in fast adapting mode as Pacinian corpuscles do through the piezoelectricity. The 3D dome-shaped architecture on the other hand allows measuring shear forces, extremely important in robotic grabbing actions.

3.9 Soft MEMS for Tactile Sensing: AlN-Based Piezoelectric/Flexoelectric MEMS on Soft Substrates

The application of tactile sensors is wide, including safe human-robot interaction, soft operation of machines in agriculture and harvesting, domotics, robotic and remote surgery, teleoperation, noninvasive diagnostics, and rehabilitation. All these applications need flexible tactile sensors able to detect static and dynamic force stimuli on both small and large areas (Carlson et al. 2006; Mannsfeld et al. 2010; Bu et al. 2009; Lees 2009; Qi et al. 2010; Dahiya et al. 2010; Eltaib and Hewit 2003). The key issue is to find a transduction mechanism able to provide very accurate tactile information (roughness, texture, stiffness, size) of the touched object.

Most transduction mechanisms have been investigated in the past (Dahiya et al. 2010; Yousef et al. 2011): optical, strain gauge, piezoresistive, magnetic, ultrasonic, capacitive, and piezoelectric. Optical tactile sensors (Yamada et al. 2005) are typically based on optical waveguides embedded in an elastomer. They detect the change of light intensity due to the force applied to the elastomer which in turn induces a modification of light path. Though flexible and sensitive, they require space and complex computation. Tactile sensors based on strain gauges exploit the elastic deformation conveyed to a long winding snake-like resistor: by applying a force, a change of resistance is generated (Xu et al. 2003). They are sensitive and have a simple electronics, but they show significant drift with temperature. Based on a similar principle, piezoresistors undergo a change of the material properties induced by the strain which in turn results in a change of resistance (Ho et al. 2009). In magnetic tactile sensors, a current is induced by the displacement under pressure of a permanent magnet embedded into silicone gel body (Takenawa 2009). Though simple, such devices suffer from magnetic interference and power consumption. Ultrasonic tactile sensors have a layer of deformable rubber and 2D array of TX and RX transducers to measure the rubber thickness: upon application of a force, the thickness changes are measured by the transducers. The main limit of ultrasonic sensors is the complex electronics. In capacitive tactile sensors, the application of the force reduces the gap between parallel plates generating a capacitance variation, and they are sensitive and low cost; however, crosstalk and hysteresis are issues when sensors are based on elastomers (Hutchings et al. 1994). Piezoelectric tactile sensors were the most investigated in the past (Dario et al. 1984). They are mainly based on PVDF (polyvinylidene fluoride) piezoelectric polymer because of its flexibility, high electromechanical coefficient ($d_{33} = -33$ pC/N), and chemical inertness. They are able to convert the applied stress into voltage due the direct piezoelectric effect, but the generated charges decay quickly with time, making these sensors only suitable for time-varying stimuli.

Piezoelectric MEMS for tactile sensing have the strong advantage of not requiring a power supply. Recently, Pang et al. have proposed a new tactile sensors (Pang et al. 2012) consisting of two polymer sheets covered by nanofibers on one side interfaced to each other. The polyurethane-based nanofibers, interlocked by Van der Waals forces, are covered by a thin layer of platinum and, being in contact, exhibit a low short circuit resistance. The resistance changes by applying pressure, torsion, and shear force, behaving similar to natural hair cells.

A new architecture, exploited to detect different types of forces, consists of a piezoelectric thin film of aluminum nitride (AlN) deposited on a soft material. AlN on polymer has several interesting characteristics with respect to PVFD: it is a polycrystalline wurtzite with a natural polarization along c-axis due to the crystal symmetry; it does not need poling treatment and the piezoelectricity is retained up to very high temperatures (1,500 °C). AlN is deposited by sputtering at medium temperatures (250–300 °C), and it grows in columnar arrangement showing a compressive stress. From the electrical point of view, AlN is very insulating, the energy gap being 6.2 eV, and it shows high breakdown voltage. The piezoelectric properties of AlN are weak ($d_{33} = 4$–5 pC/N) when compared to PVDF (−33 pC/N) and ZnO (9.9 pC/N); however, PVDF has the typical drawbacks of viscoelastic systems: lack of electrical linear behavior and hysteresis added to a low Curie temperature (120 °C). ZnO has a small energy gap 3.3 eV, which makes it less suitable for sensors because of the large current leakage. Recently, the possibility to grow AlN on polymers with a moderate crystal orientation has raised the attention of scientific community; in particular Akiyama showed that AlN deposited by low temperature sputtering on polyimide with a discrete crystal orientation manifests piezoelectricity (Akiyama et al. 2007, 2008). The inclusion of AlN/polymer structures into the family of flexible piezoelectric devices paves the way to sensors with augmented mechanical and electrical properties. Sputtered Mo/AlN/Mo heterostructures on 25 μm thick Kapton foils result in very well-oriented polycrystalline layers which can be patterned in circular shape to obtain large elastic *domes* due to the compressive stress of AlN over Kapton. The organization of the crystal in the *dome* makes the system very elastic under load, with the capability to undergo higher strains than rigid AlN thin films on silicon. The system is sensitive to two different types of mechanical stimuli: vibration through the piezoelectric effect, recorded as time-varying voltage, and pressure as capacitive variation due to the flexoelectric effect. The last contribution is due to the strain gradient generated in the crystal. By applying a pressure to the *dome*, a further polarization is generated, which is detected as capacitance variation (Fig. 3.3).

The analogy with mechanoreceptors is remarkable: the flexible AlN allows to sense time-varying stimuli as Pacinian corpuscles and Merkel disks do in human fingers (Fig. 3.4).

Despite the hybrid nature of such devices, the AlN films are crack-free and exhibit a good adhesion on the plastic Kapton film. The crystalline structure of Mo and AlN films is indeed preserved as evidenced by the X-ray diffraction patterns in the inset of Fig. 3.3.

The force transducers device can be fabricated in one lithographic step by a (SU8-25) negative photoresist. The Mo top electrode and the AlN are dry etched by inductively coupled plasma (gas mixture $SiCl_4$, N_2, and Ar). Upon detaching the device from the starting rigid substrate, a free-standing foil of circular transducers is obtained. Each transducer transforms itself into a dome-shaped 3D structure, because of the residual stress of the crystal layers on the polymer (Fig. 3.5). The structure is elastic and does not crack even under large deformations.

The piezoelectricity of AlN is well known and allows the detection of time-varying signals in a wide frequency range as the Pacinian mechanoreceptors. The application of an oscillating voltage V generates an out-of-plane deformation; the relation between the z displacement and the applied voltage depends on the piezoelectricity of the material and corresponds to d_{33}. The measured d_{33} in these devices is 4.7 ± 0.5 pm/V, which is consistent with the values reported for AlN layers grown on silicon and silicon-based substrates (Xu et al. 2001; Dubois and Muralt 2001).

In addition to piezoelectricity, the application of a load to the *dome* generates a strain gradient in the film. The strain gradient is responsible for a polarization known as flexoelectricity which manifests itself through a capacitance variation. The flexoelectric effect is the property of piezoelectric (and dielectric) materials to generate charge separation when subjected to elastic strain gradients (Tagantsev 1986). The flexoelectric polarization is described by the following equation:

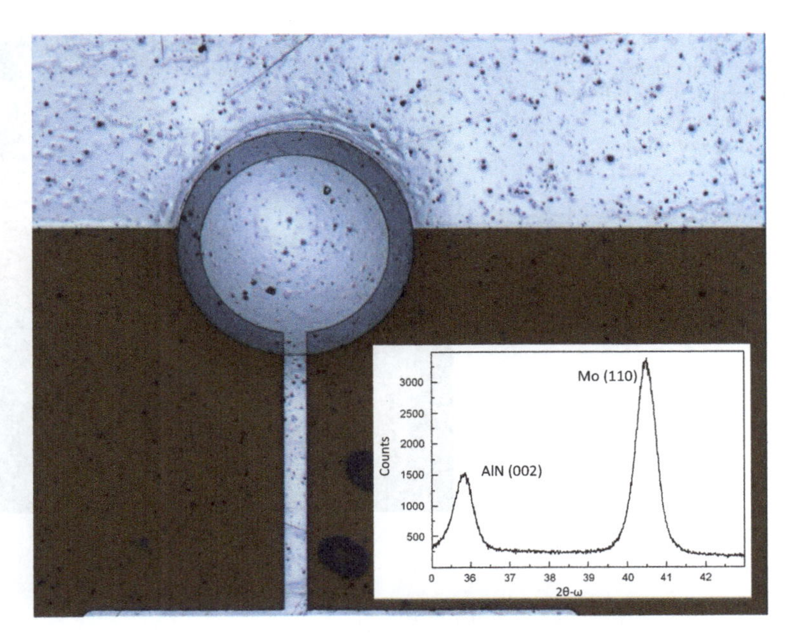

Fig. 3.3 Mo/AlN/Mo piezoelectric transducer on Kapton substrate with a circular dome and diameter of 600 μm. *Inset*: Rocking curves of the Mo/AlN/Mo structure on Kapton (FWHM is 0.55° for the AlN peak)

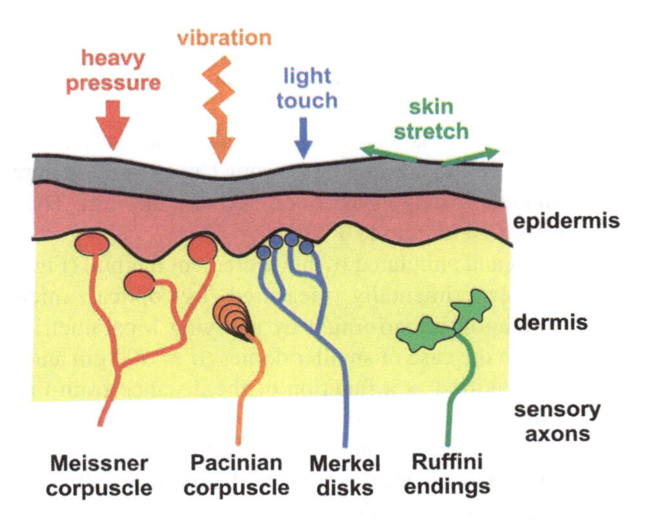

Fig. 3.4 Mechanoreceptors in human skin and different applied mechanical stimuli

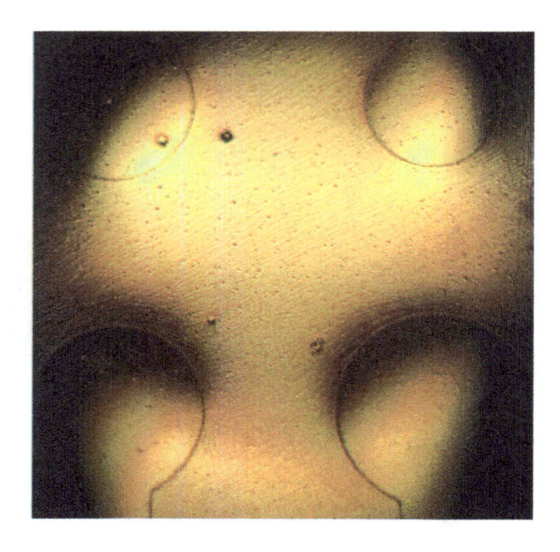

Fig. 3.5 Array 2 × 2 of piezoelectric transducers, the stress release of the AlN polycrystalline layer leads the dome shape of the circular part

$$P_l = \mu_{ijkl} \frac{\partial S_{ij}}{\partial x_k}$$

where P is the polarization, μ_{ijkl} the flexoelectric coefficient, S_{ij} the components of the elastic strain, and x_k the direction of the strain S gradient.

The flexoelectric effect is due to a discontinuity in crystal lattice, and it is experimentally observed on AlN dome since the pressure depresses the dome, thus producing a strain gradient as also confirmed by finite element method (FEM) simulations.

In Fig. 3.6a, the polarization is recorded as a capacitance variation generated by the application of a load on the dome. Loads from 1 g up to 20 g were applied for transducers with diameters d ranging between 500 and 800 μm. The investigated pressure range goes from 10 kPa up to 1 MPa.

The *dome* is designed and simulated by finite element method (Fig. 3.6b, c) with diameter and height experimentally measured by optical microscope and profilometry. The simulation is performed by applying a parametric pressure on top of the sensor *dome*. In the case of smaller domes (d = 500 μm and h = 32 μm), the x and y strains are reported as a function of the distance from the edge of the structure, and the presence of a strain gradient across the layer is confirmed (Fig. 3.6b). The strain gradient is enhanced by applying higher forces, which is consistent with the capacitance variation observed experimentally (Fig. 3.6c). The model confirms the hypothesis that AlN layer is elastically deformed under load and subjected to a growing strain.

This flexoelectric effect increases the sensitivity of flexible AlN on Kapton in sensing application for both dynamic and static forces of small medium intensity (Petroni et al. 2011, 2012). The resulting transducers are very elastic and the deformations of the substrate do not affect the electrical performances of the

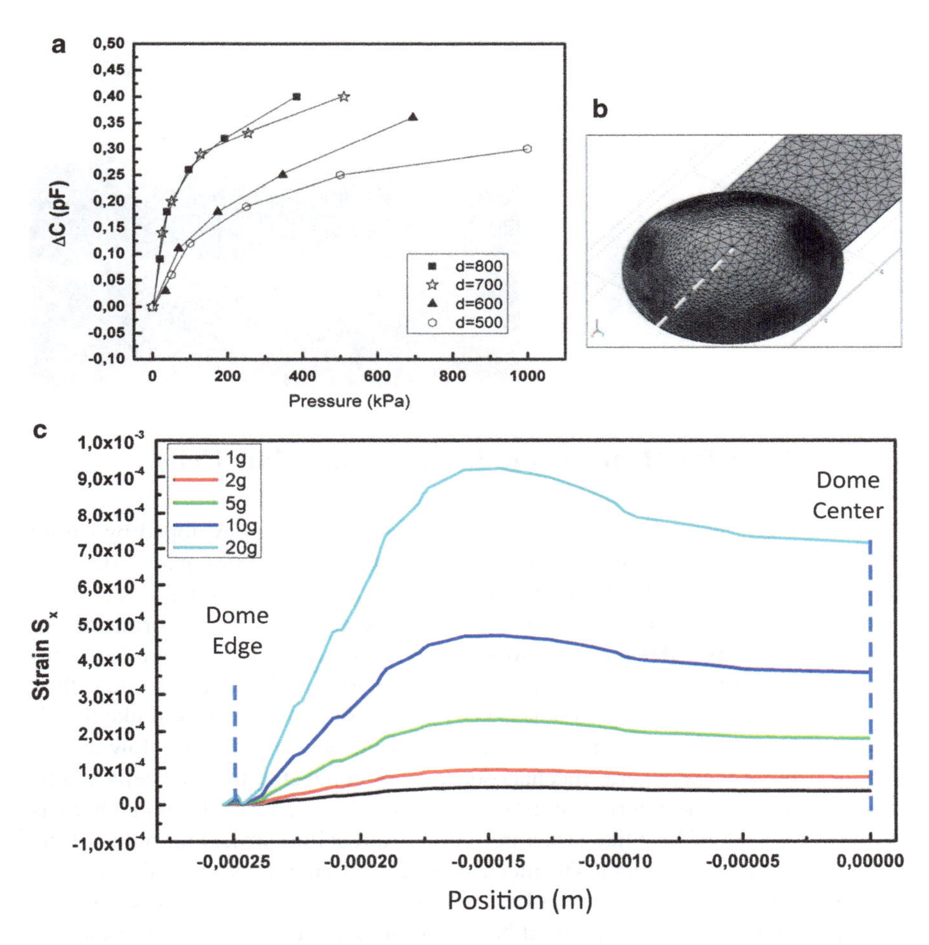

Fig. 3.6 (**a**) Capacitive variation with pressure for dome with different diameters ranging from 500 μm to 800 μm. (**b**) FEM model of the dome. (**c**) Simulated strain profile along the *dashed line* in (**b**) for the different loads on a dome with a diameter of 500 μm

devices. Devices rolled around fingerlike cylindrical surfaces (Fig. 3.7) preserve identical conductivity and capacitance behavior after many cycles, demonstrating the wearability of such structures and in perspective their potential for application to artificial tactile surfaces (Song et al. 2010). The flexoelectricity thus becomes a tool to realize multifunctional systems able to detect touch, shear forces, and vibrations as humans do in their everyday life through mechanoreceptors.

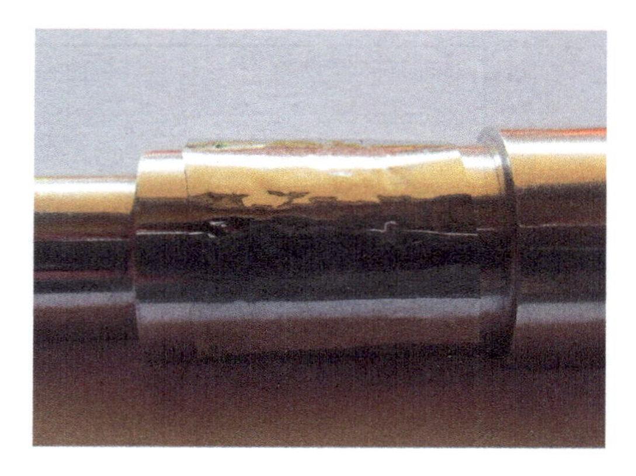

Fig. 3.7 Flexible sample of transducers lying on a fixture having different curvature radii between 5 and 10 mm

3.10 MEMS for Hearing and Flow Sensing Hair Cells

Flow sensors, vision sensors, and acoustic sensors have been developed by nature over the last billions of years to sense and perceive the environment. All these natural systems are characterized by extreme efficiency, small size, high responsivity, and high throughput, by far exceeding the performance of man-made sensors. Mechanoreceptors are very successful biological systems developed by vertebrates to sense pressure and tangential forces due to fluid flow or acoustic waves around their bodies. They consist of hairs on the skin like the air flow sensors of spiders, insects and mammals, or the neuromast water flow on fish skin. In general these natural mechanosensors are connected to "hair cells": cells developed to sense the external environment at microscopic level. Their cell body is equipped by a set of hair-like structures called stereocilia, projecting outward the external cellular environment. The mechanical deflection of these hair-like appendages produces neuro-electrical pulses transmitted to the nervous system. The relative motion of the body and fluid bends the stereocilia generating a mechanical signal converted into a neuronal stimulus by the action of the hair cells. Hair cells that feel the motion of fluids around the animals can also be found in internal organs of living systems, such as the cochlea of mammalian inner ear, where outer and inner hair cells are deflected by membrane vibrations, converting acoustic waves into electrical signals.

Hair cells show very interesting adaptation properties, especially in hearing and equilibrium organs. Adaptation is the ability of a biological system to rearrange its state when placed in a new environment (Ten Wolde 2012). In natural environments, species have to cope with different situations and adjust the way they sense the external signals, adapting to excitation to withstand relatively high external load and increasing the signal-to-noise ratio of sensing cells: they have to react to mechanical inputs from the surroundings and to be compliant to these excitations. Recent studies showed that the morphology and material properties of natural flow sensing hair cells serve to control their sensitivity by tuning their flexural stiffness (McHenry and van Netten 2007). An example of this biological system can be observed in the inner ear, where stereocilia adjust their stiffness continuously, resetting their hair bundle's range of sensitivity to respond to the position at which the bundle is held and, thereby, shifting their sensitivity in an adaptation process to prevent signal saturation (Howard and Hudspeth 1987; Hudspeth 1989; see also Hudspeth 2008). The same solution is naturally applied underwater, where fishes have developed a sensing system called "lateral line," a distributed mechanosensory array over their surface (McHenry and van Netten 2007). To a large extent, natural hair cell adaptation mechanism is relevant to recognize stimulus patterns in a chronically noisy environment.

Evolution is definitely a successful model for technical sensors, actuators, and structures. Indeed, evolutionary pressure to adapt to survive in a wide variety of environments has led to a broad variety of sensors' morphology and sensitivity. It is therefore mandatory to be inspired by nature in designing machines and microsystems working as natural systems (Bleckmann et al. 2004; Fratzl and Barth 2009). In this respect, microelectromechanical system (MEMS) technology has attracted particular attention for the production of 3D microsystems with small physical footprint, high sensitivity, and effective frequency response, such as artificial hair cells for flow sensors in underwater robotics and "active" adaptable hair cells for acoustic prosthetics. Soft probes with controlled stiffness comparable to natural hair cells cilia can be fabricated to excite a whole bundle of acoustic stereocilia, for nondestructive measurements on ex vivo hearing hair cells. On the same footing engineered biomimetic artificial hair cells (AHC) can be realized to reproduce specific natural sensors such as the natural flow sensing system of fishes or adaptive hair cells for hearing and vestibular prosthetics.

3.11 Soft Probes for Nondestructive Investigation of Adaptation Properties of Acoustic Hair Cells

Adaptation and signal amplification in natural hair cells mechanism are distinctive properties of these mechanoreceptors but their full understanding is still lacking. The need of advanced probes to study such mechanoreceptors has stimulated the development of soft probes for ex vivo measurements on hair cells to study their mechanical properties and gating process.

Hearing and equilibrium hair cells are thought to be passive transduction systems able to convert a mechanical pulse in an electrical signal (Hudspeth 1989; see also Hudspeth 2008). Mechanical stimuli are coupled to the tallest row of stereocilia by the overlying tectorial membrane in the cochlea or the vestibular otholitic membrane. The electrical signal is due to ionic current: the deflection of cilia, due to flow and acoustic waves, opens transduction gate channels in the hair cells, allowing a net flow of Ca^{2+} ions, present in the extra cellular endolymph environments (scala media of the cochlea), through the cellular membrane. This ionic current fires the nervous signal to the brain, through the hair cell and the sensory receptors of the nervous system. Hair cells have evolved force-gated ion channels that can open and close in microseconds, allowing detecting auditory frequencies up to the high kilohertz range. The channels are placed near the tips of the rodlike cilia and open, thanks to protein filaments, called gating springs, connecting adjacent cilia belonging to the same stereocilium bundle. The channels work in parallel groups of 50–100 units. By altering the mechanical tension in gating springs linked to mechanically sensitive transduction channels, this deflection changes the channels' open probability and elicits an electrical response (Martin et al. 2000).

Hearing and balance rely on the ability of hair cells in the inner ear to sense tiny mechanical stimuli, generating an electrical signal. The ionic current induced by a known displacement can be investigated, in order to study its behavior with the hair-bundle displacement. For vestibular hair cells, the displacement-current response curves show a sigmoidal shape, not symmetric with respect to the resting position or null displacement. The current shows an almost exponential current increase for slightly over half a micrometer displacement in a preferential direction (Corey and Hudspeth 1983). Displacements higher than 500 nm cause saturation in the response, suggesting a limited region of maximal sensitivity of bundle displacement. Unexpectedly, if a further short mechanical pulse is superimposed to the saturating stimulus (called adapting pulse), the curve shifts along the displacement axis in the direction of the adapting displacement (Eatock et al. 1987). This can be interpreted as the hair cell is changing its stiffness, in order to adapt its dynamic range for sensing a small stimulus over the saturating noisy stimulus. Theoretical studies indicate that the interplay between negative bundle stiffness and the biological motor responsible for mechanical adaptation produces bundle oscillation, active hair-bundle movement to amplify its mechanical inputs (Martin et al. 2000). It is believed that Ca^{2+} ions entering through open channels somehow cause them to reclose, and the protein movement associated with reclosing (about 4 nm) adds mechanical energy back to the system, making the whole bundle active (Karavitaki 2013).

All these experiments have been realized exploiting silicon microprobes which push the single kinocilium of a bundle. When the tip of a hair bundle is deflected by a sensory stimulus, the stereocilia pivot as a unit, producing a shearing displacement between adjacent tips. All stereocilia move by approximately the same angular deflection (Karavitaki and Corey 2010), but damages can happen to the spring gates. Data suggest that only stereocilia in contact with the probe will be stimulated, and the delivery of the stimulus to the remaining stereocilia will be weak and therefore not homogeneous. Therefore, to mimic the simultaneous and equal stimulus delivered by the overlying tectorial membrane to stereocilia in vivo, the stereocilium should be excited as a whole and a suitably designed (V-shaped) tip is needed. Moreover, if probes are soft enough, as in the case of small Young's modulus materials and/or soft spring constant design, their stiffness can be comparable with the stereocilium stiffness (between 1 and 10 mN/m), assuring nondestructive measurements. Figure 3.9 shows a novel soft probe realized by standard nanoimprint lithography on polydimethylsiloxane based (PDMS). The probe design

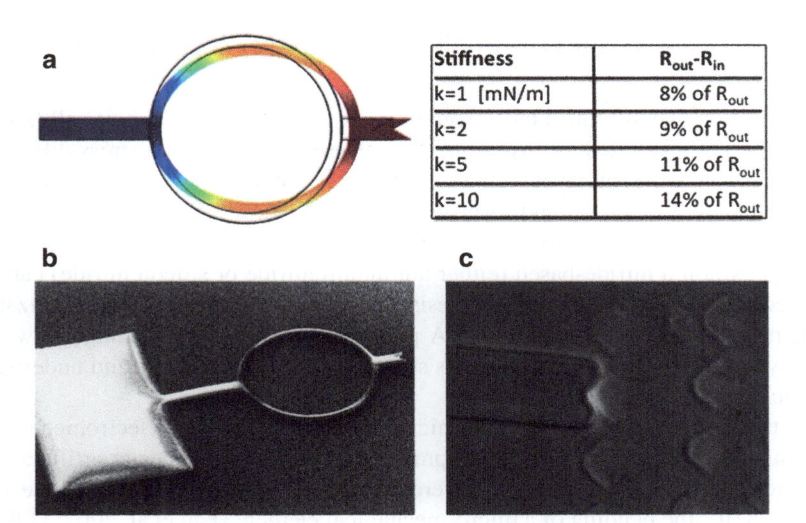

Stiffness	R_{out}-R_{in}
k=1 [mN/m]	8% of R_{out}
k=2	9% of R_{out}
k=5	11% of R_{out}
k=10	14% of R_{out}

Fig. 3.8 PDMS soft probe for stereocilia mechanical properties investigation: (**a**) finite element method based simulation showing the ring deformation by force application on the probe tip; the table shows the probe stiffness value in dependence to ring width. (**b**) A bird's eye picture of the whole probe: from *left* to *right*, attaching pad, mechanical dumping ring, the *V-shaped tip*. (**c**) Example of soft probe approaching the whole bundle of a bullfrog stereocilium

is based on circular mechanical elements (external radius is between 90 and 120 μm) able to bear high deformations (Fig. 3.8a). Tuning the geometrical dimensions of this soft ring element (table in Fig. 3.8) allows obtaining soft probes whose stiffness values match with the stereocilia bundle stiffness (Fig. 3.8b). The V-shaped tip, appropriately functionalized to be adherent to the hair bundle, pushes the stereocilium as a whole (Fig. 3.8c).

The probes have been successfully tested on Bullfrog hair cells in ex vivo experiments. The PDMS soft probes can be designed with compliance matching that of the cells to be studied, so that they can be used both to deliver stimuli and to measure forces produced by a wide variety of cells moving back to the rest position. These probes permit the identification of changes in hair cell stiffness and even small oscillations with almost no perturbations, to better understand the mechanism of adaptation and amplification of signal transduction in hair cells. The investigation of natural mechanoreceptor hair cell adaptation and amplification properties opens new opportunities to understand illness related to ear-impaired people, allowing the design for more efficient and miniaturized prostheses (Qualtieri et al. 2010).

3.12 Stress-Driven Out-of-Plane Cantilever Technology

In this section, we introduce the design of a stress-driven artificial hair cell (AHC). The technology is based on exploiting the release of the material stress difference among the constituent layers of a nitride-based cantilever beam to obtain the upward bending of its tip and to project it inside a flow stream. The beam layer characteristics (material properties and geometrical dimensions) are designed in order to exploit a nitride-based (either aluminum nitride or silicon nitride) cantilevers, equipped by a nichrome piezoresistive strain gauge read-out, for realization AHC mechanoreceptor-like sensors. A parylene waterproofing coating allows the employment in liquids for applications such as acoustic prosthetics and underwater robotics.

In the last years, advances in micro-fabrication of microelectromechanical systems (MEMS) allowed the development of several approaches to artificial hair cell mechanoreceptors based on different technological principles. In case of a passive AHC, the bending of a micro-mechanical element (Fan et al. 2002; Dijkstra et al. 2005) was the preferential approach. A strain gauge is placed on the most strained point of a mechanically deformable structure, reading-out the curvature and behaving as a mechanoreceptor for flow (liquid or air) and tactile sensing. The most investigated structure is a vertical cilium: an SU8 vertical pillar subjected to a mechanical pulse transfers its momentum to a planar cantilever (Fan et al. 2002) or a capacitive suspended membrane (Dijkstra et al. 2005). However the fragility of this approach can cause fracture upon mechanical overloading. In case of active AHC, an alternative approach was based on embedding a conductor inside a polyimide cilium. Thermally controlling the expansion of the heated aluminum conductor (Suh et al. 1996) or suspending the cilium on an ITO (indium tin oxide) electrode and applying a voltage between the two conductive layers (den Toonder et al. 2008), the system works as bimorph biomimetic cilium microactuator. An array of these cilia, each one electronically addressable, works like a micromanipulation tool. Finally, a cilium was realized by a polymeric matrix, filled by magnetic nanoparticles (iron oxide particles in this device). The switching-on of a magnetic field causes the cilium to be manipulated: an electromagnet below the device array is used to bend and move the cilia (Evans et al. 2007). These biomimetic AHC-based microactuators are interesting proof of principle devices; however, they have a few important drawbacks limiting their actual applicability to real implants. First, their response is not triggered by the input of a sensor; consequently, the switch-on of every single microactuators is driven manually and not by a natural time-varying signal. Second, their operation principle is not intrinsic to the device materials (like in a piezoelectric cantilever) but it is based on external electrostatic or magnetic fields, which might suffer the harsh physiologic liquid environments and could be detrimental for the thermal control or the external field action.

Stress-driven artificial hair cell has been recently proposed as a new and alternative approach to artificial hair cell design. A stress-driven cantilever, suspended on the substrate, keeps a curved equilibrium position, at a fixed height with respect to the substrate. If the cantilever is under the action of any type of physical force along its length direction, it bends increasing or decreasing its curvature (up to complete flattening). This approach turns out to be very robust against deformation and fast with respect to real time to external stimuli. A micro-strain gauge sensor, strongly attached on the cantilever, senses the deformation caused by an applied force: due to this variation, negative or positive, the sensor is able to distinguish the orientation of the applied force. Such architecture makes the operation of the devices very similar to the natural hair cell.

The technological principle for the realization of such artificial hair cells relies on the material properties of the constituent layers, namely, the mismatch of atomic sizes between different layered materials grown by heteroepitaxy and/or a gradient in lattice mismatch developed during single-layer material deposition or thermal cycling of the chip during micro-fabrication (Hu 1991). The generated deformation causes a release of stress in the multilayered cantilever beam which in turn induces an intrinsic upward (out-of-plane) bending of the cantilever. Previous designs related to this approach account for single-layer beam such as CVD (chemical vapor deposition) silicon nitride (Wang et al. 2007), polycrystalline silicon (Zhang et al. 2010), and silicon dioxide (Zhang et al. 2010). Noteworthy, these examples are inherent to intrinsic stress developed during growth and are hardly controlled. More recently, Qualtieri et al. (Qualtieri et al. 2011, 2012; Rizzi et al. 2013) developed a new design for stress-driven flow sensors based on multilayered cantilevers on a sacrificial layer. Once the sacrificial layer underneath is removed, the unbalanced stresses relax, bending upward the cantilever beam. The difference among internal stresses and/or crystalline lattice of each layer of the cantilever beam can be controlled through the layer thicknesses and by the lithographic patterning dimensions (beam length, beam width), resulting in a tight control of the moment and of the bending curvature and height of the device. Figure 3.9 shows the scanning electron microscope (SEM) pictures of the bent cantilevers: a 200 μm long aluminum nitride (AlN)/molybdenum (Mo) beam, equipped by a 50 μm long strain gauge on the left (Fig. 3.9a). On the right (Fig. 3.9b), the upward bending of the beam (radius of curvature and tip height) is shown to be dependent from the beam length.

For waterproofing and mechanical properties tuning, a parylene C conformal coating was deposited by room temperature chemical vapor deposition. The parylene coating has been realized on the SiN/Si cantilever beam to control directly the cantilever beam flexural stiffness and the device sensitivity. Figure 3.10 shows a SEM image of the cantilever. The upward bending through the residual stress inside the cantilever beam allows reaching a height up to 1.2 mm. The parylene coating layer, virtually unstressed (Harder et al. 2002), does not affect the bending and radius of curvature of the cantilever (i.e., the dynamic range) but the stiffness of the cantilever. Two thicknesses of parylene have been investigated (0.5 μm and 2 μm on both cantilever faces) in order to explore how a different cantilever flexural stiffness influences the sensitivity to flow sensing and the dynamic range (Rizzi et al. 2013).

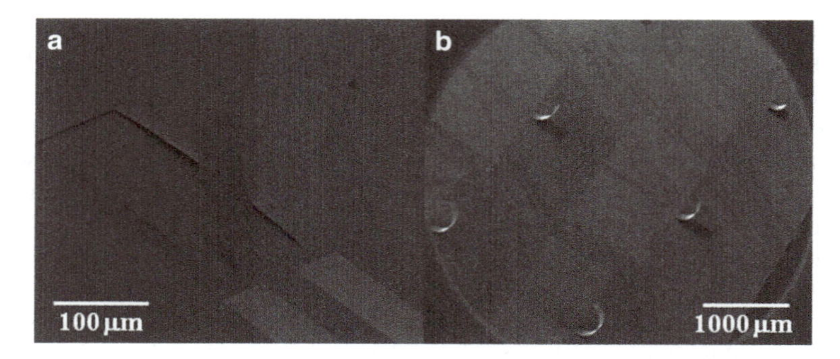

Fig. 3.9 AlN-/Mo-based cantilever. On the *left*: SEM on a bent cantilever with a 200 μm length and a 50 μm strain gauge clearly visible near the cantilever hinge. On the *right*: SEM on a cantilever array with different lengths taken at bird's eye view

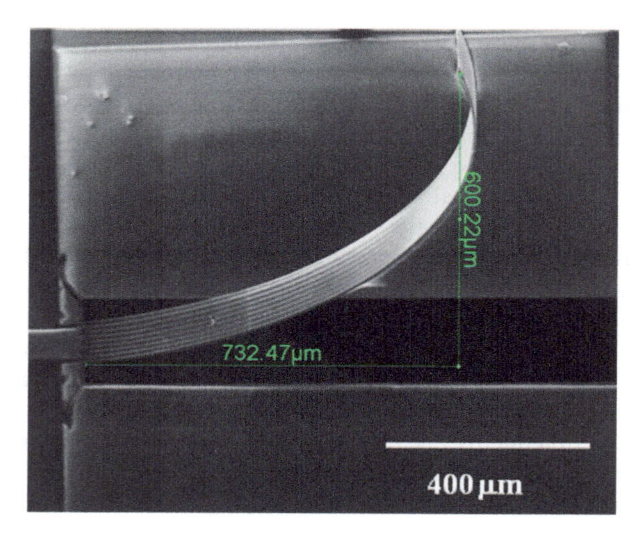

Fig. 3.10 SEM on a parylene-coated SiN/Si cantilever (tilted at 30°) with height up to 1,200 μm. The cantilever is coated by a 2 μm thick Parylene layer on both faces

Figure 3.11 shows the characterization of two SiN/Si cantilevers (denoted as sample A for 0.5 μm, and B for 2 μm thick parylene coatings on both cantilever faces) with 1.73×10^{-11} N m^2 and 2.12×10^{-11} N m^2 flexural stiffness, respectively. The specific sensor responsivity depends on the different coating thickness and related beam flexural stiffness. The thinner parylene-coated cantilever (sample A) shows a sublinear behavior as function of the water flow, while the thicker parylene-based coated sensor (samples B) shows a quadratic super-linear signal/flow velocity characteristic. When the cantilevers are flattened by high flow speed and no longer deformable, the stiffer sample B shows saturation whereas sample A shows oscillations (not shown). All the sensors return to the equilibrium positions when the flow is switched off.

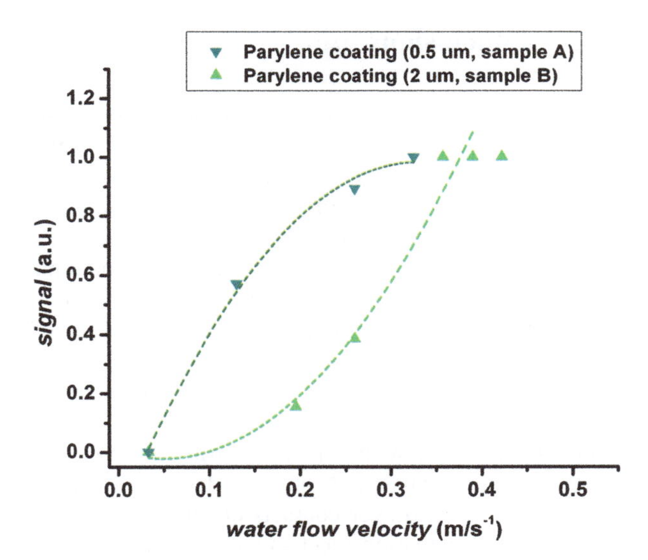

Fig. 3.11 Electrical behavior of the two coated sensors in a continuous water flow. The *dashed lines* are intended as a guide for the eye. The different coating material characteristics give a different curve shape, tuning from a sublinear to a super-linear trend. A common signal saturation region is shown

Making a biological parallel, the increase of flexural stiffness changes the behavior of the artificial hair cell from strain-hardening to strain-softening (Rizzi et al. 2013). This behavior is analogous to the hair cell mechanosensors in nature and suggests that material-based strategies in the design of artificial mechano-receptors can be further developed to optimization bioinspired sensors.

A linear array of these bioinspired flow sensors has been realized to reproduce the peculiar lateral flow sensing system of fishes. This system allows fishes to identify preys or predators without vision and schooling in ordered patterns. Phylogenetists claim the cochlear systems took its evolutionary origin from the lateral line in underwater ancestors (Manley and Koppl 1998). It has been proposed that fish lateral line afferents respond only to flow fluctuations (AC) and not to the steady (DC) component of the flow (Chagnaud et al. 2008). Therefore, it should be possible for a fish to obtain flow information using multiple afferents that respond only to flow fluctuations variations, retrieving useful information from noisy signals (Venturelli et al. 2012). A flow sensor array has been set up inside a pipeline in which airflow pulses were injected for testing the flow orientation and velocity measurements. An algorithm for cross-correlation between signals from consecutive flow sensors allowed to extract information from flow velocity fluctuations instead of a single velocity read-out, providing a more robust measurement system that is also capable of measuring events in turbulent flows. This system will be tested on underwater autonomous systems in order to mimic the natural way fishes orient underwater without vision.

3.13 Conclusions

Hair cell-based mechanoreceptors are one of the most versatile and widely spread biological sensing systems in nature. Flow sensing, hearing, and equilibrium proprioception are based on the described bending cilia, able to send electrical signals and information to the nervous system when hit by a mechanical excitation. Their adaptation to environments and signal amplification are unique properties, found specifically in acoustic and vestibular mammalian systems, able to make them highly sensitive to small signal even over high continuous noise. Bioengineers designed many sensing systems mimicking this kind of mechanoreceptors. Among those, a new flow sensor can be implemented with an active control by piezoelectricity (Qualtieri et al. 2010). A stress-driven artificial hair cell architecture can be used as an electro-active sensor in air and any fluid by combining the piezoresistivity read-out with a piezoelectric materials layer as one of the cantilever beam structural layers. A proper design of the piezoresistance and of the piezoelectrical cantilever contacts enables independent and simultaneous control of the sensing/actuation mechanisms. The piezoresistive read-out and the piezoelectric actuation mechanisms are uncoupled and independently controlled, thus making possible to control the cilium bending curvature and its elastic constant, actively increasing the dynamic range of the device.

The interplay between piezoresistance and piezoelectricity allows tuning the best sensitivity and dynamic working range for signal detection, also in the presence of a strong saturating noise in flow or inertial force application. The starting working point and dynamic range can be set by the structural and material parameters of the piezoelectric cantilever and of the strain gauge (i.e., Young's modulus, Poisson ratio, piezoelectric and piezoresistive coefficients, parylene coating thickness) and by the geometric parameters of the device (layer thickness, length, and width of the cantilever), By applying a voltage to the piezoelectric cantilever, beam curvature and working point are shifted, and, consequently, the dynamic range is increased. This kind of "active" behavior is similar to the adaptation properties of natural hair cells in the acoustic and vestibular systems, where sensory adaptation is the decay of a sensory response to a sustained stimulus, reflecting the natural importance of novel stimuli detection with respect to background stimuli or noise. Hair cells are very effective in the measurement of a small signal over a higher background noise. Similarly, the "adaptation" property of this "active" artificial hair cell device can suggest exploiting it in possible acoustic and cochlear prosthetics, setting up an array of artificial hair cells tuned to resonate to different mechanical vibrations in the acoustic range (20 Hz–20 kHz). If artificial cilia are saturated by a strong fluid flow inside the cochlear channel, they can eventually adapt for recovering further sensitivity.

References

Akiyama M, Morofuji Y, Kamohara T, Nishikubo K, Ooishi Y, Tsubai M, Fukuda O, Ueno N (2007) Preparation of oriented aluminum nitride thin films on polyimide films and piezoelectric response with high thermal stability and flexibility. Adv Funct Mater 17:458–462

Akiyama M, Morofuji Y, Nishikubo K, Kamohara T (2008) Sensitivity enhancement in diaphragms made by aluminum nitride thin films prepared on polyimide films. Appl Phys Lett 92:043509-3

Antognazza MR, Ghezzi D, Musitelli D, Garbugli M, Lanzani G (2009) A hybrid solid-liquid polymer photodiode for the bioenvironment. Appl Phys Lett 94:243501

Bareket-Keren L, Hanein Y (2013) Carbon nanotube based multielectrode arrays for neuronal interfacing: progress and prospects. Front Neural Circ 6:122

Benfenati V, Toffanin S, Bonetti S, Turatti G, Pistone A, Chiappalone M, Sagnella A, Stefani A, Generali G, Ruani G, Saguatti D, Zamboni R, Muccini M (2013) A transparent organic transistor structure for bidirectional stimulation and recording of primary neurons. Nat Mater 12:672–680. doi:10.1038/NMAT3630

Benfenati V, Martino N, Antognazza MR, Pistone A, Toffanin S, Ferroni S, Lanzani G, Muccini M (2014) Photostimulation of whole-cell conductance in primary rat neocortical astrocytes mediated by organic semiconducting thin films. Adv Healthc Mater 3:392–399

Berggren M, Richter-Dahlfors A (2007) Organic bioelectronics. Adv Mater 19:3201–3213

Blau A (2011) Prospects for neuroprosthetics: flexible microelectrode arrays with polymer conductors. In: Gargiulo GD (ed) Alistair McEwan (co-editor) Applied biomedical engineering. ISBN 978-953-307-256-2

Blau A, Murr A, Wolff S, Sernagor E, Medini P, Iurilli G, Ziegler C, Benfenati F (2010) Flexible, all-polymer microelectrode arrays for the capture of cardiac and neuronal signals. Biomaterials 32:1778

Bleckmann H, Schmitz H, von der Emde G (2004) Nature as a model for technical sensors. J Comp Physiol A 190:971–981. doi:10.1007/s00359-004-0563-y

Bolin MH et al (2009) Active control of epithelial cell-density gradients grown along the channel of an organic electrochemical transistor. Adv Mater 21:4379–4382

Bu N, Fukuda O, Ueno N, Inoue M (2009) IEEE proceedings international conference on robotics and biomimetics, pp 944–948

Carlson JA, English JM, Coe DJ (2006) A flexible, self healing sensor skin. Smart Mater Struct 15: N129

Chagnaud BP, Brucker C, Hofmann MH, Bleckmann H (2008) Measuring flow velocity and flow direction by spatial and temporal analysis of flow fluctuations. J Neurosci 28(17):4487. doi:10.1523/jneurosci.4959-07.2008

Corey DP, Hudspeth AJ (1983) Kinetics of the receptor current in bullfrog saccular hair cells. J Neurosci 3(5):962

Cramer T, Steinbrecher T, Koslowski T, Case DA, Biscarini F, Zerbetto F (2009) Water-induced polaron formation at the pentacene surface: quantum mechanical molecular mechanics simulations. Phys Rev B 79:155316

Cramer T, Campana A, Leonardi F, Casalini S, Kyndiah A, Murgia M, Biscarini F (2013a) Water-gated organic field effect transistors—opportunities for biochemical sensing and extracellular signal transduction. J Mater Chem B 1:3728

Cramer T, Chelli B, Murgia M, Barbalinardo M, Bystrenova E, de Leeuw DM, Biscarini F (2013b) Organic ultra-thin film transistor with liquid gate for extracellular stimulation and recording of electric activity of stem cell-derived neuronal networks. Phys Chem Chem Phys 15:3897–3905

Dahiya RS, Metta G, Valle M, Sandini G (2010) Tactile sensing—from humans to humanoids. IEEE Trans Robot 26(1):1–20

Dario P, De Rossi D, Domenici C, Francesconi R (1984) Ferroelectric polymer tactile sensors with anthropomorphic features. In: Proceedings of the 1984 I.E. international conference on robotics and automation, vol 1. IEEE, pp 332–340

den Toonder JMJ, Bos FM, Broer DJ, Filippini L, Gillies M, de Goede J, Mol T, Reijme MA, Talen W, Wilderbeek H, Khatavkar V, Anderson PD (2008) Artificial cilia for active microfluidic mixing. Lab Chip 8:533–541. doi:10.1039/B717681C
Dijkstra M, Van Baar JJ, Wiegerink RJ, Lammerink TSJ, De Boer JH, Krijnen GJM (2005) Artificial sensory hairs based on the flow sensitive receptor hairs of crickets. J Micromech Microeng 15:S132–S138. doi:10.1088/0960-1317/15/7/019
Dubois MA, Muralt P (2001) Stress and piezoelectric properties of aluminum nitride thin films deposited onto metal electrodes by pulsed direct current reactive sputtering. J Appl Phys 89 (11):6389–6395
Eatock RA, Corey DP, Hudspeth AJ (1987) Adaptation of mechanoelectrical transduction in hair cells of the bullfrog's sacculus. J Neurosci 7(9):2821
Eisenthal KB (1996) Liquid interfaces probed by second-harmonic and sum-frequency spectroscopy. Chem Rev 96:1343–1360
Eltaib MEH, Hewit JR (2003) Tactile sensing technology for minimal access surgery-a review. Mechatronics 13(10):1163–1177
Evans BA, Shields AR, Carroll RL, Washburn S, Falvo MR, Superfine R (2007) Magnetically actuated nanorod arrays as biomimetic cilia. Nano Lett 7:1428–1434. doi:10.1021/nl070190c
Fan Z, Chen J, Zou J, Bullen D, Liu C, Delcomyn F (2002) Design and fabrication of artificial lateral line flow sensors. J Micromech Microeng 12:655–661. doi:10.1088/0960-1317/12/5/322
Feili D, Schuettler M, Stieglitz T (2008) Matrix-addressable, active electrode arrays for neural stimulation using organic semiconductors—cytotoxicity and pilot experiments in vivo. J Neural Eng 5:68–74
Fratzl P, Barth FG (2009) Biomaterial systems for mechanosensing and actuation. Nature 462:442–448. doi:10.1038/nature08603
Gautam V, Bag M, Narayan KS (2010) Dynamics of bulk polymer heterostructure/electrolyte devices. J Phys Chem Lett 1:3277–3282
Gautam V, Bag M, Narayan KS (2011) Single-pixel, single-layer polymer device as a tri-color sensor with signals mimicking the retinal cone cells. J Am Chem Soc 133:17942
George PM, Lyckman AW, LaVan DA, Hegde A, Leung Y, Rupali A et al (2005) Fabrication and biocompatibility of polypyrrole implants suitable for neural prosthetics. Biomaterials 26:3511
Ghezzi D, Antognazza MR, Dal Maschio M, Lanzarini E, Benfenati F, Lanzani G (2011) A hybrid bioorganic interface for neuronal photoactivation. Nat Commun 2(1):166
Ghezzi D, Antognazza MR, Maccarone R, Bellani S, Lanzarini E, Martino N, Mete M, Pertile G, Bisti S, Lanzani G, Benfenati F (2013) A polymer-based interface restores light sensitivity in rat blind retinas. Nat Photon 6:400–406
Guimard NK, Gomez N, Schmidt CE (2007) Conducting polymers in biomedical engineering. Prog Polym Sci 32:876–921
Harder TA, Yao TJ, He Q, Shih CY, Tai YC (2002) Residual stress in thin-film parylene-C. In: Proceedings of the 15th IEEE international conference on micro electro mechanical systems workshop. IEEE, Piscataway, NJ, p 435. doi:10.1109/MEMSYS.2002.984296
Hassler C, Boretius T, Stieglitz T (2011) Polymers for neural implants. J Polym Sci B Polym Phys 49:18–33
Ho VA, Dao DV, Sugiyama S, Hirai S (2009) Analysis of sliding of a soft fingertip embedded with a novel micro force/moment sensor: simulation, experiment, and application. In: Proceedings of the IEEE international conference on robotics and automation (ICRA), pp 889–894
Howard J, Hudspeth AJ (1987) Mechanical relaxation of the hair bundle mediates adaptation in mechanoelectrical transduction by the bullfrog's saccular hair cell. Proc Natl Acad Sci USA 84:3064–3068
Hu SM (1991) Stress-related problems in silicon technology. J Appl Phys 70:R53–R80. doi:10.1063/1.349282
Hudspeth AJ (1989) How the ear's works work. Nature 341:397–404. doi:10.1038/341397a0

Hudspeth AJ (2008) Making an effort to listen: mechanical amplification in the ear. Neuron 59:530–545. doi:10.1016/j.neuron.2008.07.012

Humayun MS, Dorn JD, da Cruz L, Dagnelie G, Sahel J-A, Stanga PE, Cideciyan AV, Duncan JL, Eliott D, Filley E, Ho AC, Santos A, Safran AB, Arditi A, Del Priore LV, Greenberg RJ (2012) Interim results from the international trial of second sight's visual prosthesis. Ophthalmology 119:779–788

Hutchings BL, Grahn AR, Petersen RJ (1994) Multiple-layer cross-field ultrasonic tactile sensor. In: Proceedings of the 1994 I.E. international conference on robotics and automation, 1994. IEEE, pp 2522–2528

Isaksson J, Kjall P, Nilsson D, Robinson ND, Berggren M, Richter-Dahlfors A (2007) Electronic control of Ca^{2+} signalling in neuronal cells using an organic electronic ion pump. Nat Mater 6:673–679

Jimison LH, Tria SA, Khodagholy D, Gurfinkel M, Lanzarini E, Hama A, Malliaras GG, Owens RM (2012) Measurement of barrier tissue integrity with an organic electrochemical transistor. Adv Mater 24:5919–5923

Karavitaki KD (2013) Private communication

Karavitaki KD, Corey DP (2010) Sliding adhesion confers coherent motion to hair cell stereocilia and parallel gating to transduction channels. J Neurosci 30(27):9051. doi:10.1523/jneurosci.4864-09.2010

Khodagholy D, Doublet T, Gurfinkel M, Quilichini P, Ismailova E, Leleux P, Herve T, Sanaur S, Bernard C, Malliaras GG (2011a) Highly conformable conducting polymer electrodes for in-vivo recordings. Adv Mater 23:H268–H272

Khodagholy D, Gurfinkel M, Stavrinidou E, Leleux P, Hervé T, Sanaur S, Malliaras GG (2011b) High speed and high density organic electrochemical transistor arrays. Appl Phys Lett 99:163304

Khodagholy D, Rivnay J, Sessolo M, Gurfinkel M, Leleux P, Jimison LH, Stavrinidou E, Herve T, Sanaur S, Owens RM, Malliaras GG (2013a) High transconductance organic electrochemical transistors. Nat Commun 4:2133

Khodagholy D, Doublet T, Quilichini P, Gurfinkel M, Leleux P, Ghestem A, Ismailova E, Hervé T, Sanaur S, Bernard C, Malliaras GG (2013b) In vivo recordings of brain activity using organic transistors. Nat Commun 4:1575

Kotov NA, Winter JO, Clements IP, Jan E, Timko BP, Campidelli S, Pathak S, Mazzatenta A, Lieber CM, Prato M, Bellamkonda RV, Silva GA, Kam NWS, Patolsky F, Ballerini L (2009) Nanomaterials for neural interfaces. Adv Mater 21:3970–4004

Kuribara K, Wang H, Uchiyama N, Fukuda K, Yokota T, Zschieschang U, Jaye C, Fischer D, Klauk H, Yamamoto T, Takimiya K, Ikeda M, Kuwabara H, Sekitani T, Loo Y-L, Someya T (2012) Organic transistors with high thermal stability for medical applications. Nat Commun 3:723

Lanzarini E, Antognazza MR, Biso M, Ansaldo A, Laudato L, Bruno P, Metrangolo P, Resnati G, Ricci D, Lanzani G (2012) Polymer-based photocatalytic hydrogen generation. J Phys Chem C 116:10944–10949

Larsson KC, Kjäll P, Richter-Dahlfors A (2013) Organic bioelectronics for electronic-to-chemical translation in modulation of neuronal signaling and machine-to-brain interfacing. Biochim Biophys Acta 1830:4334–4344

Lees AW (2009) Smart machines with flexible rotors. J Phys Conf Ser 181:012019

Lin P, Yan F (2012) Organic thin-film transistors for chemical and biological sensing. Adv Mater 24:34–51

Lin P, Yan F, Yu JJ, Chan HLW, Yang M (2010) The application of organic electrochemical transistors in cell-based biosensors. Adv Mater 22:3655–3660

Manley GA, Koppl C (1998) Phylogenetic development of the cochlea and its innervation. Curr Opin Neurobiol 8:468

Mannsfeld SC, Tee BC-K, Stoltenberg RM, Chen CV, Barman S, Muir B, Sokolov AN, Reese C, Bao Z (2010) Highly sensitive flexible pressure sensors with microstructured rubber dielectric layers. Nature 9:859–864
Martin P, Mehta AD, Hudspeth AJ (2000) Negative hair-bundle stiffness betrays a mechanism for mechanical amplification by the hair cell. Proc Natl Acad Sci USA 97:12026. doi:10.1073/pnas.210389497
McHenry MJ, van Netten SM (2007) The flexural stiffness of superficial neuromasts in the zebrafish (Danio rerio) lateral line. J Exp Biol 210:4244–4253. doi:10.1242/jeb.009290
Moulton SE, Higgins MJ, Kapsa RMI, Wallace GG (2012) Organic bionics: a new dimension in neural communications. Adv Funct Mater 22:2003–2014
Muskovich M, Bettinger CJ (2012) Biomaterials-based electronics: polymers and interfaces for biology and medicine. Adv Healthc Mater 1:248–266
Pang, Changhyun, Gil-Yong Lee, Tae-il Kim, Sang Moon Kim, Hong Nam Kim, Sung-Hoon Ahn, and Kahp-Yang Suh (2012) A flexible and highly sensitive strain-gauge sensor using reversible interlocking of nanofibres. Nature Materials 11:795–801
Petroni S, Tegola CL, Caretto G, Campa A, Passaseo A, De Vittorio MD, Cingolani R (2011) Aluminum nitride piezo-MEMS on polyimide flexible substrates. Microelectron Eng 88 (8):2372–2375
Petroni S, Guido F, Torre B, Falqui A, Todaro MT, Cingolani R, De Vittorio M (2012) Tactile multisensing on flexible aluminum nitride. Analyst 137(22):5260–5264
Qi Y, Jafferis NT, Lyons K, Lee CM, Ahmad H, McAlpine MC (2010) Piezoelectric ribbons printed onto rubber for flexible energy conversion tissue. Nano Lett 10:524–528
Qualtieri A, Rizzi F, De Vittorio M, Passaseo A, Todaro M T, Epifani G (2010) Electro-active microelectromechanical device and corresponding detection process, Patent no. EP 2617074 A1
Qualtieri A, Rizzi F, Todaro MT, Passaseo A, Cingolani R, De Vittorio M (2011) Stress-driven AlN cantilever-based flow sensor for fish lateral line system. Microelectron Eng 88:2376–2378. doi:10.1016/j.mee.2011.02.091
Qualtieri A, Rizzi F, Epifani G, Ernits A, Kruusmaa M, De Vittorio M (2012) Parylene-coated bioinspired artificial hair cell for liquid flow sensing. Microelectron Eng 98:516–519. doi:10.1016/j.mee.2012.07.072
Richardson-Burns SM, Hendricks JL, Foster B, Povlich LK, Kim DH, Martin DC (2007a) Polymerization of the conducting polymer poly(3,4-ethylenedioxythiophene) (PEDOT) around living neural cells. Biomaterials 28:1539–1552
Richardson-Burns SM, Hendricks JL, Martin DC (2007b) Electrochemical polymerization of conducting polymers in living neural tissue. J Neural Eng 4:L6
Rizzi F, Qualtieri A, Chamber LD, Megill WM, De Vittorio M (2013) Parylene conformal coating encapsulation as a method for advanced tuning of mechanical properties of an artificial hair cell. Soft Matter 9:2584–2588. doi:10.1039/c2sm27566j
Schwartz G, Tee BC-K, Mei J, Appleton AL, Kim DH, Wang H, Bao Z (2013) Flexible polymer transistors with high pressure sensitivity for application in electronic skin and health monitoring. Nat Commun 4:1859
Sekitani T, Zschieschang U, Klauk H, Someya T (2010) Flexible organic transistors and circuits with extreme bending stability. Nat Mater 9:1015
Simon DT, Kurup S, Larsson KC, Hori R, Tybrandt K, Goiny M, Jager EW, Berggren M, Canlon B, Richter-Dahlfors A (2009) Organic electronics for precise delivery of neurotransmitters to modulate mammalian sensory function. Nat Mater 8:742–746
Song J, Noh T, Jun Y, Jung H-Y, Kang J (2010) Fully Flexible Solution-Deposited ZnO Thin Film Transistors. Moon Adv Mater 22:4308–4312
Suh JW, Glander SF, Darling RB, Storment CW, Kovacs GT (1996) Organic thermal and electrostatic ciliary micro-actuator array for object manipulation. Sensors Actuators A 58:51–60. doi:10.1016/S0924-4247(97)80224-5

Svennersten K, Larsson KC, Berggren M, Richter-Dahlfors A (2011) Organic bioelectronics in nanomedicine. Biochim Biophys Acta 1810:276
Tagantsev K (1986) Piezoelectricity and Flexoelectricity in crystalline dielectrics. Phys Rev B 34(8):5883
Takenawa S (2009) A magnetic type tactile sensor using a two-dimensional array of inductors. In: IEEE international conference on robotics and automation, 2009, ICRA'09. IEEE, pp 3295–3300
Ten Wolde PR (2012) Biophysics: The price of accuracy. Nat Phys 8:361. doi:10.1038/nphys2302
Venturelli R, Akanyeti O, Visentin F, Jezov J, Chambers LD, Toming G, Brown J, Kruusmaa M, Megill WM, Fiorini P (2012) Hydrodynamic pressure sensing with an artificial lateral line in steady and unsteady flows. Bioinspir Biomim 7:036004. doi:10.1088/1748-3182/7/3/036004
Von Holst H (2013) Organic bioelectrodes in clinical neurosurgery. Biochim Biophys Acta 1830:4345–4352
Wang YH, Lee CY, Chiang CM (2007) A MEMS-based air flow sensor with a free-standing microcantilever structure. Sensors 7:2389–2401. doi:10.3390/s7102389
White HS, Kittlesen GP, Wrighton MS (1984) Chemical derivatization of an array of 3 gold microelectrodes with polypyrrole—fabrication of a molecule based transistor. J Am Chem Soc 106:5375–5377
Xu X-H, Hai-Shun W, Zhang C-J, Jin Z-H (2001) Morphological properties of AlN piezoelectric thin films deposited by DC reactive magnetron sputtering. Thin Solid Films 388(1):62–67
Xu Y, Tai Y-C, Huang A, Ho C-M (2003) IC-integrated flexible shear-stress sensor skin. J Microelectromech Syst 12:740–747
Yamada Y, Morizono M, Umetani U, Takahashi T (2005) Highly soft viscoelastic robot skin with a contact object-location-sensing capability. IEEE Trans Ind Electron 52:960–968
Yan F, Mok SM, Yu JJ, Chan HLW, Yang M (2009) Label free DNA sensor based on organic thin film transistors. Biosens Bioelectron 24:1241
Yang SY, Kim BN, Zakhidov AA, Taylor PG, Lee J-K, Ober CK, Lindau M, Malliaras GG (2011) Detection of transmitter release from single living cells using conducting polymer microelectrodes. Adv Healthc Mater 23:H184–H188
Yousef H, Boukallel M, Althoefer K (2011) Tactile sensing for dexterous in-hand manipulation in robotics—a review. Sensors Actuators A Phys 167(2):171–187
Zhang Q, Ruan W, Wang H, Zhou Y, Wang Z, Liu L (2010) A self-bended piezoresistive microcantilever flow sensor for low flow rate measurement. Sens Actuators A Phys 158:273–279. doi:10.1016/j.sna.2010.02.002
Zhu ZT, Mabeck JT, Zhu CC, Cady NC, Batt CA, Malliaras GG (2004) A simple poly(3,4-ethylene dioxythiophene)/poly(styrene sulfonic acid) transistor for glucose sensing at neutral pH. Chem Commun: 1556
Zrenner E (2012) Artificial vision. Solar cells for the blind. Nat Photonics 6:342–343
Zrenner E, Bart-Schmidt KU, Benav H, Besch D, Brukmann A, Gabel V-P, Gekeler F, Greppmaier U, Harscher A, Kibbel S, Koch J, Kusnyerik A, Peters T, Stingl K, Sachs H, Stett A, Szurman P, Wilhelm B, Wilke R (2011) Subretinal electronic chips allow blind patients to read letters and combine them to words. Proc Biol Sci 278:1489–1497

Chapter 4
Emerging Technologies Inspired by Plants

Barbara Mazzolai, Virgilio Mattoli, Lucia Beccai, and Edoardo Sinibaldi

4.1 Introduction

Soil is a vital resource for living organisms and provides energy and precious elements for mankind. How do plants address and manage a large amount of information (which is primarily obtained from the soil) to survive extreme conditions? How can roots avoid danger if they cannot move quickly within the soil? Additionally, can science and technology take advantage of strategies to penetrate and explore soil as well as to maintain good performance in terms of energy efficiency? Biomimetics is considered as an approach to study plants and to demonstrate the improvements in technological development that can result from imitating the natural characteristics of plants. After describing some of the main characteristics of plants, specifically their roots, we focus on natural strategies that plant roots use to penetrate soil. Additionally, we describe how the elongation of the root tip apex can be studied from an engineering perspective and provide insight into the pressure required for the root to move forward. In the second part of this study, we propose robotic plant root-like systems called *Plantoids* that mimic root behavior and include distributed sensing, actuation, and intelligence for tasks such as environmental exploration and monitoring. In the final part of this study, we address bioinspiration from the motion of a plant and its materials. The active mechanism in plant movements is reviewed, and, specifically, an analytical approach to a bioinspired osmotic system is described. Finally, passive natural mechanisms and available technological actuation mechanisms are reviewed.

B. Mazzolai (✉) • V. Mattoli • L. Beccai • E. Sinibaldi
Center for Micro-Biorobotics, Istituto Italiano di Tecnologia, Pisa, Italy
e-mail: barbara.mazzolai@iit.it

R. Cingolani (ed.), *Bioinspired Approaches for Human-Centric Technologies*,
DOI 10.1007/978-3-319-04924-3_4, © Springer International Publishing Switzerland 2014

4.2 Features of Plant Roots and Their Use in the Artificial World

The term biomimetics, which is the concept of transferring ideas and principles from biology to technology, was first used by Dr. Otto Smith in 1957. Dr. Smith studied natural biological processes and developed methods and machines that replicated those actions. However, the bioinspired approach dates back much further. For example, Leonardo da Vinci studied the flight of birds and designed machines, including the first "humanoid" (a mechanical knight), but he never developed the machines, which might have been due to a lack of the appropriate technology. Nature has spent 3.8 billion years on "R&D" projects and offers many solutions that humans can use as inspiration to develop materials, devices, behavioral controls, or computing that aim to improve their quality of life. This is a continuous process. Among living organisms, plants represent valuable biological models to illustrate physical principles or develop mechanical devices. The role of plants in our ecosystems is well understood. Plants dominate every landscape and represent 99 % of the biomass on Earth. Plants are crucial for our survival because they produce oxygen, and plants are located at the lowest level in the food chain, and thus they are fundamental in the life cycle and ecosystems. Plants are also important in agriculture, entertainment, and industry. Plants are often considered to be passive organisms that are unable to move, communicate, and escape from hostile environments. This interpretation is not very different from Aristotle's classification of plants and animals in his book *De Anima*. In his classification, plants were located in the middle of the spectrum between living and nonliving organisms. Plants were considered to have a very low-level soul, called a vegetative soul, because they lack the ability to move, and thus they did not require senses. In recent years, engineers, material, and computer scientists have developed an increased interest in plants. There are many examples of technological solutions that were inspired by plants. One common example is the lotus effect, in which the leaves of water-repellent plants, such as the *Nelumbo nucifera* (lotus) and *Colocasia esculenta*, are superhydrophobic and self-cleaning due to hierarchical roughness (i.e., microstructures formed by papillose epidermal cells covered with epicuticular wax tubules) and the presence of a hydrophobic coating (Bhushan 2009). Many artificial solutions (e.g., StoColor Lotusan® and new micro- and nano-patterned polymeric- or graphene-based materials) have been developed based on the study of this plant feature (Zang et al. 2013). *Nepenthes* pitcher plants use structures to hold an intermediary liquid that acts as a repellent surface. Using this concept, Wong and colleagues (2011) recently developed "slippery liquid-infused porous surfaces" (SLIPS) that consist of a film of lubricating liquid held in place by a micro- or nanoporous substrate. Velcro is a hook-and-loop fastener used in many everyday applications and was developed in 1948 by a Swiss engineer, George de Mestral, who observed that the hooks in plant burrs (*Arctium lappa*) adhered to the fur of his dog. In 1955, he patented Velcro, which represents one of the most successful bioinspired products.

These are only some of the examples of artificial solutions that were inspired by plants. This chapter gives a brief overview of some attempts to translate various plant features into artificial solutions, including plant root-like robotic devices and actuators.

4.2.1 Plant Root Sensory Systems and Tropisms

For efficient uptake, plant roots must move toward mineral ions and water in soil. For this reason, plant roots must sense and respond to a variety of environmental (both biotic and abiotic) stimuli as they move through soil. A plant's root system adapts itself morphologically to explore and penetrate the soil, which results in the capillary exploration of the entire volume of soil. Plant roots can perform these complex actions by using a large number of tips (apices) that contain many different types of sensors (e.g., for touch, humidity, gravity, and ions) so that various parts of the plant can communicate information and implement complex, adaptive behaviors. Sensory capabilities allow roots to develop specific growth responses (tropisms) to react to changes in their environment. In general, a tropic movement is the directional movement of a plant or part of a plant that results in the curvature of plant organs toward or away from certain stimuli. Tropisms can be positive (the plant will bend toward a stimulus) or negative (the plant will bend away from a stimulus). To form a curvature toward or away from a directional stimulus, plant roots use a differential growth response in which cells in one region actively elongate at a faster rate than those located in the opposite region. Signal transduction pathways of tropic sensing result in a differential redistribution of auxin in the responding plant organ (Esmon et al. 2005). Current models of tropic responses are primarily based on the Cholodny–Went theory, which states that tropic stimuli induce lateral redistribution of auxin, which results in unequal accumulation between opposing sides of a responding organ and promotes differential growth (Esmon et al. 2006). A wide range of tropisms exists in plants, including phototropism (light; Hohm et al. 2013), gravitropism (gravity; Blancaflor and Masson 2003), thigmotropism (touch; Hart 1990), thermotropism (temperature; Ding and Pickard 1993), chemotropism (chemicals; Estabrook and Yoder 1998; Van Norman et al. 2004; Loreto et al. 2006), and hydrotropism (water or humidity gradient; Takahashi et al. 2009; Esmon et al. 2005; Eapen et al. 2005). In a root apparatus, a single root must move through a substrate by orienting along the gravity vector, negotiating obstacles, and locating resources.

4.2.2 Strategies of Plant Roots for Soil Penetration

Plant roots are excellent natural diggers, and their characteristics such as adaptive growth, energy movements, and the capability of penetrating soil at any angle are

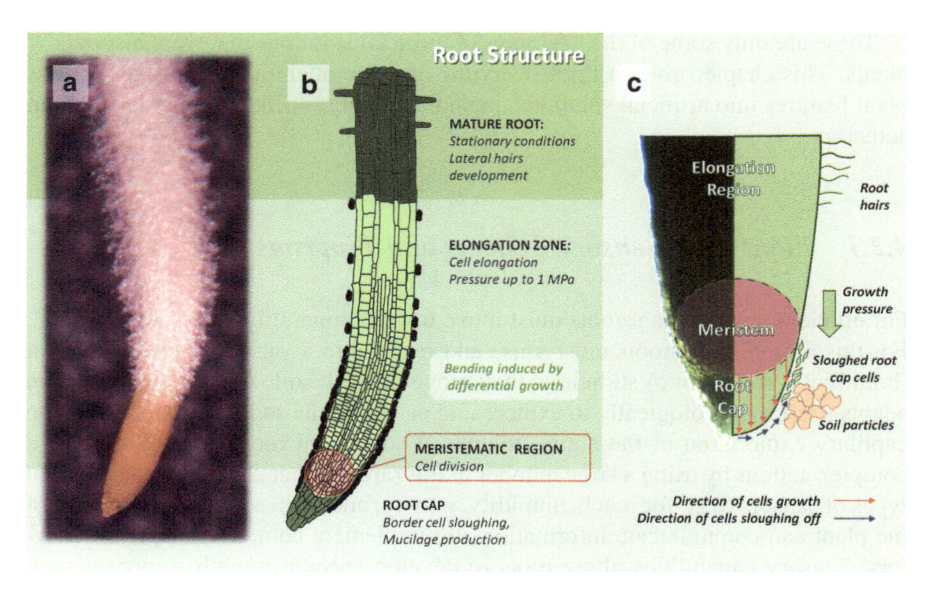

Fig. 4.1 An overview and schematic representation of a plant root and its regions. (**a**) Plant root apex of *Zea mays*. (**b**) The exploration capability of plant root arises from the root apex, i.e., the plant root moves and penetrates soil by growing at the apical region by adding new cells at the level of the meristematic region. Then, newly generated cells move from the meristematic region to the elongation region, where they axially expand because of the water absorbed by osmosis and the directional loosening of the cell wall. This action allows the root to penetrate soil with only a small part of its structure (the apex), while the remainder of the structure is stationary and in contact with the soil (the mature region). The lateral formation of hairs permits to increase surface for absorbing water and nutrients and anchoring the structure to the soil. (**c**) Root cap cells are continually produced in the meristematic region. These cells move to the root cap and then slough off from its outer surface while producing mucus. In this way, the cap cells create an interface between the soil and root apex. The root cap protects the delicate cells in the meristematic region, and the mucus promotes root penetration by reducing friction

interesting from an engineering perspective. Roots grow from the tip with a velocity of 1–3 mm/h (Clark et al. 2003), and root development is driven by two continuous processes: (1) cell division at the level of the meristem region (MR, which is located in the apex) and (2) cell elongation in the elongation region (ER, which is just behind the meristem) (Fig. 4.1). The meristem is covered by a root cap, which protects the meristem and newly generated cells from pathogenic agents and from mechanical damage during soil penetration (Iijima et al. 2008). The elongation from the tip (EFT) reduces the resistance because only a small part of the body (the root apex) moves, whereas the remainder of the body is fixed.

Most of the newly generated cells move from the MR to the ER, where they expand in the axial direction due to water uptake and the loosening of the directional cell wall, which results in axial pressures up to 1 MPa (Clark et al. 2003). This process provides the pressure required for forward movement of the apex.

This pressure is dissipated into the expansion of a soil cavity and into the frictional resistance of the soil to advance the root.

As the root cap moves through the soil, cells are sloughed off, and the structure constantly needs to be replaced. The root cap is covered with a thick layer of mucilage, which is secreted by the root tip and helps lubricate the root as it pushes through the soil. Mature cells (located behind the apex) are anchored to the soil to allow the apex to move forward. This anchoring is achieved by using root hairs, secondary roots, and root waving. While the mature root is anchored to the soil, root growth from the tip represents both the development and movement of this organ (Fig. 4.1). This process enables roots to adapt their morphology and organ development to environmental conditions, even in hard soil, because the cell division and morphology are directly influenced by the surrounding environment. Additionally, EFT results in the reduction of dynamic frictional resistance during penetration due to the movement of only a limited part of the root body, the apex.

An estimation of the EFT strategy to increase the efficiency of the root during soil penetration is difficult to calculate. Additionally, these biological strategies are not immediately applicable to new engineering solutions. The development of dedicated bioengineering tools to quantify mechanical and physical biological properties can offer some support in studies related to penetration capabilities and in biomimetic approaches. To quantify the relevance of EFT in penetration with respect to the entire body insertion, two sets of penetration tests were performed in granular substrates by using a probe (Tonazzini et al. 2013). These tests demonstrated that the amount of penetration energy required for EFT was less than the energy required for NoEFT for all of the initial depths that were considered. There was a significant difference between the results achieved for different initial depths. The reduction increased from approximately 20 % at an initial depth of 100 mm to 50 % at an initial depth of 250 mm. These results indicate that increasing the penetration depth could reduce the energy consumption by more than 50 % by using penetration with EFT. Therefore, EFT in plant roots represents an efficient solution for penetrating deep soils and is a source of inspiration for designing a robotic system to explore soil.

4.3 Plant Root-Like Robotic Artifacts: The PLANTOIDS

The plant root features that were previously mentioned can be considered in the design and development of a new generation of hardware and software technologies. These technological solutions are called "PLANTOIDS," which are robotic systems equipped with distributed sensing, actuation, and intelligence to perform environmental exploration and monitoring tasks.

PLANTOIDS were inspired by an attempt to reproduce the penetration, exploration, and adaptation capabilities of plant roots. Using a biomimetic approach, this technology has two major goals: (1) to detail and synthesize principles that enable plant roots to effectively and efficiently explore and adapt to underground

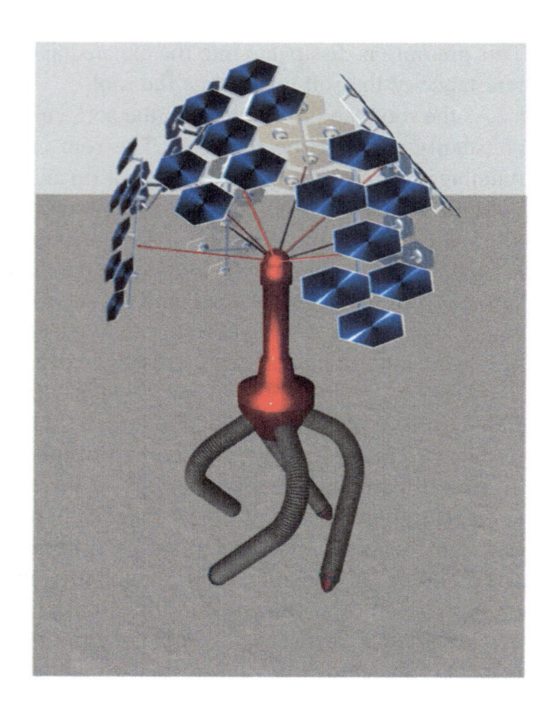

Fig. 4.2 A sketch of a PLANTOID, the plant-like robot. The PLANTOID is endowed with distributed sensing, actuation, and intelligence for tasks of environmental exploration and monitoring. Analogously to the biological counterpart, the robotic roots grow by adding new material at the level of the tip (apex). The apex embeds physical (e.g., gravity, humidity, touch, temperature, etc.) and chemical (e.g., nitrate, phosphate, pH, sodium, potassium, etc.) sensors, which are crucial to implement tropic behaviors. Bending allows robotic roots to follow or escape from hostile environments

environments with robotic artifacts and (2) to formulate hypotheses and models of unknown aspects of the plant roots that can be evaluated using the bioinspired platform (Fig. 4.2).

An initial technological implementation (Sadeghi et al. 2013) was addressed, which was inspired by the growth and sloughing of cells from the tip, as well as by the soil anchoring that was achieved through the root hairs (as previously described). The bioinspired concept and robotic implementation are shown in Fig. 4.3.

The core parts of the system are a hollow, rigid cylindrical shaft, a soft and flexible skin, and an actuation system for the skin, which is external to the soil. The skin is stored inside the shaft and can traverse the hole to the external surface of the shaft. The outward movement of skin from the tip imitates the sloughing behavior of root border cells and provides a low-friction interface between the shaft and soil. The robotic system is designed such that soil does not enter the tip, and adhesion of the skin to soil is guaranteed. As the tip adheres to the soil during its outward movement and pushes aside the soil, the shaft moves inside the skin. In the flank zone, the skin remains adhered to the soil and avoids slippage and backward movement. This mechanism is activated by a motor on top of the shaft that pulls the skin upwards as the hollow shaft moves downwards with respect to the skin.

To achieve proper soil penetration, a second aspect was implemented that mimics the anchoring achieved by the natural root hairs that grow laterally and perpendicularly to its wall. If the skin is anchored to the soil, then the shaft also

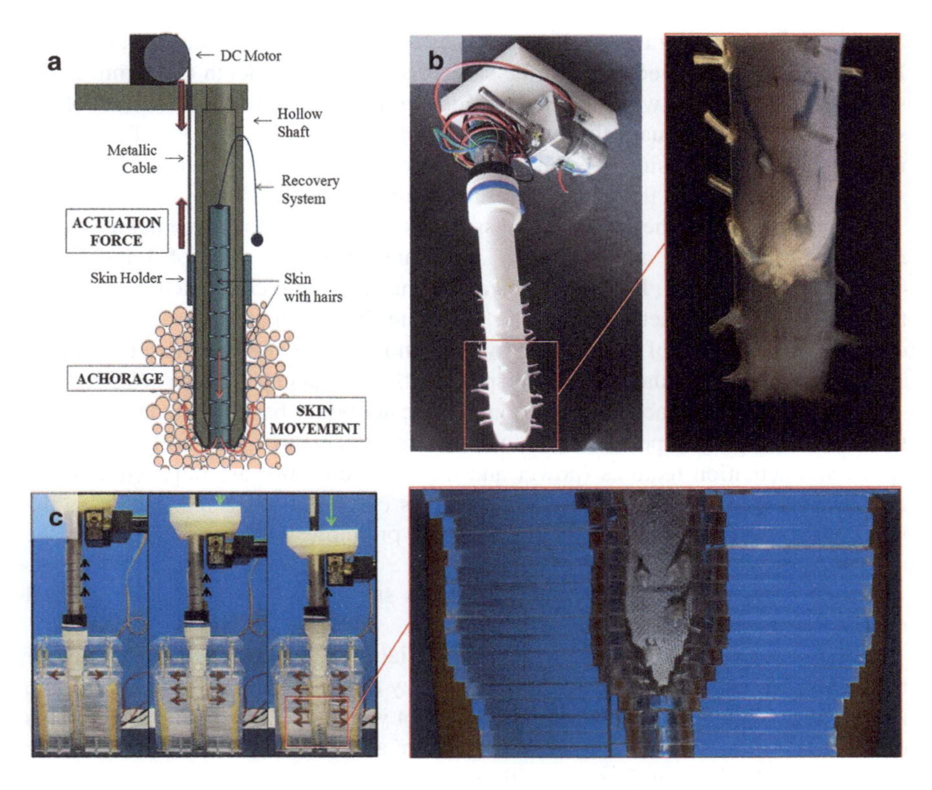

Fig. 4.3 View of a prototype inspired by the sloughing phenomenon that occurs at the level of the apex. (**a**) Sketch of the system that shows its components: a hollow cylindrical shaft, a DC motor that pulls metallic cables, and a flexible skin that embeds hairs. (**b**) Picture of the bioinspired prototype. A virtual effect made by stroboscopic photography shows the movement of the artificial root. (**c**) How the artificial sloughing mechanism works. Detail of the flexible skin released from the tip for implementing the sloughing mechanism: this mechanism greatly decreases the force required by the artificial root for the penetration in the artificial soil. Lateral hairs are visible

moves with respect to the soil and the system penetrates into the soil. Therefore, artificial hairs that resemble the root hairs were integrated on the external part of the skin that makes contact with the soil. The static frictional resistance increases as the interaction with the substrate grains increases.

In the prototype shown in Fig. 4.3, a hollow aluminum cylinder (∅ 20 mm) and a textile skin with silicone hairs (∅ 1.5 ± 0.6 mm average, length 5 ± 1 mm) were combined with a DC motor that was coupled to a gearbox. The robotic system was able to penetrate the substrate using the movement of the soft skin without adding any external force, and the system was validated for its skin characteristics, type of granular substrate, and skin displacement speed (Sadeghi et al. 2013). The system was tested during free penetration up to 40 mm in depth by using three different hair densities (0, 0.006, and 0.012 hairs/mm^2) and two different granular substrates (glass spherical beads with diameters of 0.5 mm and 5 mm), which were representative of the granular characteristics of fine and coarse sand, respectively. Penetration was achieved in all of the cases that started at a depth of 50 mm in the substrate. The ratio between the penetration depth and upward displacement of the skin was used to evaluate the performance of the actuation system. The results indicate that by increasing the hair density from 0 to 0.012, more anchoring in the soil was achieved, and the ratio increased to approximately 30 %.

Upon actuation of the skin mechanism, the axial penetration force decreased by maximum amounts of approximately 30 % and 50 % for rates of 1 mm/s and 0.5 mm/s, respectively. In this investigation, the tests were conducted by assisting the perpendicular penetration in the substrate by using a load cell that was connected to the top of the robotic system and moving downwards at a rate of 1 mm/s, which was equal to the skin speed in the free penetration test (0.5 mm/s).

This artificial approach provided some of the necessary benchmark data required to build a system that penetrates efficiently. Improvements in the soil penetration speed and actuation features (power and transmission ratio) are required, and the influence of soil types and skin characteristics can be investigated further as the system is optimized. However, two of the basic principles that were observed in the natural root behavior were validated.

The bending movement of plant roots was studied to account for the natural mechanism of differential elongation.

In the process of identifying possible artificial solutions, the implementation of soft movement characteristics in the root is a key aspect. The bending motion is the result of a growth of cells on one side of the root with respect to the other side. This differential mechanism allows for slow, smooth, and well-defined movement in the soil that results in a preferred position that is beneficial for the continued root development process. An attractive artificial solution to create this bending motion is based on hydraulic actuation using electro-rheological fluids (ERF), which are smart materials that are used in soft robotics. These fluids consist of dielectric microparticles that are suspended in a nonconducting carrier liquid, and they can shift from a liquid to solid-like phase (similar to a gel) in a reversible and repeatable manner by applying an electric field that modifies their rheological properties (viscosity, yield stress, and other properties) (Gast and Zukoski 1989). Electro-rheological (ER) fluids have been used in new valve designs to provide a soft structure, which can selectively (and in different positions) transform into more rigid structures (Sadeghi et al. 2012). In this design, the movement of each soft joint produces a flow of ER fluid between two connected vessels that pass through an ER valve. By activating the ER valve, the flow, and subsequently, the degree of freedom (DoF) of the joint, is blocked. Similarly, a robotic platform prototype with a soft bending motion in the tip of a root was developed, as shown in Fig. 4.4. In this system, a fluid actuator controlled by ER valves was implemented such that if the pressure increases in one of the three flexible fluid chambers, then the chamber stretches in its axial direction. As a result, the system bends in the opposite direction. A conical tip was also integrated. The bending of the system is triggered by a touch event at the tip of the device. Three normal force sensors were embedded at the tip such that if a contact force is externally applied, then the sensor signal

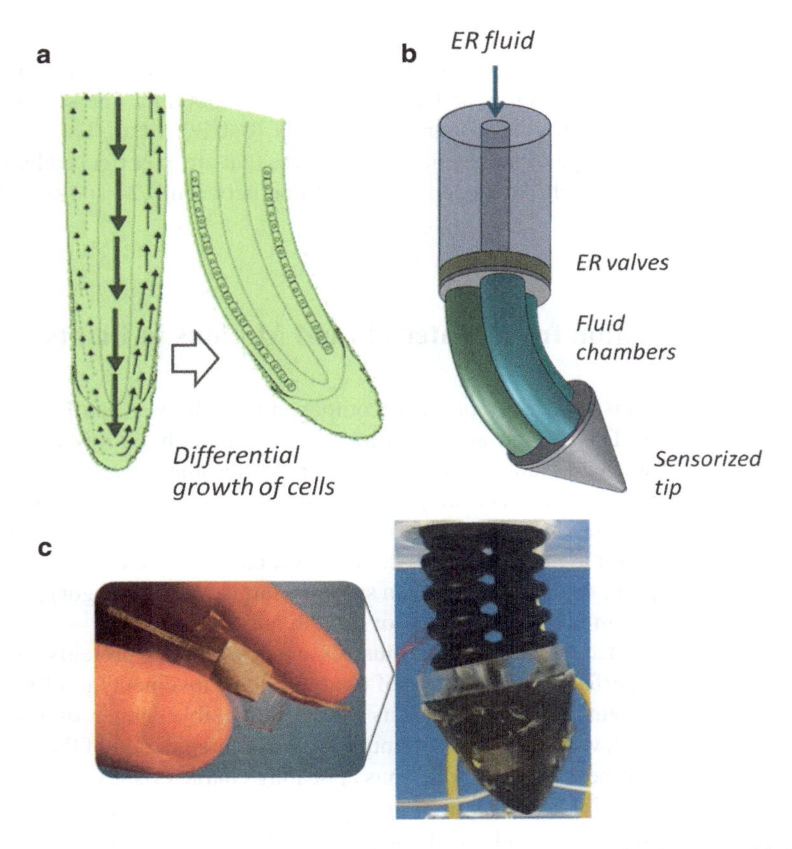

Fig. 4.4 A schematic representation of the differential growth response in plant roots (**a**) due to the elongation at faster rates of cells in the region opposite to the direction of a stimulation in the soil (hardness, water, temperature, etc.). In (**b**) a 3D representation of an artificial soft bending mechanism with a tip is depicted. The system is actuated through the electrical control of three fluid-filled chambers by means of ad hoc valves integrated at their back. The prototype is shown in (**c**) where the right inset image depicts the soft flexible 8 mm $\times$ 8 mm tactile sensor integrated at the tip. Three of these tactile sensors are integrated in the artificial tip at 120°; when they are touched, the bending movement is triggered so that the tip moves away from the mechanical stimulus (Images courtesy of A. Sadeghi and C. Lucarotti)

provides feedback to the external control system that drives the ER valve, which then controls the ER fluid-based bending.

The tactile sensors were developed to mimic the tactile sensitivity of the root. The sensors are normal force soft sensors, which can adapt and conform to the 3D structure of the root. Upon an external force, a change in the capacitance is induced by the decreased dielectric layer between two opposite electrodes. The building materials were elastomers for the dielectric layer and conductive textiles for the electrodes. The sensitivity can be optimized based on a balance between the electrode area and dielectric thickness as well as a balance between the electrical and mechanical characteristics of the constitutive materials. The sensors must be sensitive to a suitable range of forces but sufficiently robust to operate in soil. The sensors had an area of 8 × 8 mm and a total thickness of 500 μm. The sensors had the ability to detect a force in the range of 0–20 N (0–0.32 MPa). This range is representative of the range of mechanical impedances that are experienced by some types of plant roots, which have been reported to be between 0.24 and 0.58 MPa (Clark et al. 2003).

4.4 Bioinspiration from Materials and Motions in Plants

Plant cell walls consist of four primary components: cellulose, hemicelluloses, lignin, and pectin. This design and variations in the hierarchical microstructure are responsible for a wide range of mechanical properties and movements. Cellulose is the main structural fiber in plants. Cellulose molecules align to form microfibrils (with a diameter of 3–4 nm), which are aligned and bound together into macrofibrils (with a diameter of 10–25 nm) by a matrix of hemicelluloses and either pectin or lignin. A plant cell wall can sustain a large internal (turgor) pressure (up to 10 atm) and can vary its stiffness for growth and motion.

Despite the absence of animal-like muscles and contractile proteins in their tissues, plants can perform a wide range of nonmuscular movements to efficiently explore an environment, search for nutrients and avoid possible danger, or to spread their genetic material, which ensures continuation and diversification of the species. These types of movements exhibit numerous appealing characteristics: high energy efficiency (gained during the evolution process over approximately half a billion years), high actuation force, and a wide range of motion (a successful strategy that increases survivability in different challenging conditions). As a result of these considerations, and since the pioneering work of Darwin (1875, 1880), the question of how plants move without using muscles has attracted the interest of many scientists. From a biological perspective, the physiology of plant movements is important to understand plant development and plant responses to environmental stimuli, such as light and gravity (Gilroy and Masson 2008; Moulia and Fournier 2009). Additionally, an adequate understanding of these nonmuscular movements has potential for developments in applied sciences and engineering, in particular, the creation of new biomimetic actuation strategies related to high energy efficiency and low power consumption (Taya 2003; Burgert and Fratzl 2009; Martone et al. 2010).

Movements in plants can be characterized according to the following categories: their nastic (movement that is independent of the spatial direction of a stimulus) or tropic (the response of plant is influenced by the direction of a stimulus) character and their active (live plant cells activate and control the response by moving ions and by changing the permeability of membranes based on potential actions) or passive (movements that are based on dead tissue that is suitable to undergo predetermined modifications upon changes in environmental conditions) character.

These passive systems do not require control or a supply of energy from the organism once their growth completes and includes dead tissues that can be activated by swelling or drying of the plant cell walls without any metabolism. The cellulose fibril orientation and its interaction with changing external environmental conditions also control the deformation of plant organs.

These properties are interesting from a biomimetic perspective and could be translated into engineering mechanisms and principles.

4.4.1 Active Mechanisms in Plants

4.4.1.1 Osmosis-Based Mechanisms

Osmosis is important for the active movement (both slow and rapid) of plants and is a driving force that generates actuation in plant organs. Osmosis is a chemo-physical phenomenon based on solvent transport that is commonly present in living beings. The term "osmosis" originates from the Greek "ωσμος" (osmos), which means a "push or impulsion." Osmosis drives solvent flows through an osmotic membrane from a less concentrated solution to a concentrated solution. From a functional perspective, natural osmotic systems rely on four primary elements: an osmotic membrane, a rigid structure, a compliant transducer, and a suitable osmotic power reservoir. The osmotic pressure is built owing to a stiff plant cell wall, which is composed of highly organized cellulose microfibrils embedded in a pectin matrix (Preston 1974; Taiz and Zeiger 2002; Baskin 2005). From a biomechanical perspective, without considering any active transport and gate proteins, this complex polymeric system serves two functions:

- It constitutes most of the natural osmotic membrane (which exhibits good solute rejection properties and good water permeability).
- It serves as a first-level transducer for actuation power through pressure-driven deformation (Dumais and Forterre 2012).

Additionally, the isotropic turgor pressure inside the plant cell can be converted in directional movement at the cellular/tissue/organ level, thanks to inhomogeneity and anisotropy of the cell wall/tissue/organ. For instance, directional actuation can be obtained by using additional stiff elements (e.g., lignin-rich structure, death tissue, in root growing) of metastable structures or by using specific biochemical mechanisms (e.g., the auxin mechanism, special osmotic metabolism, and osmotic agent active transport) (Dumais and Forterre 2012). Clearly, in this type of framework, water can be an osmotic power reservoir in close tissue or in soil (if it is in contact) (Steudle and Peterson 1998).

Additionally, although osmosis generally drives slow plant movements such as root growth, it also contributes to several fast and reversible movements, such as those of *Mimosa pudica* and *Dionaea muscipula* (Venus flytrap).

Mimosa pudica has the ability to quickly react to external mechanical stimuli by quickly folding its leaves. The closing motion is rapid (it requires only a few seconds) and is driven by motor cells (i.e., extensor cells) on one side of the pulvinus (a joint-like thickening at the base of a plant leaf) that change the turgor pressure upon stimulation (Samejima and Sibaoka 1980). As a result, the hinge loses its bending stiffness, deflects, and produces a folding movement. Conversely, osmosis drives leaf opening, although this is a slower process.

Another example of quick plant movement is the Venus flytrap, which is named for its ability to capture insects by a quick closing motion of the leaves, which occurs in approximately 100 ms (Forterre et al. 2005). The closing mechanism is triggered by mechanical stimuli induced by prey touching dedicated leaf sensory hairs; this stimulus is converted into an action potential via a change in membrane permeability and a decrease in turgor pressure (Hodick and Sievers 1989). When the leaves are open, they exhibit concave plane folding, which is maintained in a metastable state by means of highly turgorized cells. If the cell turgor decreases, then the volume change of the leaves induces an instability that triggers the elastic relaxation of the concave folding. This relaxation results in a convex folding motion that closes the trap (Forterre et al. 2005). In this case, the opening phase is much slower than the closing phase, which is affected by the metastable mechanism and thus requires a large amount of energy.

4.4.1.2 Basic Models for Osmosis

Understanding osmosis-based actuation strategies used in plants provides a source of inspiration for developing innovative, low power consumption actuation devices. The development of a simplified mathematical model can explain the role of the involved parameters by including their characteristic values for effective actuation to occur. Equations that describe osmosis are strongly related to the chemical nature of osmolytes.

By considering a simple example such as strong electrolytes with ideal behavior, osmosis can be modeled (as a first approximation) using Van't Hoff's law:

$$\Pi = iMRT, \tag{4.1}$$

where M is the molarity of the electrolytes in the solution, R is the universal gas constant, T is the absolute temperature (in K), and i is the Van't Hoff coefficient, which accounts for the particle effect in the presence of electrolytes (Atkins and de Paula 2006). In the case of strong common electrolytes, deviations from this law are generally less than 2 %, and they can be estimated by introducing a correction factor as

$$\Pi = \phi iMRT, \tag{4.2}$$

where ϕ is considered to be the osmotic equivalent of the real gas compressibility factor and can be estimated from literature if needed. In a more complex system, similar to the actual pool of osmolytes active in plant tissue, we can use a more general equation, such as a virial expansion, which is normally used to account for the deviation from the ideal polymer solution. An example relation is given by

$$\Pi \approx c_1 M + c_2 M^2 + O(M^3). \tag{4.3}$$

This simple model can be used to calculate the pressure of an osmotic solution from the concentration of the osmolytes (Atkins and de Paula 2006). From the osmotic pressure calculation, the net water flux through the osmotic membrane, maximum force of the actuator, and energy density can be calculated as well as the characteristic time, which is described below.

Osmotic pressure causes the flow of water from a dilute to a concentrated solution according to the following equation:

$$\dot{q} = S_{\mathrm{OM}} \alpha_{\mathrm{OM}} (\Pi + p_{\mathrm{d}} - p_{\mathrm{c}}), \tag{4.4}$$

where $\dot{q}$ is the solvent flux across the osmotic membrane; S_{OM} and α_{OM} denote the surface area and permeability of the osmotic membrane, respectively; and p_{d} and p_{c} denote the pressure of the dilute and concentrated solution, respectively.

In actual osmotic phenomena, the total flux $\dot{q}_{\mathrm{tot}}$ is also influenced by external concentration polarization phenomena (ECP) and internal concentration polarization phenomena (ICP). The ECP results in a decrease in the osmotic pressure due to the formation of a bilayer of ions on the face of an osmotic membrane. The ICP results in a decrease in the osmotic pressure, due to the formation of a double layer of ions on different faces of the membrane.

4.4.1.3 Bioinspired Osmotic Systems

The osmotic principle, which is used by plants for their movements, has been considered for actuating artificial systems. Most of the related studies were developed in a biomedical context (particularly for controlled drug release). Starting from a study by Theeuewes and Yum (1976), numerous small pumping systems were developed based on forward osmosis with the goal of achieving a constant drug release rate over a prolonged period (Herrlich et al. 2012). Most of these systems were developed for intracorporeal applications, and their miniaturization strongly relies on a simple design based on the osmotic principle, because of the availability of water (as a solvent) in bodily fluids and because no external power source is required for operation. Two types of devices can be identified, depending on whether the drug is used as an osmotic agent or not. If the drug is used as an osmotic agent, then it is possible to maximize drug storage, but the solubility of the drug strongly affects the release performance, and it is difficult to use an osmotic pump with different drugs. If the drug is not used as an osmotic agent, then a release rate is achieved independent of the drug properties by introducing an additional compartment that stores the osmotic agent and a movable wall that pushes the drug outwards in response to an increase in volume of the osmotic agent compartment. The design is more complex for the second type of system, which results in a reduced amount of drug storage. In all of the cases, a constant release rate is attained as long as the solution containing the osmotic agent remains saturated. Additionally, the design of the drug outlet is important to guarantee that the drug release is effectively driven by the osmotic process rather than by diffusive phenomena. This also applies to the case in which tiny catheters are added to the outlet to achieve localized release to targeted zones. Additionally, all of these systems were developed with biocompatible materials, which are suitable for implants even if the biodegradable materials (degradation would be designed to occur after the operational time interval) would avoid the explantation phase. Additional devices that include a solvent reservoir were proposed that were suitable for extracorporeal usage. However, this increases the complexity of the system, and the performance of these systems can be affected by additional factors such as environmental temperature. Additional details on these types of osmotic pumps can be found in Herrlich et al. (2012). Most of the previously discussed systems are commercially available and are used in clinical development; however, they have not reached a stable position within the biomedical market. Within the biomedical sector, a miniature osmotic actuator was proposed in Li and Su (2010), which combines drug release and mechanical actions that focused on bone distraction. In particular, the distraction force (less than 10 N over nearly 200 h) was generated by an osmosis-driven piston mechanism in which the design and fabrication steps were carefully studied to avoid solution leakages.

Outside of the medical field, an osmotic actuator was proposed to steer the tip of a mechatronic system inspired by the apex of the plant roots (Mazzolai et al. 2011), which has applications in soil exploration and monitoring. This type of actuator was based on electroosmosis because of its potential for reversibility. In particular, the steering concept was based on three cells that were separated by pairs of semipermeable osmotic membranes and ion-selective membranes and individually coupled with a piston mechanism. Technical issues primarily related to the degradation of the ion-selective membranes during the electroosmotic process (lead acetate was used as salt) encouraged the development of an alternative actuation strategy based on forward osmosis. By adopting a bioinspired approach, a modeling study was performed (Sinibaldi et al. 2013) to extract preliminary design guidelines based on targeted performance metrics such as the characteristic time of actuation or the maximum force. A dynamic model of the osmotic actuation concept was developed based on the following key elements: an osmotic membrane, an actuation chamber that contains the osmotic agent and both a rigid and a deformable boundary, and a solute reservoir chamber. These elements should also be accounted for when considering osmotic actuation in plants. The elastic deformation of the movable boundary of the actuation chamber (which acted as a force transducer) was modeled in more detail by assuming that energy storage occurred either through an external elastic load (a spring-piston system) or membrane bulging (see Fig. 4.5).

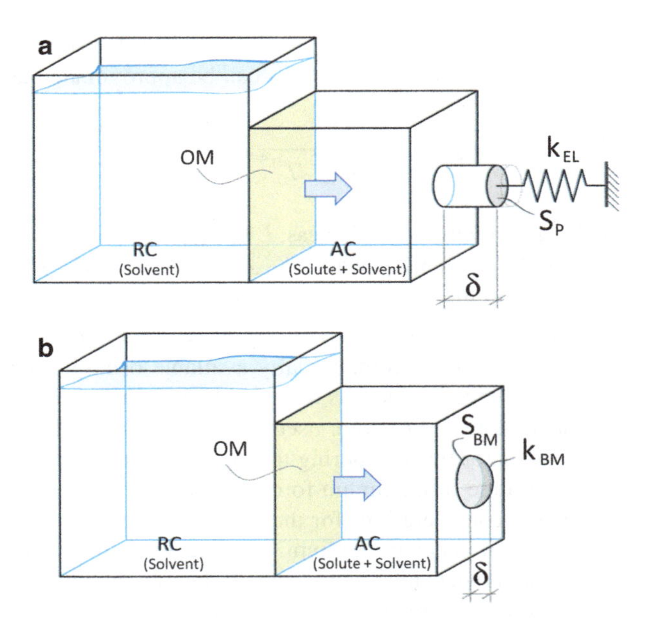

Fig. 4.5 Schematics of the osmotic actuator. Solute flux crosses the osmotic membrane (OM), from the reservoir (RC) to the actuation chamber (AC). A corresponding increase in the AC pressure results in the displacement of a piston (**a**) or membrane bulging (**b**). The surface areas of the piston and the bulging membrane are denoted by S_P and S_{BM}, respectively. The actuation work is stored through an elastic deformation, either of the spring (**a**), with stiffness k_{EL}, or of the bulging membrane (**b**) with stiffness k_{BM}. Piston displacement and bulge height are denoted by δ [Adapted from Sinibaldi et al. (2013)]

In both cases, analytical expressions were obtained for the actuation dynamics. For example, for the piston implementation, the actuation chamber volume V at time t is given by the following expression:

$$\begin{aligned} 2\frac{t}{\bar{t}} &= \log_e\left[\frac{\Psi(1;C)}{\Psi(v;C)}\right], \text{ with} \\ \Psi\ (\xi;C) &:= \left(\frac{(1+\omega)}{2}-\xi\right)^{1+1/\omega}\left(\xi-\frac{(1-\omega)}{2}\right)^{1-1/\omega}, \end{aligned} \tag{4.5}$$

where $v = V/V_0, \omega = \sqrt{1+4C}, C = \Pi_0 S_p^2/(V_0 k_{EL})$, and $\bar{t} = S_p^2/(k_{EL} S_{OM} \alpha_{OM})$. The terms V_0 and Π_0 denote the initial value of V and the osmotic pressure difference, respectively; S_p is the piston base area; k_{EL} is the spring stiffness; S_{OM} is the osmotic membrane surface area; and α_{OM} is the permeability coefficient. Similar equations were derived for the implementation of the bulging membrane. Using these equations, formal expressions for the quantities of interest were developed (the characteristic actuation time, maximum force, peak power, power density, cumulated work, and energy density) in terms of the physical parameters that were included in this actuation strategy. For instance, for small bulge deformations, the characteristic actuation time $t_{c,BM}$ can be approximated as follows:

$$t_{c,BM} \cong \frac{1}{3\alpha_{OM}k_{BM}^{1/3}\Pi_0^{2/3}}\beta^{5/3}L^{4/3}, \tag{4.6}$$

where k_{BM} is the bulging membrane stiffness, $L = S_{OM}{}^{1/2}$ is the characteristic size of the actuator, and $\beta = S_{BM}/S_{OM}$, where S_{BM} is the base area of the bugling membrane. Similarly, both the actuator energy and power density can be increased by decreasing the design parameter $\lambda = V_0/S_{OM}^{3/2}$, which represents the volume-to-surface-area aspect ratio. After a commercially available osmotic membrane was identified and a fixed reference value was used for the bulging membrane stiffness, then scaling laws such as Eq. (4.6) were used to estimate the preliminary dimensions of the osmotic actuator by considering the design targets and constraints (the characteristic actuation time or maximum force). In addition to theoretical derivations, there are practical considerations for the fabrication of the osmotic actuator, such as material selection (because sodium chloride was chosen as the solute, corrosion is an issue) and mechanical constraints to be implemented (e.g., affixing the osmotic membrane to minimize deviations from the ideal working behavior). Based on this study, new osmotic actuators characterized by reduced power consumption and high energy and power density can be developed that exhibit more rapid dynamics (on order of minutes) compared to previously developed actuators.

4.4.2 Passive Mechanisms in Plants

Osmotic pressure is only one of many actuation mechanisms in plants. Dead tissues can be actuated as a result of changes in environmental conditions to accomplish functional movement (Burgert and Fratzl 2009; Dumais and Forterre 2012). Passive movements in plants are essentially driven by humidity gradients between the cell and ambient air. The water potential of air (Ψ_{vap}) is a function of the partial pressure of water vapor P_{vap} and can be calculated using the Van't Hoff equation:

$$\Psi_{vap} = (RT/V_w)\ \ln\left[P_{vap}/P_{sat}(\mathrm{T})\right], \tag{4.7}$$

where $V_w \approx 18\ \mathrm{cm}^3\ \mathrm{mol}^{-1}$ is the partial molar volume of liquid water and $P_{sat}(\mathrm{T})$ is the saturation pressure of water (Atkins and de Paula 2006).

Under certain conditions, variations in the water potential gradient on dead cells (sclerenchymal tissue) can result in actuation at the tissue level (Jost and Gibson 1907). This actuation occurs because sclerenchymal tissue typically consists of fiber cells with walls that are composed of several layers of oriented cellulose fibrils. When absorbing or expelling water in response to changes in air humidity, the tissue expands or shrinks anisotropically (perpendicular to the orientation of the

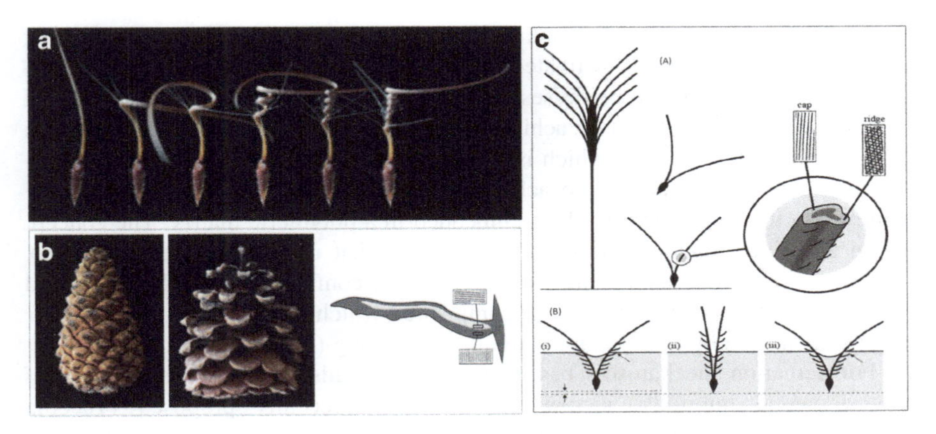

Fig. 4.6 (**a**) The drilling motion of Erodium awns (Evangelista et al. 2011). (**b**) The opening motion of conifer cones as a function of wetting and drying transients (*left*) [adapted from Dumais and Forterre (2012)]. Schematic of a pine cone cut along its longitudinal axis (*right*): the cellulose fibril orientations in the cell walls of fibers on the upper (*white*) portion and on the lower (*gray*) portion are indicated by the *inclined lines* in each rectangle. The relative fibril orientation is responsible for the opening of the pine cone, which is driven by the absorption of moisture [Adapted from Burgert and Fratzl (2009)]. (**c**) A schematic of the structure and function of wheat awns. (A) The structure of a wheat awn dispersal unit. The actuating portion of the awn (magnified in the *circle*) is composed of an outer active portion (ridge) and a passive portion (cap) that faces inwards. The cellulose fibril orientations are indicated by the *inclined lines* in each rectangle. (B) The daily cycle of dispersal unit movement, which results in a soil penetration: (i) day, (ii) night, and (iii) day [from Burgert and Fratzl (2009)]

fibrils (Fahn and Werker 1972; Burgert and Fratzl 2009). Asymmetry in the orientation of the fibrils at the organ level then converts this local swelling or shrinking to a global bending motion.

Some interesting examples of this movement include the opening and closing of a pine cone (Dawson et al. 1997; Reyssat and Mahadevan 2009), the drilling motion of *Erodium* awns (Evangelista et al. 2011), and the swelling and drying mechanisms of the seed dispersal units of wild wheat (Elbaum et al. 2007) (see Fig. 4.6).

4.4.2.1 Smart Materials for Passive Mechanisms

In materials science, a large amount of research is being conducted to develop polymeric materials that can react to external stimuli or change in environmental conditions by modifying their shape or other properties. As a result, these materials are commonly called smart polymers. Among the numerous classes of polymeric materials and composites, some candidates that are inspired by plants exhibit a potential to be used in biomimetic applications.

For example, hydrogels, which are three-dimensional polymer networks filled with aqueous solutions, have some potential in this regard because they can mimic the swelling and shrinking behavior of plant cells and produce macroscopic actuation upon swelling and shrinking (Ionov 2013). This swelling and shrinking behavior can be reversibly activated by a number of stimuli (including pH, temperature, and biochemical processes), and inhomogeneous deformations that result in changes to its shape can be achieved by modifying the material properties. In addition to planar bending, which is commonly achieved using bilayer structures, complex shape changes can be achieved by using material anisotropy, e.g., by controlling the orientation of fibers embedded in a polymeric matrix. The concept of an adaptive structure was recently proposed that uses fluidic flexible matrix composite (F^2MC) cells that were inspired by the configuration of plant cells and cell walls. The development of these composites, which are based on different fiber angles connected by internal fluid circuits, is ongoing (Li and Wang 2013).

For actuation mechanisms based on reversible adsorption and desorption of environmental humidity, a new approach was recently proposed (Taccola et al. 2013a) that combines the possibility to achieve active and passive actuation with a single composite material. This approach is based on the use of poly (3,4-ethylenedioxythiophene):poly(styrenesulfonate) (PEDOT:PSS), a well-known conjugated conducting polymer that exhibits a unique water absorption capability (due to the hydrophilic PSS) which can be used for sensing (e.g., humidity sensing (Taccola et al. 2013b) and actuation. Actuation can be obtained by coupling an ultrathin film of PEDOT:PSS (a thickness of several hundreds of nm) with a passive elastomeric layer (a thickness of hundreds of μm) in a bilayered fashion. If the humidity in the ambient air increases, then the PEDOT:PSS layer adsorbs water vapor and increases in volume, which results in bending of the structure due to the constraints of the passive layer. Figure 4.7a shows this effect with a leaf-shaped actuator that passively bends when a finger approaches its surface, because of humidity released from the skin, which demonstrates a remarkable sensitivity.

Additionally, the advantage of this hygromorphic actuator is that the bending due to electrical stimuli is easily controlled. The application of an electrical current to the PEDOT:PSS layer generates localized heating that causes the desorption of water vapor in the film at equilibrium with the air environment, which causes a reversible contraction of the PEDOT:PSS layer and an actuation (Fig. 4.7b shows an example of a flower-shaped, electrically controlled actuator). This technology, which has potential for bioinspired applications, can be further improved with the addition of material anisotropy via a hierarchical fiber structure at the level of a conducting polymer.

4.5 Conclusions

Exactly replicating nature is worthless but great advantages can be brought to science and technology when it is deeply studied and its underlying principles translated in functional and useful artificial solutions. Living plants provide this opportunity that can be carefully undertaken.

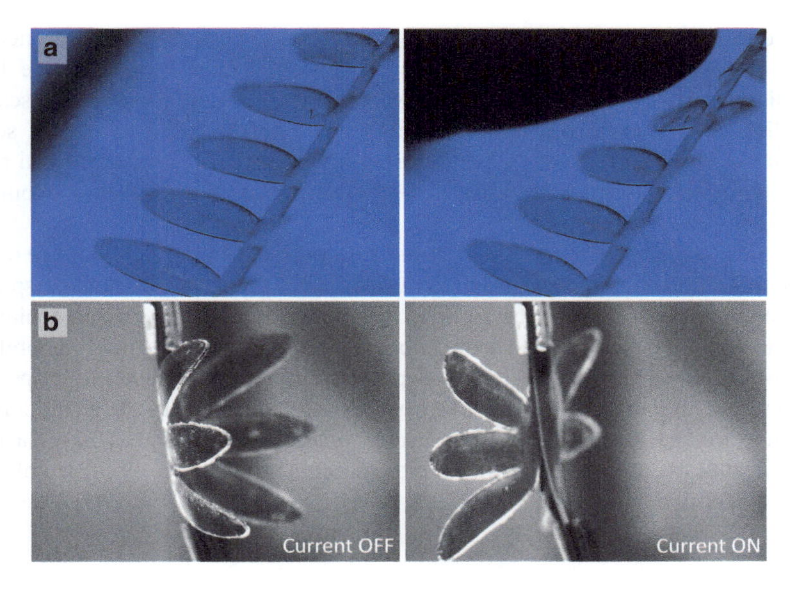

Fig. 4.7 (**a**) A PEDOT:PSS/PDMS leaf-shaped actuator (*left*) that passively bends when a finger approaches their surface (*right*) (image courtesy of Massimo Brega). (**b**) A PEDOT:PSS/PDMS *flower-shaped actuator* (*left*) that bends when an electrical current is applied (image courtesy of Silvia Taccola)

We review state-of-the-art examples of how plant root features can be exploited in the artificial world. Some of the lessons learned in studying their movements from an engineering viewpoint are detailed. These encompass, for example, the possibility of building systems that penetrate the soil by elongating their structures at the tip region, instead of using energy to produce a penetration in the soil by pushing the remaining top part of their body. Preliminary results in this area are reported demonstrating an effective reduction of energy consumption of more than 50 %.

Currently, the engineering and biological scientific communities are discussing the best approaches toward robotic systems that aim at mimicking the amazing penetration, exploration, and adaptation capabilities of plant roots. We report some of the interdisciplinary platforms, the PLANTOIDS, built both to study plant biological principles that are still unknown and to fabricate enabling technologies for future markets and applications. We report about the implementation of a system that achieves penetration and anchorage to the soil imitating the growth and cells that are sloughed off at the level of the natural root apex. The artificial skin used in this system allows for a significant reduction of the axial force penetration of the artifact. Moreover, a soft bending system, built following the differential elongation mechanism of the plant root, is also depicted. The soft robotic approach of this implementation is such that tactile sensory feedback can be provided with sensors that adapt to the soil mechanical stimulation and trigger a bending motion of the overall system. Indeed, one of the major contributions that scientists can provide in this field is related to the implementation of new materials and mechanisms directly inspired from the plant movements. Here, we emphasize how osmosis plays a key role in the active movements of plants, at different timescales, providing several examples on how it has been fruitfully used to actuate some artificial systems. In pursuing a fully bioinspired mechanism for an artificial root, we show how a forward osmosis-based system can be carefully designed to build a microscale actuator.

The final aim of this research is to invent systems that can perform because of the biomimetic structures of sensing, actuation, and body parts. A bioinspired-integrated approach reduces the complexity of control that is needed to achieve a fully bioinspired behavior of an artificial root. Therefore, we indicate some preliminary work related to novel design concepts and different approaches to shape soft materials for implementing plant-like passive mechanisms. This is an important challenge for the material and engineering communities: the quest is for a new vision in investigating and exploiting bioinspired approaches to bring simple but highly performing solutions.

References

Atkins PW, de Paula J (2006) Physical chemistry, 8th edn. Oxford University Press, New York, NY

Baskin TI (2005) Anisotropic expansion of the plant cell wall. Annu Rev Cell Dev Biol 21:203–222

Bhushan B (2009) Biomimetics: lessons from nature—an overview. Phil Trans R Soc A 367 (1893):1445–1486

Blancaflor EB, Masson PH (2003) Plant gravitropism. Unraveling the ups and downs of a complex process. Plant Physiol 133(4):1677–1690

Burgert I, Fratzl P (2009) Actuation systems in plants as prototypes for bioinspired devices. Philos Trans R Soc A 367(1893):1541–1557

Clark L, Whalley WR, Barraclough PB (2003) How do roots penetrate strong soil? Plant Soil 255:93–104

Darwin C (1875) Insectivorous plants. Murray, London

Darwin C (1880) The power of movement in plants. Murray, London

Dawson C, Vincent JFV, Rocca AM (1997) How pine cones open. Nature 390:668

Ding JP, Pickard BG (1993) Modulation of mechanosensitive calcium-selective cation channels by temperature. Plant J 3(5):713–720

Dumais J, Forterre Y (2012) "Vegetable Dynamicks": the role of water in plant movements. Annu Rev Fluid Mech 44:453–478

Eapen D, Barroso ML, Ponce G, Campos ME, Cassab GI (2005) Hydrotropism: root growth responses to water. Trends Plant Sci 10(1):44–50

Elbaum R, Zaltzman L, Burgert I, Fratzl P (2007) The role of wheat awns in the seed dispersal unit. Science 316(5826):884–886

Esmon CA, Pedmale UV, Liscum E (2005) Plant tropisms: providing the power of movement to a sessile organism. Int J Dev Biol 49(5–6):665–674

Esmon CA, Tinsley AG, Ljung K, Sandberg G, Hearne LB, Liscum E (2006) A gradient of auxin and auxin-dependent transcription precedes tropic growth responses. Proc Natl Acad Sci USA 103:236–241

Estabrook EM, Yoder JI (1998) Plant-plant communications: rhizosphere signaling between parasitic angiosperms and their hosts. Plant Physiol 116(1):1–7

Evangelista D, Hotton S, Dumais J (2011) The mechanics of explosive dispersal and self-burial in the seeds of the filaree, Erodium cicutarium (Geraniaceae). J Exp Bot 215(2):521–529
Fahn A, Werker E (1972) Anatomical mechanisms of seed dispersal. In: Kozlowski TT (ed) Seed biology. Academic, New York, NY, pp 151–221
Forterre Y, Skotheim JM, Dumais J, Mahadevan L (2005) How the Venus flytrap snaps. Nature 433:421–425
Gast AP, Zukoski CF (1989) Electrorheological fluids as colloidal suspensions. Adv Colloid Interface Sci 30:153–202
Gilroy S, Masson PH (2008) Plant tropisms. Blackwell, Oxford
Hart JW (1990) Plant tropisms and other growth movements. Unwin Hyman, London
Herrlich S, Spieth S, Messner S, Zengerle R (2012) Osmotic micropumps for drug delivery. Adv Drug Deliv Rev 64:1617–1627
Hodick D, Sievers A (1989) On the mechanism of trap closure of Venus flytrap (Dionaea muscipula Ellis). Planta 179(1):32–42
Hohm T, Preuten T, Fankhauser C (2013) Phototropism: translating light into directional growth. Am J Bot 100:47–59
Iijima M, Morita S, Barlow WP (2008) Structure and function of the root cap. Plant Prod Sci 11:17–27
Ionov L (2013) Biomimetic hydrogel-based actuating systems. Adv Funct Mater 23:4555–4570
Jost L, Gibson RJH (1907) Lectures on plant physiology. Clarendon, Oxford
Li Y-H, Su Y-C (2010) Miniature osmotic actuators for controlled maxillo-facial distraction osteogenesis. J Micromech Microeng 20:065013
Li S, Wang KW (2013) On the synthesis of a bio-inspired dual-cellular fluidic flexible matrix composite adaptive structure based on a non-dimensional dynamics model. Smart Mater Struct 22:014001
Loreto F, Barta C, Brilli F, Nogues I (2006) On the induction of volatile organic compound emissions by plants as consequence of wounding or fluctuations of light and temperature. Plant Cell Environ 29:1820–1828
Martone PT, Boller M, Burgert I, Dumais J, Edwards J, Mach K, Rowe NP, Rueggeberg M, Seidel R, Speck T (2010) Mechanics without muscle: biomechanical inspiration from the plant world. Integr Comp Biol 50:888–907
Mazzolai B, Mondini A, Corradi P, Laschi C, Mattoli V, Sinibaldi E, Dario P (2011) A miniaturized mechatronic system inspired by plant roots for soil exploration. Trans Mechatron IEEE/ASME 16:201–212
Moulia B, Fournier M (2009) The power and control of gravitropic movements in plants: a biomechanical and systems biology view. J Exp Bot 60:461–486
Preston R (1974) The physical biology of plant cell walls. Chapmann and Hall, London
Reyssat E, Mahadevan L (2009) Hygromorphs: from pine cones to biomimetic bilayers. J R Soc Interface 6(39):951–957
Sadeghi A, Beccai L, Mazzolai B (2012) Innovative soft robots based on electro-rheological fluids. In: Proceedings of the IEEE/RSJ international conference on intelligent robots and systems, IROS 2012, Vilamoura, Algarve, 7–12 October 2012
Sadeghi A, Tonazzini A, Popova L, Mazzolai B (2013) Innovative robotic mechanism for soil penetration inspired by plant roots. In: Proceedings of the 2013 I.E. international conference on robotics and automation, ICRA2013, Karlsruhe, 6–10 May 2013
Samejima M, Sibaoka T (1980) Changes in the extracellular ion concentration in the main pulvinus of Mimosa pudica during rapid movement and recovery. Plant Cell Physiol 21 (3):467–479
Sinibaldi E, Puleo GL, Mattioli F, Mattoli V, Di Michele F, Beccai L, Tramacere F, Mancuso S, Mazzolai B (2013) Osmotic actuation modelling for innovative biorobotic solutions inspired by the plant kingdom. Bioinspir Biomim 8(2):025002
Steudle E, Peterson CA (1998) How does water get through roots? J Exp Bot 49:775–788

Taccola S, Zucca A, Greco F, Mazzolai B, Mattoli V (2013) Electrically driven dry state actuators based on PEDOT:PSS nanofilms. In: EuroEAP 2013, international conference on electromechanically active polymer (EAP) transducers & artificial muscles, Duebendorf, 25–26 June 2013

Taccola S, Greco F, Zucca A, Innocenti C, de Julián Fernández C, Campo G, Sangregorio C, Mazzolai B, Mattoli V (2013b) Characterization of free-standing PEDOT:PSS/iron oxide nanoparticles composite thin films and application as conformable humidity sensors. ACS Appl Mater Interfaces 5(13):6324–6332

Taiz L, Zeiger E (2002) Plant physiology. Sinauer Associates, Sunderland

Takahashi H, Miyazawa Y, Fujii N (2009) Hormonal interactions during root tropic growth: hydrotropism versus gravitropism. Plant Mol Biol 69:489–502

Taya M (2003) Bio-inspired design of intelligent materials. Proc SPIE 5051:54–65

Theeuewes F, Yum SY (1976) Principles of the design and operation of generic osmotic pumps for the delivery of semisolid or liquid drug formulations. Ann Biomed Eng 4:343–353

Tonazzini A, Sadeghi A. Popova L, Mazzolai B (2013) Plant root strategies for robotic soil. In: Lepora N, Mura A, Holger K, Verschure P, Prescott T (eds) Biomimetic and biohybrid systems. Second international conference, living machines 2013, London, 29 July–2 August 2013. Lecture notes in artificial intelligence, vol 8064. Springer, Heidelberg, p 447

Van Norman JM, Frederick RL, Sieburth LE (2004) BYPASS1 negatively regulates a root-derived signal that controls plant architecture. Curr Biol 14:1739–1746

Wong TS, Kang SH, Tang SKY, Smythe EJ, Hatton BJ, Grinthal A, Aizenberg J (2011) Bioinspired self-repairing slippery surfaces with pressure-stable omniphobicity. Nature 477:443–447

Zang J, Wang Q, Tu Q, Ryu S, Pugno N, Buehler M, Zhao X (2013) Multifunctionality and control of the crumpling and unfolding of large-area graphene. Nat Mater 12:321–325

Chapter 5
Mechanism and Structures: Humanoids and Quadrupeds

Darwin G. Caldwell, Nikos Tsagarakis, and Claudio Semini

5.1 Introduction

The world, both natural and man-made, is a **complex, unstructured, cluttered and dynamically changing environment** through which humans and animals move with consummate ease, adapting to changing environments, terrains and challenges. Wheeled robots are increasingly able to work in some of these terrains, particularly those that have naturally or artificially smoothed surfaces, but there are, and will continue to be, many scenarios where only human-/animal-like levels of **agility, compliance, dexterity, robustness, reliability** and **movement/locomotion** will be effective. These domains will create new opportunities for legged locomotion (both bipedal and quadrupedal), but these new challenges will demand increased functionality in the legged robots, moving from the current domain dominated by simple walking and balance maintenance, to address key whole-body interaction issues during physical contact with humans, other robots and the environment (Fig. 5.1). This will require the development of robots that are able to exploit:

- ***Multiple Adaptive Locomotion Formats***:
  - Walking on smooth, undulating and cluttered surfaces
  - Crawling on two, three or four limbs and even with the torso in contact with the ground
  - Using external supports to assist and augment locomotion (handrails, crutches, desks, walls, etc.)
  - Manoeuvring through small, cramped and confined spaces (e.g. entering narrow corridors, reaching between objects, etc.)
  - Grasping and manipulating objects while moving—picking up objects 'in passing'

D.G. Caldwell (✉) • N. Tsagarakis • C. Semini
Central Research Laboratory, Istituto Italiano di Tecnologia, Genova, Italy
e-mail: Darwin.Caldwell@iit.it

R. Cingolani (ed.), *Bioinspired Approaches for Human-Centric Technologies*,
DOI 10.1007/978-3-319-04924-3_5,

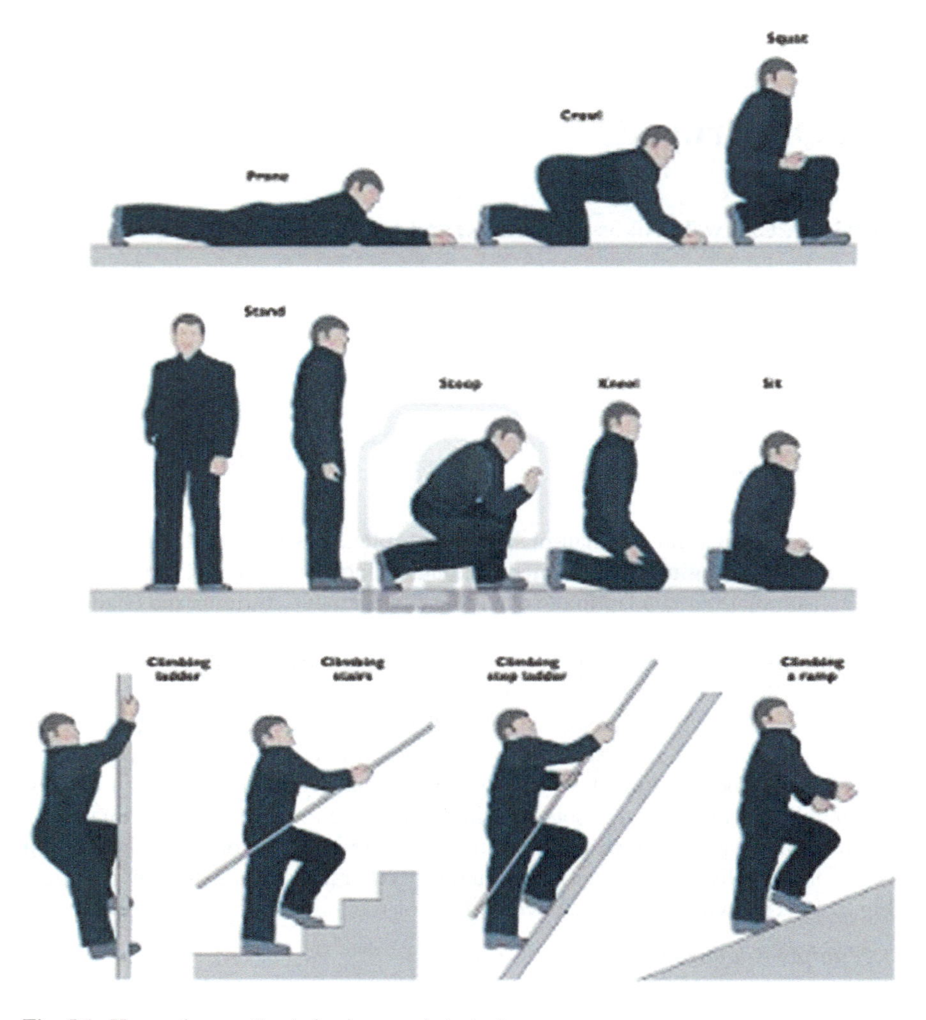

Fig. 5.1 Human locomotion behaviours and strategies

- Jumping to reach or catch an object
- Climbing steep stairs or ladders
- Pushing objects blocking a path and opening heavy doors
- Climbing debris piles

Legged robots can dramatically increase the range of terrains and situations in which an autonomous machine can be useful. The actions outlined above are crucial as we seek to develop robots to operate in such unstructured environments that have not been specifically built for the usage of machines. It is in these environments that legged robots will have particular advantages.

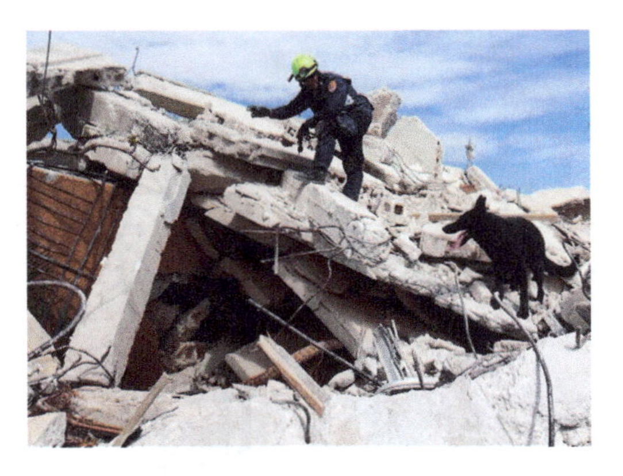

Fig. 5.2 Highly unstructured "disaster" environments require dynamic mobile responses

5.2 Operational Scenarios for Legged Robots

5.2.1 Disaster-Relief Scenario

Recent natural disasters such as the 2011 earthquake and tsunami in Japan, Fig. 5.2, and the subsequent human-centred problems at the Fukushima nuclear power plant have dramatically highlighted the need for effective and efficient robotic systems that can be deployed rapidly after the disaster, to assist in tasks too hazardous for humans to perform. Unfortunately, despite the developments in robotics, current state-of-the-art systems still do not demonstrate a capability to operate in such unstructured and unpredictable environments.

The importance of this field of research has been highlighted by the latest DARPA Robotics Challenge (DRC) (Darpa 2013; Fig. 5.3).

Although the DRC certainly sets daring and worthwhile targets, it is by no means unique and further specifications will come from other independent agencies, such as the Japanese Project on Disaster Response Robots of the Council on Competitiveness or on-going European projects.

5.2.2 Robots Working in Hazardous Industries

But it is also important to note that the use of legged systems need not only be considered in extreme disaster scenarios. In a less destructive but not unrelated context, humans are often required to work in plants that potentially pose a high level of risk to life and/or health. This will occur in nuclear, chemical, petroleum, etc., facilities and in advanced scientific facilities such as accelerators, synchrotrons, etc. These environments are characterised by the presence of steps and stairs, elevators and sometimes also ladders, narrow platforms and spaces with steps and various kinds of obstacles such as cables on the floor. In some instances (Electra 2011),

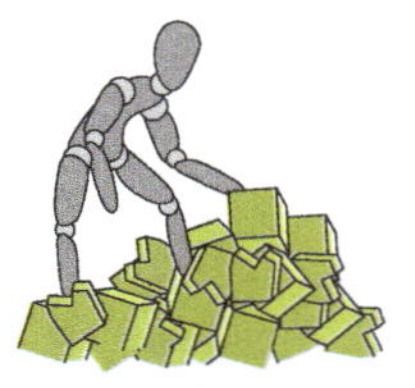

1. Walking/Moving across rubble.

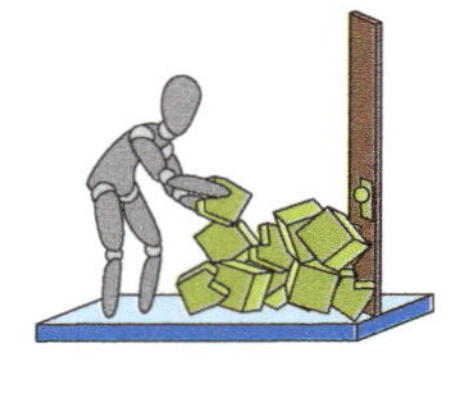

3. Remove debris blocking an entryway.

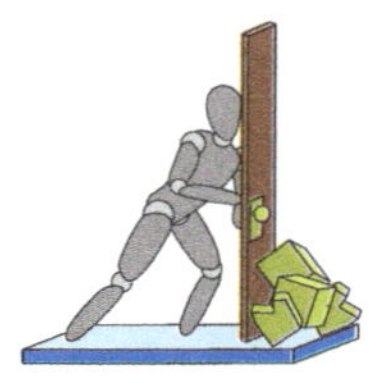

4. Open a door and enter a building.

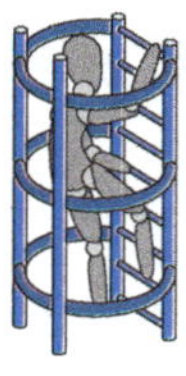

5. Climb an industrial ladder.

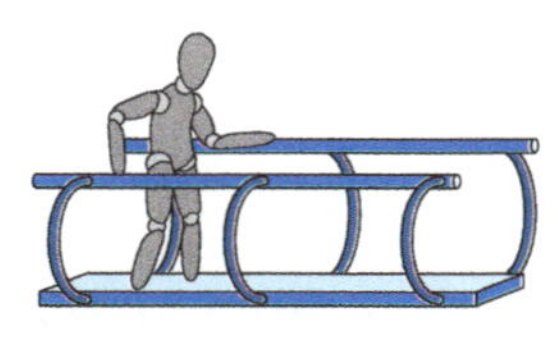

6. Traverse an industrial walkway.

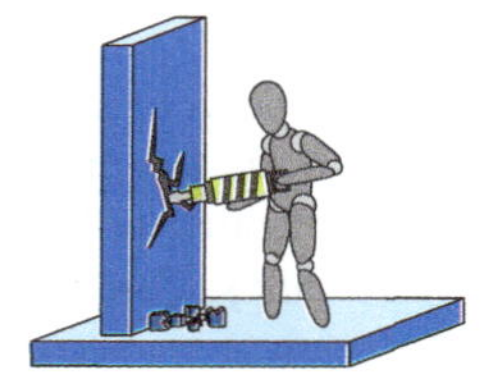

7. Use a tool to break through a concrete panel.

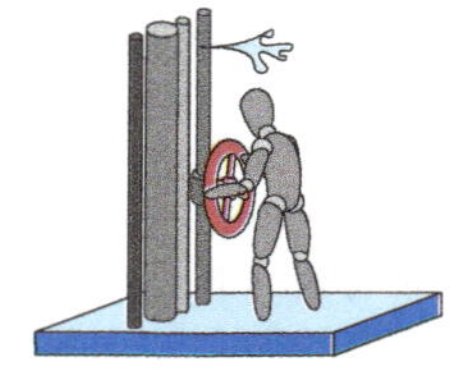

8. Locate and close a valve near a leaking pipe.

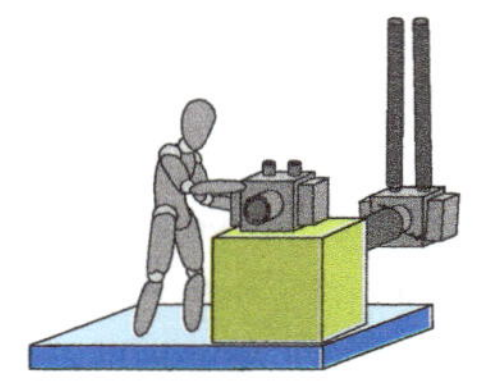

9. Replace a component such as a cooling pump.

Fig. 5.3 Tasks of the DARPA Robot Challenge were defined after a careful investigation and analysis of the dramatic events that unfolded in the first 24 h at Fukushima, when human workers attempted but ultimately failed to fix one of the crippled reactors

wheeled robots have been deployed and can pass with difficulties, yet many key areas still remain completely inaccessible to traditional wheeled robots requiring intervention by human personnel with the associated hazard risk or requirement to have a costly shutdown of plant operation or both. To operate within infrastructures originally designed for humans, but which are or have become hostile or dangerous, a robot should possess a rich repertoire of human-like skills and probably a humanoid or animal-like form. Any robot operating in such conditions should also exhibit physical power, agility and robustness, manipulation and locomotion capability and ultimately have the capacity to reach and physically interact with a harsh environment (Fig. 5.4).

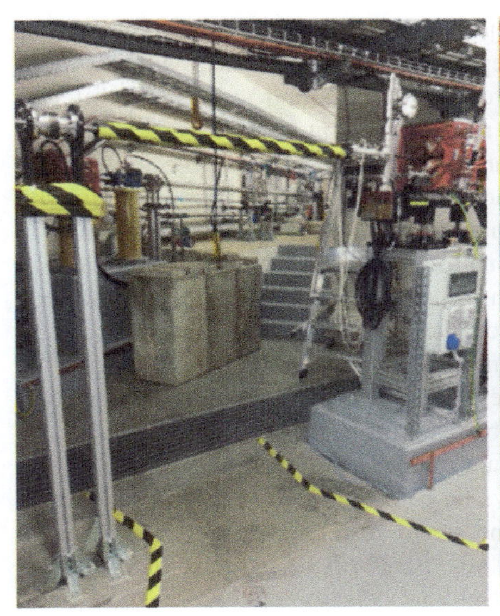
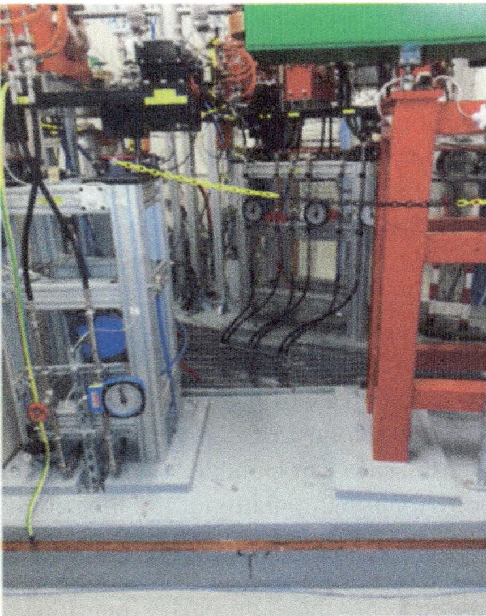

Fig. 5.4 Operating environment within industrial plant

5.2.3 Robots Working in Construction, Forestry and Farming

While the previous potential applications have focused on hazardous domains, there are also good technical reasons to consider legged robots for applications in less physically risky areas. Typical examples include construction, forestry and farming where there could be a demand for machines that can move across the often very uneven terrains to assist workers or to work autonomously.

In applications such as forestry and farming, this could have environmental and ecological benefits in addition to operational advantages. For instance, in delicate environments such as tundra, marshlands and shorelines, wheeled and tracked vehicles essentially plough up the land causing damage that can take years and in extreme cases decades to recovery. With legged platforms the footfall is much more confined and can be made environmentally friendlier similar to the motion of animals.

5.3 State of the Art

In a working or domestic scenario, tasks can typically be separated into locomotion and manipulation subtasks, which can be executed by controlling the legs, arms or hands. This requires the performance of several tasks at the same time, such as balancing, walking and manipulating objects while satisfying constraints such as avoiding joint and actuator limits or keeping appropriate contacts with the environment. Most of the time, these different constraints and tasks have different priorities. For example, generally it is more important to maintain balance or appropriate contacts with the environment rather than to grasp an object. However, multiple contacts are not necessarily a bad feature, and indeed, **humans naturally and efficiently perform heavy tasks by using their legs, arms, head and trunk in a coordinated whole-body movement producing locomotion and manipulation while keeping equilibrium**. Contacts on the more proximal limb parts are often intentionally sought, because their reduced mobility turns into an advantage in terms of stronger and more robust grasping.

Although clearly advantageous, the use of the whole body for loco-manipulation introduces a host of completely new problems on the modelling and control side. These issues can be addressed by compliant interaction modelling to make whole-body loco-manipulation a real possibility. To empower a humanoid or quadruped with the necessary adaptability, robustness and resilience to be deployed and effectively used in a disaster scenario, a key asset will be the technology of *soft robotics*. In this approach, traditional rigid robots are replaced by compliant structural elements and elastic actuators, to withstand large force peaks, contact uncertainties and energy exchange with the environment, but also permit safe interaction with humans. These are key features of the robots (e.g. COMAN and HyQ) under development in the Department of Advanced Robotics at IIT (Fig. 5.5).

5.3.1 State of the Art: Humanoid and Quadrupeds

For humanoids the development in 1973 of WABOT-1, the first multi-DOF (>20) fully actuated humanoid robot represented a ground-breaking achievement, forming the design template for most subsequent humanoids and particularly for those robots that originated in Japan. From this inspiration, the Honda series of robots was developed from E0 (1986), E1-E2-E3 (1987–1991), E4-E5-E6 (1991–1993), P1-P2-P3 (1993–1997), through to the original ASIMO (2000) and the new ASIMO (2005) (Hirai et al. 1998; Hirose and Takenaka 2001). The P3 prototype unveiled in 1998 (Hirose and Ogawa 2007) was one of the most critical designs, proving the viability of free moving humanoid platforms and spurring research on other platforms such as the Humanoid Robot Platform (HRP) which subsequently lead to HRP-2 L/2P/2/3/4 (Akachi et al. 2005; Kaneko et al. 2008). At the same time at Waseda University, the WABOT evolved through many generations to the Wabian robot (Ogura et al. 2006).

Encouraged by the developments in Japan, researchers at KAIST designed and built KHR-1/2/3 which ultimately became Hubo (Park et al. 2007), which is now one of the first commercial humanoid products. In Europe the iCub formed a concerted effort to produce a “child-like” humanoid platform for understanding and development of cognitive systems (Tsagarakis et al. 2007; Metta et al. 2008),

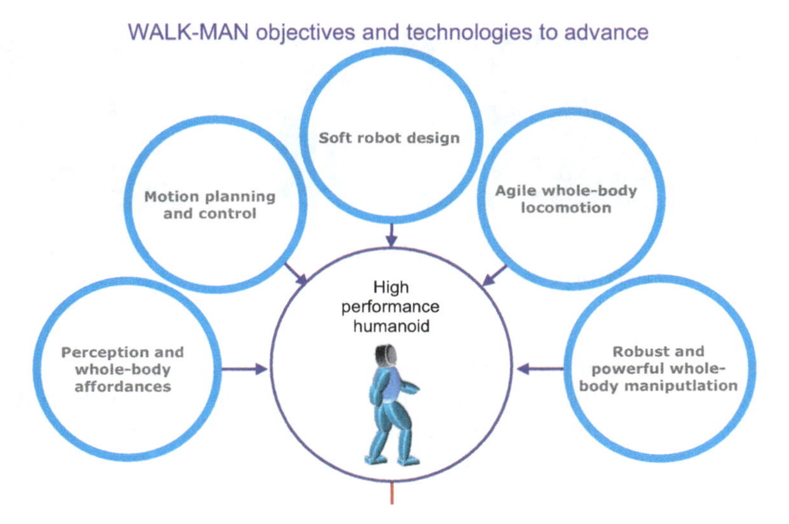

Fig. 5.5 Technologies for a humanoid capable of walking inside human-oriented infrastructures while manipulating human tools and interfaces

but although it is perhaps the best known of the European platforms, it is not unique and the TU Munich Johnnie and later LOLA robots showed excellent technical abilities. (Lohmeier et al. 2006). While the preceding robots are marked by the performance of their legged systems, upper body performance is also critical and ARMAR-III (Asfour et al. 2008) formed an autonomous system able to perform sophisticated grasping and manipulation tasks in human-centred environments, e.g. placing objects on the table, fetching objects from the refrigerator, loading the dishwasher and interacting with humans using natural speech (Fig. 5.6).

Yet in spite of the advances in humanoids/bipeds, significant barriers remained preventing robot hardware (physical structure and actuation) from equalling the performance of human in locomotion and full-body motion agility. Among the most critical issues was the large mechanical impedance of most traditional systems that made them inherently unsafe during human interaction, and reduced their adaptability and capacity to absorb impacts, making them susceptible to damage during interactions. Essentially, **the natural dynamics of such humanoids more closely resembled a stiff industrial robot arm** than anything natural.

The past two decades have seen considerable progress in the mechatronic development of legged robots (humanoids, bipeds, quadrupeds, etc.), with designs ranging from entirely passive units to systems with one and sometimes two motors per joint. Yet, the traditional approach taken during this period delivered machines where the key performance parameters were speed and positional accuracy, and under these operating conditions, large, heavy, rigid robots with accurate positional control of the (almost always) highly geared electric servo drives were the norm. This use of position controlled as opposed to torque-controlled actuation means the robots must rely on kinematically planned trajectories. The recently presented

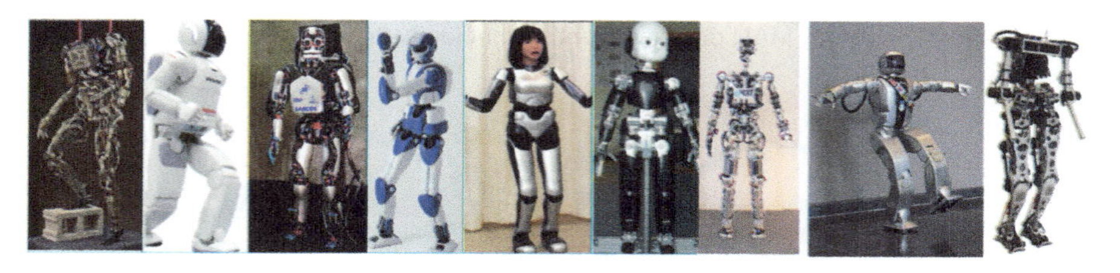

Fig. 5.6 "Stiff" full-body humanoids: the PetMan, ASIMO, CB, HRP-4 and HRP4c and iCub and ARMAR-4, HUBO and LOLA

ASIMO is a good example of the performance that can be achieved with such hardware by pushing the kinematic planning approach to its limits. Robust locomotion on truly rough terrain, however, has not been achieved yet.

Although position control was the standard during this period, there was growing realisation that compliance regulation and torque control could yield some interesting results. Work on passive dynamic walking and developments in torque sensing, actuator design (Series Elastic Actuators and Variable Impedance Actuators) and control have meant that it became possible (and certainly in some instances desirable) to introduce compliance into the drive chain to create robots that have both accurate positional and, more importantly, torque-controlled joints.

There are currently two main approaches to use of compliance and torque in legged systems.

The first approach, used in the bipeds PETMAN, ATLAS, CB (Sang-Ho et al. 2007), the DLR Biped and the quadruped HyQ (Semini et al. 2011), seeks to use actuators that have a high torque control bandwidth to improve the dynamic performance and external perturbation (impact/interaction) rejection. With the exception of the DLR biped, most robots of this form are hydraulic robots, with high power weight performance and mechanical robustness; nonetheless, they still rely on sensing and software to regulate their very high mechanical impedance and replicate compliant behaviours. There is no inherent compliance. At the same time the very high power means that safety is a very real concern making them unsuitable when operating in human-centred environments. Finally, although pumps and hydraulic power can be very efficient, the energy efficiency is a major hurdle due to the power lost in various transmission stages, which can lead to overall efficiencies of less than 20 % loss.

The second common actuation approach used to provide controlled power while reducing the intrinsic mechanical impedance uses physically compliant actuation systems. Here, elasticity is introduced between the load and the actuator to effectively decouple the high inertia of the actuator from the link side. The Series Elastic Actuator (SEA) (Pratt and Williamson 1995) which has a fixed compliance element between a high impedance actuator and the load was one of the earliest of these designs, and state-of-the-art robots powered by SEAs include the M2V2 bipedal robot (Pratt et al. 2012), the FLAME humanoid from Delft and the MABEL biped (Hurst and Rizzi 2008; Hurst 2011).

Finally, there is the IIT compliant humanoid COMAN which uses a combined active and passive approach (Tsagarakis et al. 2009, 2011b; Li et al. 2012).

The following sections will explore the design and construction of two robots developed at IIT that have compliance at their heart: the electrically power passive/active compliant humanoid COMAN and the actively compliant hydraulic quadruped HyQ.

5.4 Humanoid and Quadruped Design and Construction

5.4.1 COMAN Humanoid Robot

The COMAN is derived from previous work on the lower body of the iCub humanoid and the compliant biped cCub (Tsagarakis et al. 2007, 2011a, 2013), Fig. 5.7. The height, at the neck, is 945 mm, although with a head this increases to 1.1 m (approx. the size of a 4-year-old child). The width and depth at the hips is 147 mm and 110 mm, respectively, and the distance between the centres of the shoulders is 312 mm. The total weight of the robot is 34 kg with the legs/waist weighing 18.5 Kg and the torso and the arms weighing 15.5 Kg.

COMAN has 31 DOF distributed across the body. Each leg has 6 DOF: 3 DOF at the hip, 1 DOF at the knee level and 2 DOF at the ankle. For the trunk there is a 3 DOF waist, which gives greater flexibility than that provided by 1 or 2 DOF waist mechanisms used in the majority of humanoids. Each arm has currently 7 DOF: 3 DOF at the shoulder, 1 DOF at the elbow level and 3 DOF at the wrist/forearm (Table 5.1; Figs. 5.8 and 5.9).

Previous generations of humanoids have been position controlled robots with excellent accuracy in the control of joint motions. This means that with accurate models of carefully controlled environments, it is possible to achieve highly effective walking and even running, but when the contacts are unexpected or poorly modelled, which are the prevailing conditions in most aspects of daily activity, the robot can be unstable leading to damage to the robot or the environment (including people). COMAN has the traditional high-fidelity joint position sensing but in addition has high-fidelity torque sensors integrated in the motors of every joint giving full active torque (compliance) regulation. This means that the robot can respond precisely to the unmodelled contacts and collisions, but the use of active torque sensing means that there are control bandwidth limitations which can still cause impact problems. To further enhance the interaction capacity, passive compliance based on series elastic actuation (SEA) is incorporated in 14 of the 25 DOF including all flexion/extension DOF of the legs, the 3 DOF of the waist, the flexion/extension of the shoulder and elbow and the shoulder abduction/adduction. This gives COMAN unequalled tolerance to single and multiple, sequentially and simultaneously impacts and disturbances over all of the body [Li12]. The current system does not have a head although a 2 DOF powered neck is included within the torso.

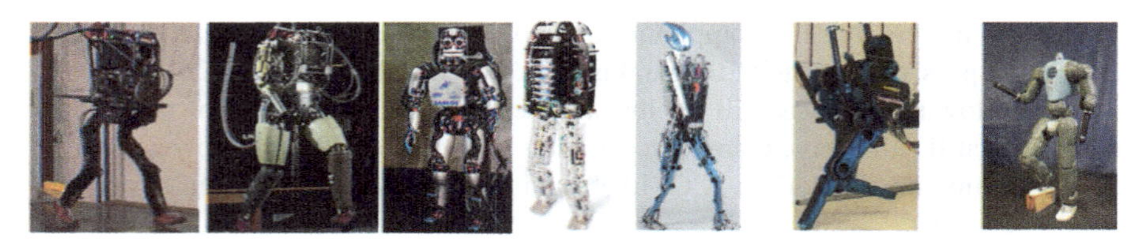

Fig. 5.7 PetMan, Atlas, SARCOS CB, M2V2, FLAME, MABEL and COMAN

Table 5.1 COMAN Specifications

Property	Value
Dimensions	110 cm tall
Weight	34 kg
Degrees of freedom	31 DOF Leg 2 × 6 DOF Waist 3 DOF Arms 2 × 7 DOF Neck 2 DOF
Compliance	Active compliance in all joints Passive compliance Legs (ankle, knee and hip) Waist (roll, pitch and yaw) Arm (all joints)
Actuators and gearing	DC brushless motors (Kollmorgen) 55 Nm peak torque Harmonic gear (100:1 ratio)
Battery	Lithium polymer ion (29 V 10 Ah)
Construction	• Body (aluminium 7075) • Shell (ABS) • High stress sections (steel or titanium)
Body housing	All internal electrical wiring Fully covered—no exposed components/wires No cable transmissions
Onboard sensing and perception	Position (relative and absolute encoder) Joint torque 2 × 6 axis force/torque sensor in ankle Inertial measurement unit (IMU)
Onboard computer	PC104 Pentium with real-time Linux (Xenomai)
Control frequency	100 Hz—fully torque controlled

5.4.1.1 Materials

Most of the mechanical components (motor and bearing housing and link structures) are machined from aluminium alloy 7075 (Ergal), while heavily stressed units such as joint shafts and torque sensors were produced from stainless steel 17-4PH which gives an excellent combination of oxidation and corrosion resistance together with high strength. The body covers were made of ABS plastic, while the

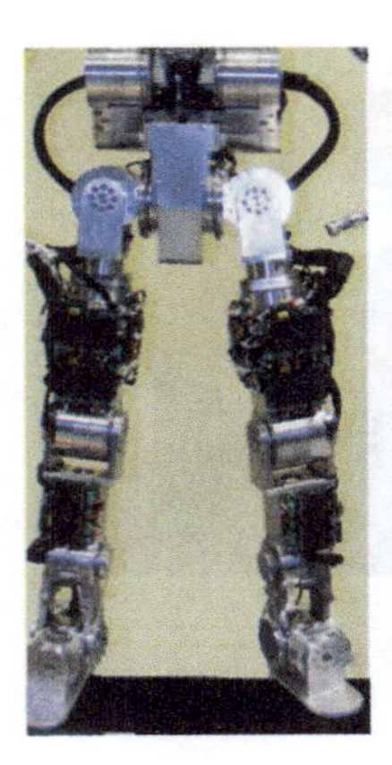
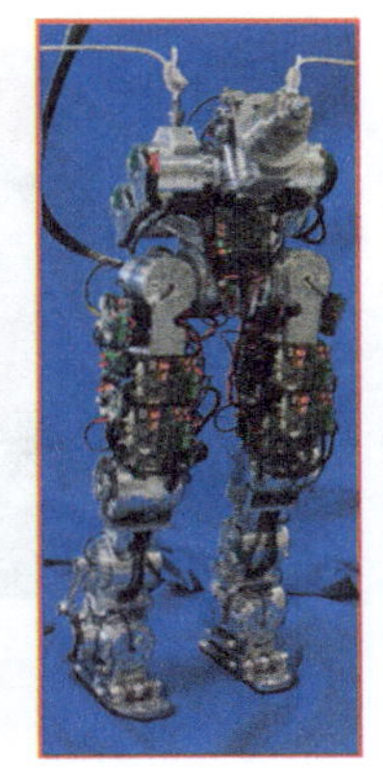
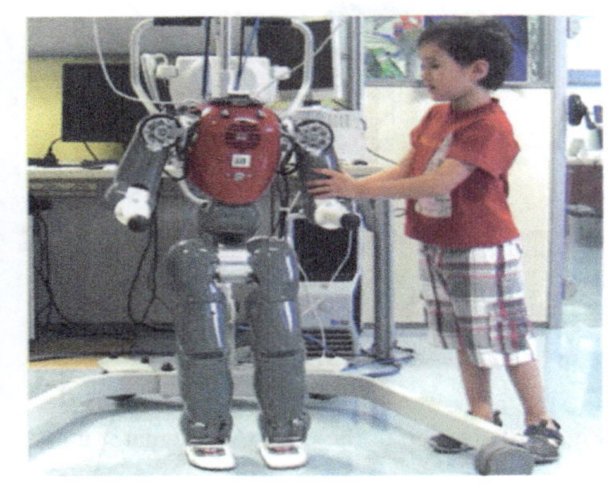

Fig. 5.8 Evolution from iCub legs through the cCub biped to the COMAN humanoid

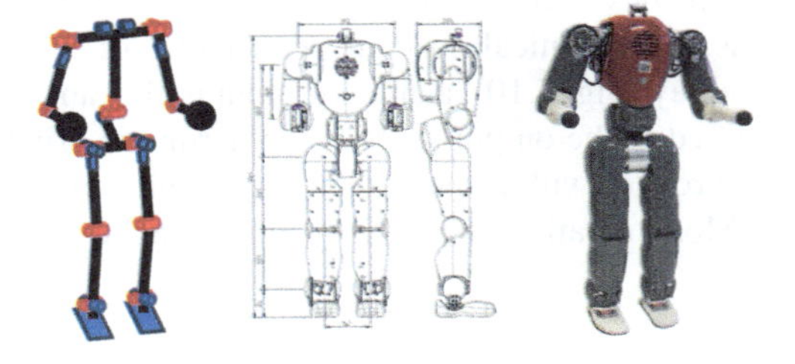

Fig. 5.9 COMAN kinematics

core of the torso used as the mounting for the battery, electronics systems and the support for the shoulders and neck is made from titanium for strength and low mass.

5.4.1.2 Compliant Actuation Unit

Based on prior experience with iCub and cCub, particular attention was paid to optimising the size, weight and modularity of the mechanical assembly of the actuation units to ensure "easy" integration of the SEA units into multi-DOF body of COMAN (Tsagarakis et al. 2009). The highly integrated technology within COMAN relies on a novel rotary series elastic element formed into compliant actuation module (CompAct), Fig. 5.10. This assembly uses high-performance and low mass frameless brushless motor with a patented rotational series elastic element (CompAct) (Tsagarakis et al. 2011b). This element can within millisec. provide compliance variation over a range of over 60:1 (10 Nm/rad to 600 Nm/rad). This is greater than the compliance range variation of human muscle (typically

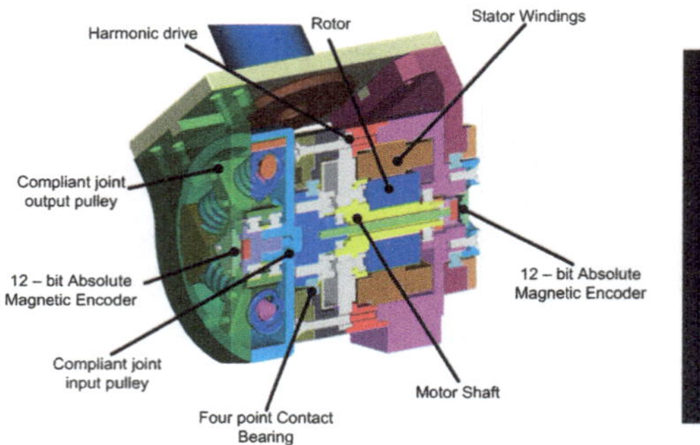

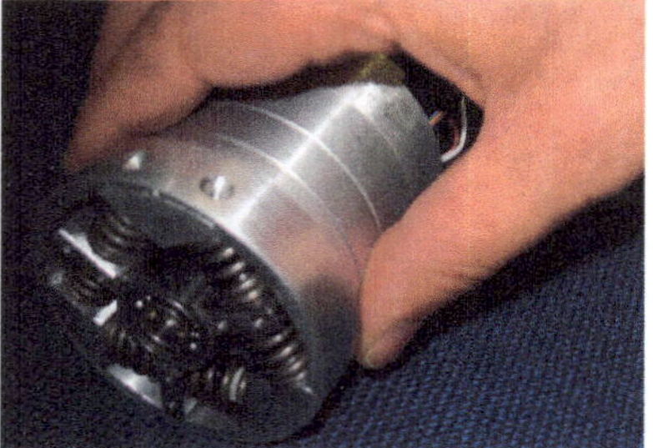

Fig. 5.10 Design of the CompAct Actuator unit

20:1). Each CompAct actuator unit weighs 0.52 Kg, with a maximum output torque of 40 Nm, a peak output speed 10.7 rad/s and a nominal power 190 W.

To minimise dimensions while achieving high rotary stiffness, the compliant module is formed as a mechanical structure consisting of a three spoke output component (output pulley (Fig. 5.10), a circular input pulley and six linear springs). The input pulley is fixed to the output shaft of the harmonic drive. The output link (three spoke element) rotates with respect to the input pulley and is coupled to it by six linear springs. More details on the SEA unit can be found in Tsagarakis et al. (2009).

5.4.1.3 Leg Mechanical Design

COMAN's legs have an anthropomorphic kinematic structure with hips, a thigh with integrated knee joints, a calf with integral ankle joints and a foot. The design of leg is based on the "cCub" prototype developed in Tsagarakis et al. (2011a), although several joint modules were radically redesigned to improve the assembly process, profile and compactness while incorporating an additional passive compliance in the hip flexion joint. The hip joint is constructed as a cantilever structure with a pitch-roll-yaw assembly providing a large range of motion, Table 5.2. The hip pitch motion is driven by the compliant actuation module introduced before (peak torque of 55 Nm), while the roll and yaw motion actuators are conventional stiff modules (Kollmorgen Brushless DC motor combined with a 100:1 Harmonic reduction drive giving a peak torque of 55 Nm). The hip roll motor is placed below the hip centre transmitting its torque to the hip (around the hip centre) using a four bar mechanism. This permits integration of the CompAct SEA module at the hip pitch actuator without increasing the distance between the two hip centres. The hip yaw motion is powered by an actuator enclosed inside the thigh structure.

The knee joint is directly driven by a CompAct compliant actuator (peak torque of 55 Nm) at the centre of the knee joint, Fig.5.11. The ankle pitch motion is driven

Table 5.2 Range of motion of joints

Joint	Range of motion ()
Hip flexion/extension	+45, –110
Hip abduction/adduction	+60, –25
Thigh rotation	+50, –50
Knee flexion/extension	+110, –10
Ankle flexion/extension	+70, –50
Ankle inversion/eversion	+35, –35
Ankle twist	Not implemented
Waist pitch	+50, –20
Waist roll	+30, –30
Waist yaw	+80, –80
Shoulder flexion/extension	+95, –195
Shoulder abduction/adduction	+120, –18
Upper arm rotation	+90, –90
Elbow flexion/extension	+135, 0

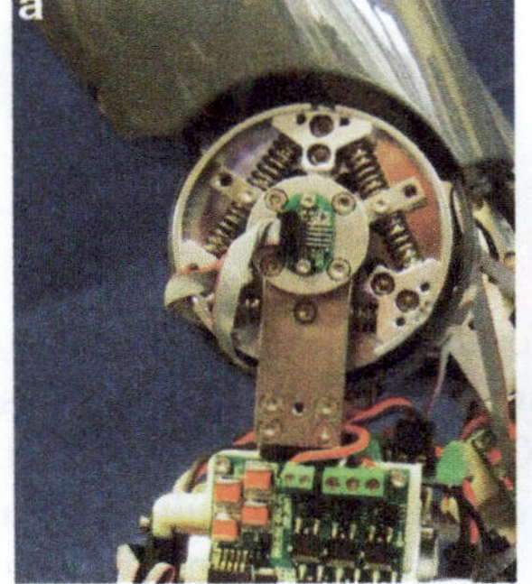

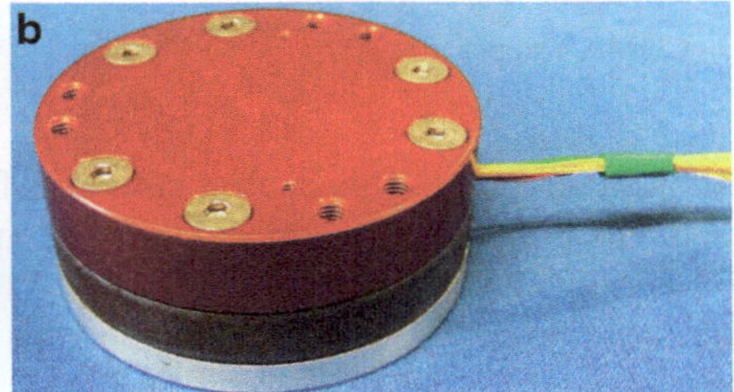

Fig. 5.11 (**a**) Knee joint and (**b**) custom design force torque sensor

by CompAct actuator (peak torque of 55 Nm) that is placed at the calf section. Torque to the ankle pitch motion is transferred through a four bar link transmission. The last DOF which produces ankle inversion/eversion uses a stiff actuator (peak torque of 55 Nm) located on the foot plate and directly coupled to the ankle roll joint.

In addition to the torque sensing in the individual joints, there are custom-designed DOF force/torque sensors integrated below the ankle joint to measure the interaction forces between the foot and the ground, Fig. 5.11.

5.4.1.4 Torso and Arm Design

The torso serves as a housing for the onboard processing unit and power autonomy system which includes the batteries and the battery management system. The core of the torso is made in titanium to give stiffness, strength and low weight to this

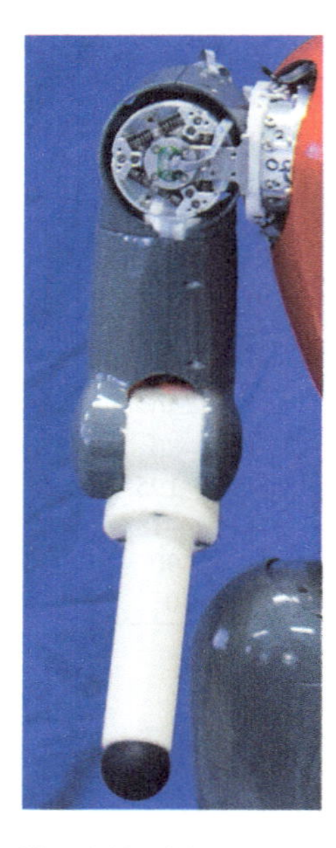

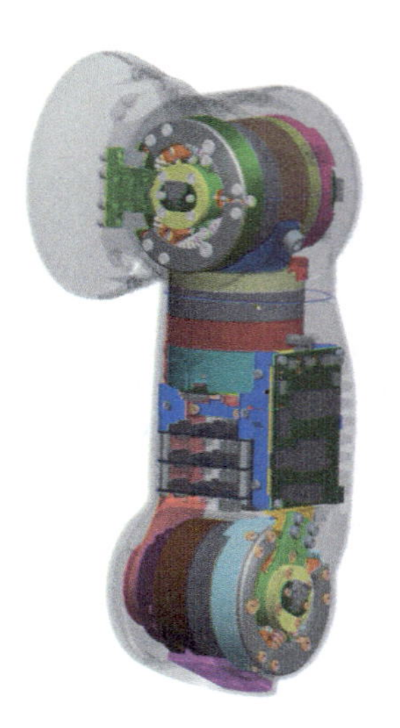

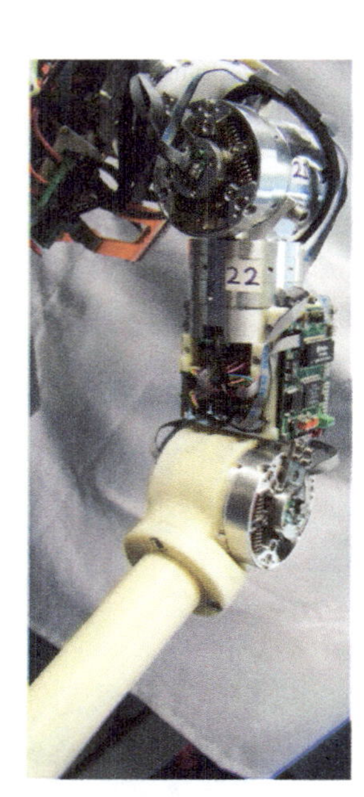

Fig. 5.12 COMAN upper arm

critical central structure. This central core also forms the mounting support of the shoulder flexion DOF in each arm and the neck modules. The onboard processing is based on an embedded dual core Pentium PC104 unit running at 2.5 GHz. The computational environment provides onboard computation (multi onboard PC modules combined with GPUs) connected via an EtherCAT network to distributed DSPs located at each joint. The battery is a custom 29 V lithium ion polymer battery with a gravimetric energy density of 180 Wh/Kg.

The upper arms have 4 DOF providing a typical pitch-roll-yaw shoulder kinematic arrangement and an elbow flexion/extension joint, Fig.5.12. The shoulder flexion/extension unit is entirely housed within the torso and is actuated by the SEA unit (peak torque of 55 Nm) described previously. The shoulder abduction/adduction (roll) is also powered by a similar SEA unit located at the centre of the shoulder joint. The final shoulder DOF (upper arm rotation) is actuated by a stiff actuator (with active compliance regulation ability) mounted within the forearm structure. The elbow is directly driven by a compliant (SEA) module (peak torque of 55 Nm) at the centre of the elbow joint, Fig.5.12. No forearm hand is mounted on this variant of the COMAN, although units for this have previously been shown in Davis et al. (2008).

The torque-controlled COMAN offers a unique opportunity to implement and test such novel controllers.

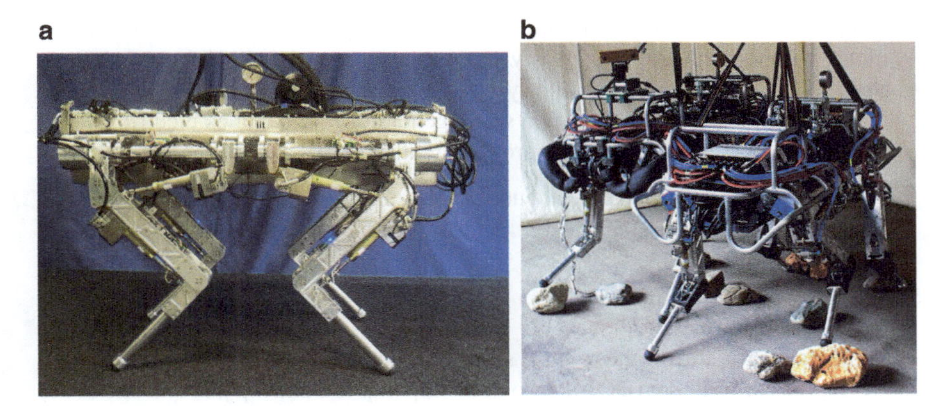

Fig. 5.13 (**a**) The hydraulically actuated quadruped robot HyQ, (**b**) Two naked HyQs showing mechanical parts (Semini et al. 2011)

5.4.2 HyQ Quadrupedal Robot

5.4.2.1 Goal and Specifications

The HyQ (hydraulic quadruped) robot shown in Fig. 5.13a, b is a versatile and high-performance quadruped robot that has been developed at the IIT during the past 7 years (Semini et al. 2011; Barasuol et al. 2012; Ugurlu et al. 2013). The main goals of developing HyQ are as follows:

- The creation of a robotic platform able to perform highly dynamic tasks such as running and jumping and able to move autonomously (in terms of energy and control) in difficult terrain, where wheeled robots cannot go
- To study biologically inspired locomotion focusing on dynamic running gaits and the importance of (adjustable) joint compliance, energy efficiency, gait pattern generation, gait transitions and robot balancing skills
- To study and test the applicability of hydraulic actuation to power legged robots. Furthermore, to evaluate low-level control algorithms and new system configurations and to test novel propulsion systems to increase the robot's energy-autonomous operating time

One of HyQ's goals is energy-autonomous operation for several hours. Since today's battery technology is not yet capable of providing energy for extended operating times in mobile robots, combustion engines (energy stored in fuel) are a better choice than electric motors (energy stored in batteries). The disadvantages of such engines are the noise and exhaust emissions although these are more acceptable for outdoor machines.

HyQ's development process has been divided into three stages:

- **Stage 1** has external supply of hydraulic pressure and flow and therefore does not carry a pump unit on board (approx. weight: 80 kg).

- **Stage 2** has an onboard hydraulic system with a pump actuated by an electric motor with external electric energy supply (approx. weight: 110 kg).
- **Stage 3** has an onboard hydraulic system whose pump is powered by an onboard internal combustion engine with a small generator that supplies electric energy to the motors and electronics (approx. weight: 90 kg).

To date stage 1 and 2 have been successfully tested.

5.4.2.2 Robot Kinematics

The kinematic structure of the robot is shown in Fig. 5.14. Each leg consists of three active degrees of freedom (DOF): Two in the hip (*hip a/a* and *hip f/e*) and one in the knee (*knee f/e*). In some early versions of the HyQ, there was a fourth passive DOF at the ankle joint consisting of a mechanical spring located on the lower leg segment. In later versions, the compliance offered by the spring was provided by the torque-controlled software and was no longer needed. This helped to reduce the mass at the foot. The leg configuration is based on the skeletal configuration of cursorial mammals.

5.4.2.3 Performance Specifications

For a quadruped robot, performance is typically determined by the desired locomotion gaits (walk, trot or gallop/bound), maximum running speed, jumping height, etc.

As it is not trivial to express these specifications in numbers, inspiration was taken from both the animal kingdom and existing robots. In nature, several quadruped running gaits can be observed, depending on the timing of leg touchdown and the coupling of the diagonal or lateral pair of legs. It has been generally accepted that quadruped animals choose the gait and preferred forward velocity to minimise energy consumption and to avoid injuries created by excessive musculoskeletal forces at foot touchdown (Hoyt and Taylor 1981; Farley and Taylor 1991).

The trot, which pairs diagonal legs, exhibits good energy efficiency over a wide range of running speeds and shows no significant pitch or roll motion during each strides. It is often seen in nature (Nanua and Waldron 1995). Several robots with similar dimensions and mass to HyQ, such as KOLT (Nichol et al. 2004) and BigDog have successfully demonstrated trotting. Furthermore, the trot gait can be used even at zero forward velocity which was useful in early trials as a wide range of velocities can be tested without implementing walk/trot gait transition. Heglund and Taylor studied a large range of running quadruped animals and concluded that common trotting speeds and stride frequencies are related to the animal's body mass (Heglund and Taylor 1988). Table 5.3 lists these results for HyQ's estimated weights during the two stages of development. Trotting was selected as the baseline dynamic gait.

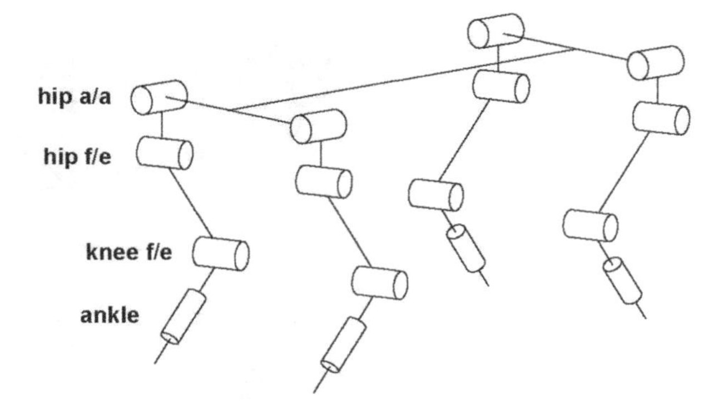

Fig. 5.14 Kinematic structure of the 16-DOF robot: each leg consists of three active joints, hip a/a, hip f/e and knee f/e. The fourth DOF is a passive ankle joint

Table 5.3 Trotting speed and stride frequencies of quadrupeds

Quadruped's mass	50 kg	90 kg
Minimum trotting gait	1.57 m/s 1.70 Hz	1.82 m/s 1.61 Hz
Preferred trotting gait	2.6 m/s 2.01 Hz	2.96 m/s 1.87 Hz
Maximum trotting gait	3.56 m/s 2.33 Hz	4.07 m/s 2.13 Hz

We used the above considerations and estimates as a base for the robot component sizing and mechanical design.

5.4.2.4 Robot Leg Design

Based on the design and experimental study of a first prototype 2 DOF leg (Semini et al. 2008), an improved version with 3 active DOF (*Leg V2*) was constructed, Fig. 5.15. Table 5.4 lists the most important specifications of the leg.

Due to the cylinder attachment geometry [reported in Semini (2010)], the hydraulic joints have a non-linear torque vs. stroke length characteristic. An estimate of the required flow is provided in Semini et al. (2011).

5.4.2.5 Quadruped Robot Design

In the following sections full quadruped robot with its system components, list the robot's key specifications, show its mechanical structure and describe the hydraulic power and sensory systems. Table 5.5 lists the key specifications of the robot.

The total mass of HyQ (stage 1) is 80 kg. The mass of all four legs (including the cylinders and feet) is 21 kg, which is 23.3 % of the total robot mass. This corresponds well to animals with a comparable body weight (dogs and small horses), which have a relative leg mass of 19–26 % (Fedak et al. 1982).

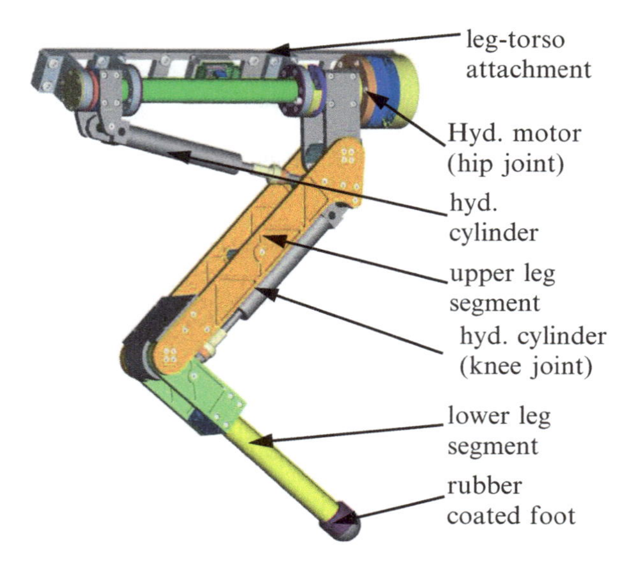

Fig. 5.15 CAD model of the improved robot leg design (*Leg V2*, 2011) (Semini et al. 2011)

Table 5.4 Specifications of the HyQ robot leg V2 (2011)

Description	Value
Active DOF	3 (2 hydraulic, 1 electric)
Joint range of all joints	120°
Electric motor gear reduction	1:100
Hydraulic cylinder stroke	80 mm
Piston area/Piston ring area	2.01 cm^2/1.23 cm^2

Table 5.5 Key specifications of HyQ (2013) robot

Description	Value
Dimensions (fully stretched legs)	1.0 m × 0.5 m × 0.98 m (Length × Width × Height)
Weight (2013)	80 kg (stage 1), 110 kg (stage 2)
Number of active DOF	12—(Hydraulic cylinders, four hydraulic rotary motors)
Joint range of motion	120°
Maximum torque (hydraulic)	145 Nm
Maximum hydraulic pressure $P_{\max}$	16 MPa
Onboard sensors	Joint position and torque, cylinder pressure, IMU, stereo cameras, Lidar
Onboard computer	PC104 Pentium, real-time Linux (low-level hardware control)
	Intel i7, Linux and ROS (high level processes eg state estimation, localization, mapping foothold computation)
Control frequency	1 kHz (position and torque)

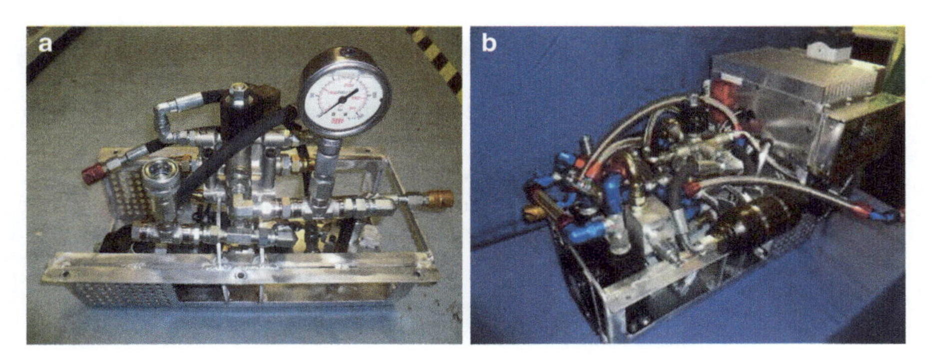

Fig. 5.16 (**a**) Hydraulic components for external power, (**b**) Full onboard hydraulic system

5.4.2.6 Mechanical Structure

Figure 5.13 shows the mechanical structure of HyQ. All mechanical parts are fabricated either in *Ergal*, a strong aluminium alloy (type 7075), or in stainless steel (39NiCrMo3) for the heavily stressed parts. The torso is formed from folded Ergal sheet (thickness 3 mm) with internal ribbing to increase torsional robustness. This design is simple, rigid, (comparatively) light-weight, easy to manufacture and leaves space to mount and accommodate secondary components.

5.4.2.7 Hydraulic System

The hydraulic system consists of a pump powered by an 8–9 kW ac electric motor (stage 2), oil 0.5 L tank, heat exchanger, accumulator, filter, central manifold with relief and vent valve, 12 MOOG E024 valves, pressure sensors, 8 hydraulic cylinders (Hoerbiger LB6-1610), 4 rotary hydraulic motors (Hydro-hips), fittings and tubing/hosing. Figure 5.16 shows the hydraulic system as mounted within the robot torso.

5.4.2.8 Sensory System

The robot is equipped with a network of over 50 sensors for low- and high-level control, system state monitoring and diagnostics, comprising the following: a relative (high resolution) and an absolute encoder on each active joint, compression/tension load cells they are removed since the upgrade with the MOOG valves for each hydraulic cylinder, IMU on robot torso and several sensors to measure the state of the hydraulic system. For external perception some variants have stereo vision (bumble bee), RGBD colour and depth sensor (Microsoft Kinect) and lidar (Velodyne), together with custom-built force/torque sensing in the feet.

5.5 Conclusions

While legged robots certainly in the short term to medium term will be restricted to relatively specialised domains, it is clear that there are emerging specific tasks for which these robots are best suited, and with the developments in the applications, the confidence and the technical know-how, the prospects for legged robots (both bipedal and quadrupedal) have never been better.

References

Akachi K, Kaneko K, Kanehira N, Ota S, Miyamori G, Hirata M, Kajita S, Kanehiro F (2005) Development of humanoid robot HRP-3P. In: 2005 5th IEEE-RAS international conference on humanoid robots. IEEE, pp 50–55

Asfour T, Azad P, Vahrenkamp N, Regenstein K, Bierbaum A, Welke K, Schroeder J, Dillmann R (2008) Toward humanoid manipulation in human-centred environments. Robot Auton Syst 56:54–65

Barasuol V, Buchli J, Semini C, Frigerio M, De Pieri ER, Caldwell DG (2012) A reactive controller framework for quadrupedal locomotion on challenging terrain. In: IEEE international conference on robotics and automation (ICRA)

Darpa (2013) http://www.darpa.mil/Our_Work/TTO/Programs/DARPA_Robotics_Challenge.aspx

Davis S, Tsagarakis NG, Caldwell DG (2008) The initial design and manufacturing process of a low cost hand for the robot iCub. In: IEEE humanoids 2008. Daejean, Korea, December 2008, pp 40–45

Electra (2011) http://www.elettra.trieste.it/lightsources/labs-and-services/scientific-computing/sincrobot.html

Farley C, Taylor C (1991) A mechanical trigger for the trot-gallop transition in horses. Science 253 (5017):306–308

Fedak MA, Heglund NC, Taylor CR (1982) Energetics and mechanics of terrestrial locomotion. Kinetic energy changes of the limbs and body as a function of speed and body size in birds and mammals. J Exp Biol 79:23–40

Heglund NC, Taylor CR (1988) Speed, stride frequency and energy-cost per stride—how do they change with body size and gait. J Exp Biol 138:301–318

Hirai K, Hirose M, Haikawa Y, Takenaka T (1998) The development of Honda humanoid robot. In: Proceedings of the 1998 I.E. international conference on robotics and automation. IEEE, pp 1321–1326

Hirose M, Ogawa K (2007) Honda humanoid robots development. Philos Trans A Math Phys Eng Sci 365:11–19

Hirose R, Takenaka T (2001) Development of the humanoid robot ASIMO. Honda R&D Tech Rev 13:1–6

Hoyt D, Taylor R (1981) Gait and the energetics of locomotion in horses. Nature 292:239–240

Hurst J (2011) The electric cable differential leg: a novel design approach for walking and running. Int J HR 8(02):301–321

Hurst JW, Rizzi AA (2008) Series compliance for an efficient running gait. IEEE Trans Robot Autom 15(3):42–51

Kaneko K, Harada K, Kanehiro F, Miyamori G, Akachi K (2008) Humanoid robot HRP-3. In: IEEE/RSJ international conference on intelligent robots and systems (IROS 2008), September 2008, pp 2471–2478

Li Z, Tsagarakis N, Caldwell DG (2012) A passivity based cartesian admittance control for stabilizing the compliant humanoid COMAN. In: 2012 IEEE-RAS international conference on humanoid robots, IEEE Humanoids'12, Osaka, Japan, November 2012, pp 44–49

Lohmeier S, Buschmann T, Ulbrich H, Pfeiffer F (2006) Modular joint design for performance enhanced humanoid robot LOLA. In: IEEE international conference on robotics and automation (ICRA 2006), May 2006, pp 88–93

Metta G, Sandini G, Vernon D, Natale L, Nori F (2008) The iCub humanoid robot: an open platform for research in embodied cognition. In: Proceedings of the 8th workshop on performance metrics for intelligent systems, 2008. ACM, pp 50–56

Nanua P, Waldron KJ (1995) Energy comparison between trot, bound, and gallop using a simple model. J Biomed Eng 117(4):466–473

Nichol JG, Singh SPN, Waldron KJ, Palmer LR, Orin DE (2004) System design of a quadrupedal galloping machine. Int J Rob Res 23(10–11):1013–1027

Ogura Y, Aikawa H, Shimomura K, Kondo H, Morishima A, Ok Lim H, Takanishi A (2006) Development of a new humanoid robot WABIAN-2. In: IEEE international conference on robotics and automation (ICRA 2006), May 2006, pp 76–81

Park IW, Kim JY, Lee J, Oh JH (2007) Mechanical design of the humanoid robot platform, HUBO. Adv Robot 21:1305–1322

Pratt GA, Williamson MM (1995) Series elastic actuators. In: IEEE/RSJ international conference on intelligent robots and systems—workshop on 'human robot interaction and cooperative robots', Pittsburg, PA, pp 399–406. D:\Dropbox\MyPhDThesis\ReferenceArticles\SEA_mattw_ms_thesis.pdf

Pratt J, Koolen T, De Boer T, Rebula J, Cotton S, Carff J, Johnson M, Neuhaus P (2012) Capturability-based analysis and control of legged locomotion, part 2: application to M2V2, a lower-body humanoid. Int J Rob Res 31:1117–1133

Sang-Ho H, Hale JG, Cheng G (2007) Full-body compliant human-humanoid interaction: balancing in the presence of unknown external forces. IEEE Trans Robot Autom 23:884–898

Semini C (2010) HyQ – design and development of a hydraulically actuated quadruped robot. Ph.D. thesis, Italian Institute of Technology, University of Genoa, Italy

Semini C, Tsagarakis NG, Vanderborght B, Yang Y, Caldwell DG (2008) HyQ—hydraulically actuated quadruped robot: hopping leg prototype. In: IEEE BioRob, pp 593–599

Semini C, Tsagarakis NG, Guglielmino E, Focchi M, Cannella F, Caldwell DG (2011) Design of HyQ – a hydraulically and electrically actuated quadruped robot. Proc Inst Mec Eng Part I J Syst Eng Control 225(6):831–849

Tsagarakis NG, Metta G, Sandini G, Vernon D, Beira R, Santos-Victor J, Carrazzo MC, Becchi F, Caldwell DG (2007) iCub—the design and realisation of an open humanoid platform for cognitive and neuroscience research. Int J Adv Robot 21(10):1151–1175

Tsagarakis NG, Laffranchi M, Vanderborght B, Caldwell DG (2009) A compact soft actuator unit for small scale human friendly robots. In: ICRA 2009, Kobe, Japan, May 2009, pp 4356–4362

Tsagarakis NG, Zhibin Li, Saglia JA, Caldwell DG (2011) The design of the lower body of the compliant humanoid robot "cCub". In: IEEE international conference on robotics and automation, ICRA 2011, Shanghai, China, May 2011, pp 2035–2040

Tsagarakis N, Sardellitti I, Caldwell DG (2011) A new variable stiffness actuator (CompAct-VSA) design, implementation and modelling. In: IEEE/RSJ proceedings of international conference on intelligent robots and systems, IROS'11, San Francisco, CA, September 2011, pp 378–383

Tsagarakis NG, Morfey S, Medrano-Cerda GA, Li Z, Caldwell DG (2013) Development of compliant humanoid robot COMAN: body design and Stiffness Tuning. In: IEEE international conference on robotics and automation 2013 (ICRA 2013), Karlsruhe, Germany, pp 665–670

Ugurlu B, Havoutis I, Semini C, Caldwell DG (2013) Dynamic trot-walking with the hydraulic quadruped robot—HyQ: analytical trajectory generation and active compliance control. In: IEEE/RSJ international conference on intelligent robots and systems (IROS)

Chapter 6
Sensorimotor Coordination in a Humanoid Robot: Building Intelligence on the iCub

Lorenzo Natale, Francesco Nori, Alberto Parmiggiani, and Giorgio Metta

6.1 Introduction

Sensorimotor coordination in humanoid robots is the key to accomplish realistic human behavior. Paradigmatic tasks in sensorimotor coordination include force and impedance control, whole-body coordination during physical interaction with the environment, point-to-point reaching movements, and grasping visually identified objects. To tackle these problems a variety of sensors and methods have to be integrated, including vision, force and touch, hand-coded models, and machine learning. This requires a careful balance of the a priori design effort in order to properly manage the complexity of data collection for learning and the overall performance of the robotic system. In this chapter we treat the implementation of these techniques on the well-known iCub humanoid robot.

It is the case that humanoid robots are becoming increasingly complex and, to a certain extent, they can now imitate human behavior. One of the greatest challenges in designing controllers for humanoid robots is the implementation of interfaces that allow humans to collaborate, communicate, and teach robots as naturally and efficiently as they would with other human beings (Lallee et al. 2010). This line of inquiry follows a twofold approach by drawing on our knowledge of natural cognition and, simultaneously, by instantiating plausible models of cognitive skills on humanoid robots (Metta et al. 2010; Vernon et al. 2007). The hallmark of cognition, according, e.g., to developmental psychologists (von Hofsten 2004), is the ability to predict the behavior of the environment and the consequences of the interaction with the body, simulating and evaluating the possible outcomes of actions before they are actually executed. In the brain, this is thought to happen through the activation of appropriate sensorimotor schemas (Gallese et al. 1996) that effectively function to couple sensory and motor signals in planning sensible

L. Natale (✉) • F. Nori • A. Parmiggiani • G. Metta
Central Research Laboratory, Istituto Italiano di Tecnologia, Genova, Italy
e-mail: lorenzo.natale@iit.it

R. Cingolani (ed.), *Bioinspired Approaches for Human-Centric Technologies*,
DOI 10.1007/978-3-319-04924-3_6, © Springer International Publishing Switzerland 2014

actions. Sensorimotor schemas have been long posited to be a functional explanation of the brain's direct and effortless perception of the environment and its properties leading to efficient action execution (Gibson 1977; Arbib 1981). The literature abounds of computational and robotic models of these sensorimotor schemas as, for example, the work of Miyamoto et al. (1996).

In this chapter we consider a variety of basic sensorimotor coordination problems which are typically encountered in the domain of humanoid robotics. These make up the baseline to address larger applications such as the already mentioned human-robot collaboration scenario. In particular, we focus on the problem of force and impedance control, whole-body coordination during physical interaction with the environment, point-to-point reaching movement, and finally grasping visually identified objects. Our reference platform is the iCub (Metta et al. 2010), a humanoid robot shaped as a three-and-half-years-old child. The iCub, by design, only uses "passive" sensors as, for example, cameras, gyroscopes, pressure, force and contact sensors, microphones, and so forth. We excluded the use of lasers, sonars, and other esoteric sensing modalities.

In these conditions and in an unstructured environment where humans can freely move and work (our laboratory space in the daily use of the iCub), it is unlikely that the robot obtains any accurate model of the environment for accurate impact-free planning of movements. One common solution (Villani and De Shutteer 2008) is to control the robot's mechanical impedance and, simultaneously, minimize impacts by using, for example, vision and trajectory planning. The possibility of impedance control lowers the requirements on visual accuracy and guarantees a certain degree of safety in case of unexpected contacts with the environment—though, strictly speaking, the robot can still be potentially dangerous and cause damage if moving fast.

The lowest level component of the control architecture described in this chapter is not very different, in principle, from a standard computed torque approach (Sciavicco and Siciliano 2005) in that it compensates for the robot dynamics and linearizes the system. Because of the communication bus of the iCub microcontrollers, bandwidth requirements, and various implementation constraints (e.g., CPU speed), it has been designed to operate in joint space only. The robot dynamics can be computed either from a simple Newton-Euler formulation or via nonparametric function approximation as shown later.

Force control is the starting point to implement more sophisticated controllers that use knowledge of contact forces to, e.g., simultaneously balance the robot and achieve useful tasks (e.g., grasp an object, open a door, etc.). This is addressed via a control approach called "prioritized motion-force control" which in our specific formulation can take into account hybrid motion and force control, soft and rigid contacts, and free (floating base) and constrained robots. This opens up the possibility of executing tasks that involve the robot moving in the environment to retrieve an object, lift, and carry it to a different location. It also allows manipulating the environment; opening drawers, doors, etc.; and interacting physically with people as in the case of human-robot cooperation tasks.

Reaching and pointing belong to a special class of movements which deserves a dedicated study. They are fundamental in learning about the environment enabling object interaction and manipulation as, e.g., pushing, grasping, tapping, swiping, etc. For this reason a separate section in the following deals with the case of arm-hand point-to-point movements. With respect to the prioritized motion-force controller described above, reaching can be seen simply as the specification of a trajectory of the hands in space, i.e., the reference signals or reference force/ impedance profiles depending on the exact formulation of the task. Finally, in order to be useful, the robot needs to manipulate the object that has just been reached. For this reason vision is employed to estimate the shape of the object and plan the placement of the fingers in such a way to guarantee grasp stability.

6.2 Experimental Platform: The iCub

The iCub is one of the humanoid robotic platforms developed at the Italian Institute of Technology (IIT). The project was launched by RobotCub (Metta 2010), a joint IIT-EU endeavor to create a common platform for researchers interested in embodied artificial cognitive systems.

The initial specifications of the robot aimed at replicating the size of a three-and-a-half-year-old child. In particular, it was required that the robot be capable of crawling on all fours and possess fine manipulation abilities. For a motivation of why these features are important, the interested reader is referred to Metta et al. (2005).

Dimensions, kinematic layout, and range of movement were drafted by considering biomechanical models and anthropometric tables (Tilley 2002). Rigid body simulations were used to determine the crucial kinematic features in order to perform the set of desired tasks and motions, i.e., reaching, crawling, etc. (Tsagarakis et al. 2007). These simulations also provided joint torque requirements. Data were then used as a baseline performance indicator for the selection of the actuators. The final kinematic structure of the robot is shown in Fig. 6.1c. The iCub has 53 degrees of freedom (DoF). Its kinematics has several special features which are rarely found in other humanoid robots: e.g., the waist has three DoFs which considerably increase the robot's mobility; the three DoF shoulder joint is constructed to have its axes of rotation always intersecting at one point.

To match the torque requirements, we employed rotary electric motors coupled with speed reducers. We found this to be the most suitable choice in terms of robustness and reliability. Motor groups with various characteristics were developed (e.g., 40 Nm, 20 Nm, and 11 Nm) for different placements into the iCub. We used the Kollmorgen-Danaher Motion RBE-type brushless frameless motor (BLM) and a CSD frameless Harmonic Drive as speed reducer. The use of frameless components allowed further optimization of space and reduced weight. Smaller motors for moving the fingers, eyes, and neck are from Faulhaber in various sizes and reduction gear ratios.

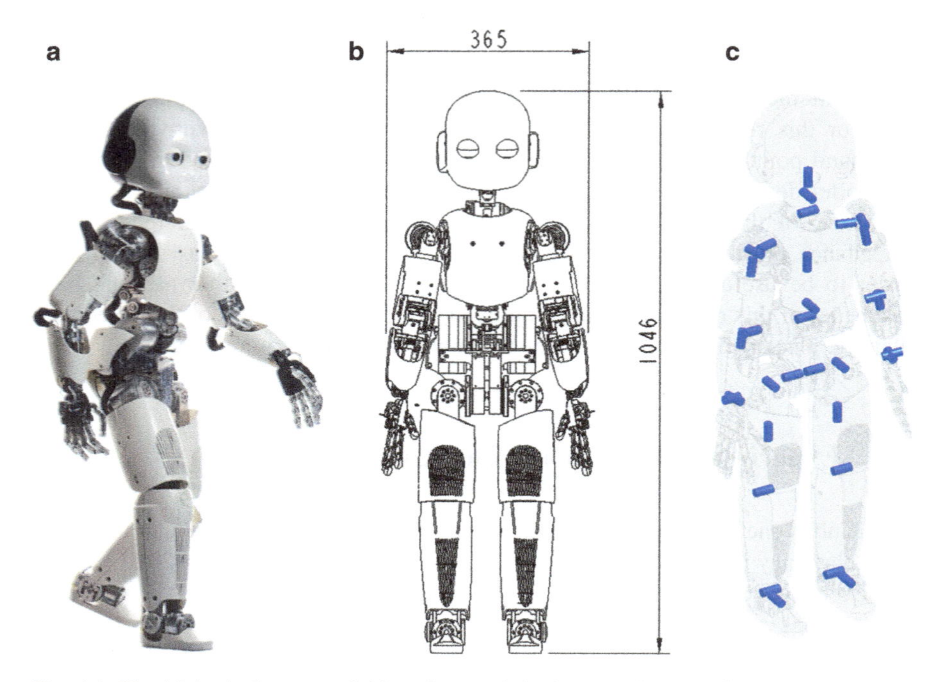

Fig. 6.1 The iCub platform: panel (**a**) a picture of the latest realization of the iCub; panel (**b**) approximate dimensions height × width; and panel (**c**) the kinematic structure of the major joints

Cable drives were used almost everywhere on the iCub. Most joints have relocated, motors as, for example, in the hand, shoulder (but the first joint), elbow, waist and legs (apart from two joints). Cable drives are efficient and almost mandatory in order to optimize the motor locations and the overall "shape" of the robot. All joints in the hand are cable driven. The hand of the iCub has 20 joints which are moved by nine motors: this implies that some of the fingers are under-actuated and their movement is obtained by means of the cable couplings. Similar to the human body, most of the hand actuation is in the forearm subsection. The head is another particular component of the iCub enabling independent vergence movements supported by a three DoFs neck for a total of six DoFs.

By design we decided to only use "passive sensors" and in particular cameras, microphones, gyroscopes and accelerometers, force/torque (FTS), and tactile sensors as well as the traditional motor encoders. Of special relevance is the sensorized skin which is not easily found in other platforms as well as the force/torque sensors that are used for force/impedance control (see later). No active sensing is provided as, for example, lasers, structured light projectors, and so forth.

The iCub mounts custom-designed electronics which consists of programmable controller cards, amplifiers, DACs, and digital I/O cards. This ecosystem of micro-controller cards relies on multiple CAN bus lines (up to 10) for communication and synchronization and then connects with a cluster of external machines via a Gbit/s

Ethernet network. Data are acquired and synchronized (and time stamped) before being made available on the network. We designed the software middleware that supports data acquisition and control of the robot as well as all the firmware that operates on the microcontrollers which eventually drive each single transistor that moves the motors.

The software middleware is called YARP (Fitzpatrick et al. 2008). YARP is a thin library that enables multi-platform and multi-IDE development and collaboration by providing a layer that shields the user from the quirks of the underlying operating system and robot hardware controllers. The complete design of the iCub (drawings, schematics, specifications) and its software (both middleware and controllers) is distributed according to the GPL and LGPL licenses.

6.2.1 iCub 2.0

More recently we released an updated version of the iCub which shares some of the advanced mechatronic solutions for the bodyware already described in Chap. 5 for the compliant robot Coman (such as the new legs with series-elastic actuators—SEAs), a new industrially viable version of the skin sensors, and a new version of the microcontroller cards with Ethernet connectivity [for a complete description, see Parmiggiani et al. (2012b)]. Almost all subsystems were affected including a new head design, a consistent revision of the hands especially in the routing of the cables for improved durability, a new version of the skin, and electronics with Ethernet connectivity. Simultaneously we "ported" certain features of Coman, more specifically the SEAs, to the iCub. We included a SEA joint at the knee and ankle, high-resolution encoders in the SEA for torque control, the removal of the cable at the ankle, and an overall improvement by simplifying the design with respect to both the original iCub and Coman.

Previous experiments with Coman allowed determining a suitable value for the torsional stiffness of the elastic modules. The optimal value was found to be in the range of 300–350 [Nm/rad]. Being the maximum leg actuator torque in the ballpark of 40 [Nm], the required passive angular deflection of the SEA which permits the delivery of the peak torque within the elastic deflection range is in the order of 0.1333 [rad]. The elastic module of Coman however did not allow to obtain such torsional stiffness values. During experimentation, the elastic deflection limit was reached at about 50 % of the maximum torque, canceling the benefits of the integration of the SEA modules. We therefore considered possible alternative designs of the elastic components. As described in Tsagarakis et al. (2011), the elastic module of Coman comprises three pairs of opposing helical springs. We considered the substitution of the springs with a different set of helical springs, disk springs, and volute springs while keeping the overall mechanics as close as possible to the original size. We considered a different design comprising leaf springs. The "stiffness envelopes" of the different alternatives are represented in Fig. 6.2 panel (a). None of them allowed obtaining the desired torsional rigidity. The selection of

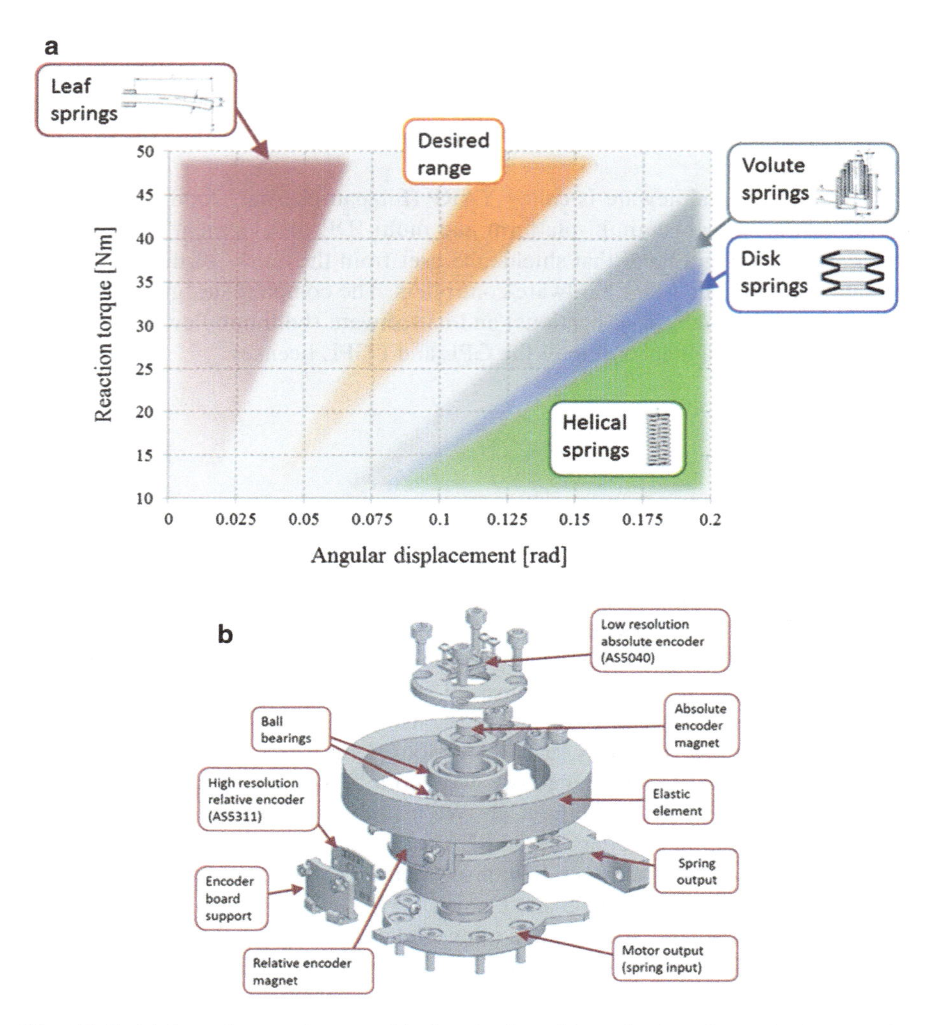

Fig. 6.2 In (**a**) the spring envelopes used in the selection of the technology for the SEA actuator's "C-spring" described in text, (**b**) the exploded view of the SEA mechanical design; not the "C-shaped" spring

the springs represents a very delicate trade-off. In general only springs with a diameter < 12 [mm] were compliant enough to achieve the desired stiffness levels in the available volume. Unfortunately these springs would reach their yield point well before the maximum loads. On the other hand, springs capable of withstanding these loads would be too big to be integrated in the elastic mechanical components.

The original solution we devised consists of a "curved beam" spring that we call "C-spring," somewhat similar to the Robonaut torsional spring (Ihrke et al. 2010). By means of analytical calculations, it is shown to be a viable design alternative. We first designed the spring shape via standard calculations and then verified the results both through FEM analysis and later experimentally on the robot. The experimental results yielded about 30 % lower stiffness than expected, a fact to be corrected in the future, although it was not critical for the current release of the iCub (i.e., our design safety margins were large enough to accommodate this variation). For a complete description and evaluation of the SEAs, the reader is referred to the Parmiggiani et al. (2012a) paper and a more recent comparison of SEA vs. stiff actuation in Eljaik et al. (2013).

6.3 Torque Control

Torque control lays at the lowest level in the hierarchy of sensorimotor problems since it results in the calculation of the joint reference torques that drive the motors. Torque control requires the computation of the body dynamics to separate internal from external wrenches. In its simplest possible version, the microcontroller cards implement a 1 ms feedback loop relying on the error e defined as

$$e = \tau - \tau_{\mathrm{d}}, \tag{6.1}$$

where τ is the vector of joint torques and τ_{d} its desired value. We do not know τ directly on the iCub but we have access to estimates through the force/torque sensors (FTSs). They are mounted as indicated in Fig. 6.3 in the upper part of the limbs and can therefore be used to detect wrenches at any location in the iCub limbs and not only at the end-effector as it is more typical for industrial manipulators.

We show that τ can be estimated from the FTS measurements of each limb (equations repeat identical for each limb). Let's indicate with w_{s} the wrench measured by the FTS and assume that it is due to an actual external wrench at a known location (e.g., at the end-effector) which we call w_{e}. We can estimate w_{e} by propagating the measurement on the kinematic chain of the limb (changing coordinates):

$$\hat{w}_{\mathrm{e}} = \begin{bmatrix} I & 0 \\ -[\overline{r}_{\mathrm{se}}]_{\times} & I \end{bmatrix} \cdot (w_{\mathrm{s}} - w_{\mathrm{i}}), \tag{6.2}$$

with $[\overline{r}_{\mathrm{se}}]_{\times}$ the skew-symmetric matrix representing the cross product with the vector $\overline{r}_{\mathrm{se}}$, $\hat{w}_{\mathrm{e}}$ the estimate of w_{e}, and w_{i} the internal wrench (due to internal forces and moments). Note that $[\overline{r}_{\mathrm{se}}]_{\times}$ is a function of q, the vector of joint angles. w_{i} can be estimated from the dynamics of the limb (either with the Lagrange or Newton–Euler formulation). To estimate τ_{e} we only need to project $\hat{w}_{\mathrm{e}}$ to the joint torques using the transposed Jacobian, i.e.:

$$\hat{\tau}_{\mathrm{e}} = J^{\mathrm{T}}(q) \cdot \hat{w}_{\mathrm{e}}. \tag{6.3}$$

We can then use this estimate in a control loop by defining the torque error e as

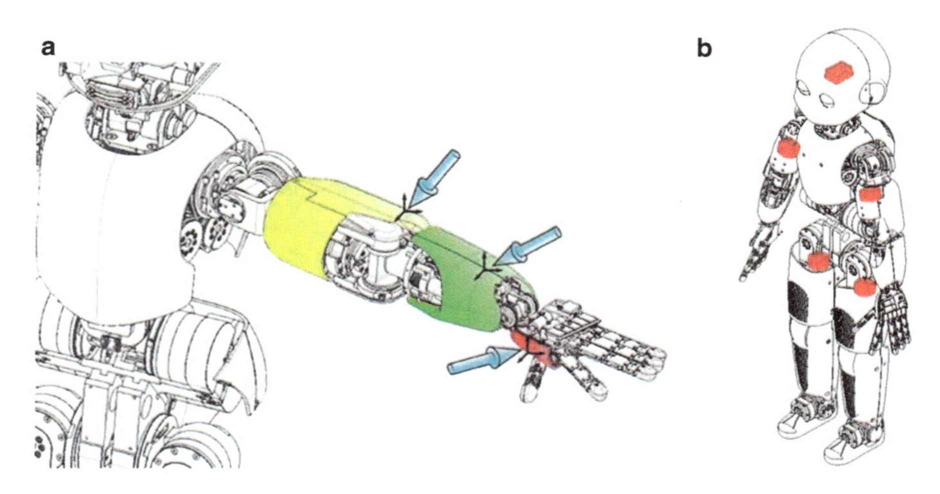

Fig. 6.3 In (**a**) a typical interaction of the iCub arm with the environment exemplified here with a number of wrenches at different locations and in (**b**) the location of the four FTSs of the iCub in the upper part of the limbs (proximal with respect to the reference frame of the robot kinematic chains) and of the inertial sensors mounted in the head

$$e = \hat{\tau}_{\mathrm{e}} - \tau_{\mathrm{d}}, \tag{6.4}$$

where $\hat{\tau}_{\mathrm{e}}$ is an estimate of τ regulated by a PID controller of the form:

$$u = k_{\mathrm{p}} \cdot e + k_{\mathrm{d}} \cdot \dot{e} + k_{\mathrm{i}} \cdot \int e, \tag{6.5}$$

where k_{p}, k_{d}, and k_{i} are the usual PID gains and u the amplifier output (the PWM duty cycle which determines the equivalent applied voltage at the motor). Similarly we can build an impedance controller in joint space by making τ_{d} of the form

$$\tau_{\mathrm{d}} = K \cdot (q - q_{\mathrm{d}}) + D \cdot (\dot{q} - \dot{q}_{\mathrm{d}}), \tag{6.6}$$

which can be implemented at the controller card level if K and D are diagonal matrices. Furthermore, we can command velocity by making

$$q_{\mathrm{d}}(t) = q_{\mathrm{d}}(t - \delta t) + \dot{q}_{\mathrm{d}}(t)\delta t, \tag{6.7}$$

with δt the control cycle interval (1 ms in our case). This latter modality is useful when generating whole trajectories incrementally. The actual computation of the dynamics and kinematics is based on a graph representation which we detail in the following. Other control laws can be easily designed as described later in Sect. 6.4.

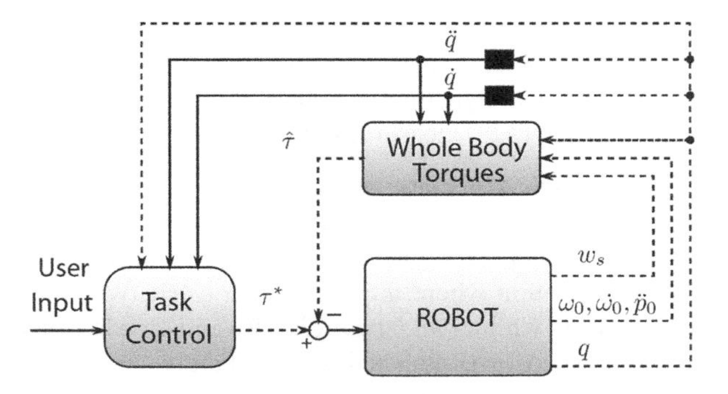

Fig. 6.4 The torque controller of the iCub. See text for details

6.3.1 iCub Dynamics

We start by considering an open (single or multiple branches) kinematic chain with n DoF composed of $n + 1$ links. Adopting the Denavit-Hartenberg notation (Sciavicco and Siciliano 2005), we define a set of reference frames $\langle 0 \rangle$, $\langle 1 \rangle$, ..., $\langle n \rangle$, attached at each link. The ith link of the chain is described by a vertex v_i (sometimes called node), usually represented by the symbol $\textcircled{i}$. A hinge joint between the link i and the link j (i.e., a rotational joint) is represented by an oriented edge $e_{i,j}$ connecting v_i with v_j: $\textcircled{i} \rightarrow \textcircled{j}$;. In an n DoF open chain, each vertex (except for the initial and terminal, v_0 and v_n, respectively) has two edges. Therefore, the graph representation of the n-link chain is an oriented sequence of nodes v_i, connected by edges $e_{i-1,i}$. The orientation of the edges can be either chosen arbitrarily (it will be clear later on that the orientation simply induces a convention) or it can follow from the exploration of the kinematic tree according to the *regular numbering scheme* (Featherstone and Orin 2008), which induces a parent–child relationship such that each node has a unique input edge and multiple output edges. We further follow the classical Denavit-Hartenberg notation, we assume that each joint has an associated reference frame with the z-axis aligned with the rotation axis; this frame will be denoted $\langle e_{i,j} \rangle$. In kinematics, an edge $e_{i,j}$ from v_i to v_j represents the fact that $\langle e_{i,j} \rangle$ is fixed in the ith link. In dynamics, $e_{i,j}$ represents the fact that the dynamic equations will compute (and make use of) $w_{i,j}$, i.e., the wrench that the ith link exerts on the jth link, and not the equal and opposite reaction—$w_{i,j}$, i. e., the wrench that the jth link exerts on the ith link. In order to simplify the computations of the inverse dynamics on the graph, kinematic and dynamic measurements have been explicitly represented. Specifically, the graph representation has been enhanced with a new set of graphical symbols: a triangle to represent kinematic quantities (i.e., velocities and acceleration of links—$\omega, \dot{\omega}, \dot{p}, \ddot{p}$) and a rhombus for wrenches (i.e., force sensors measurements on a link $- f, \mu$). Moreover these symbols have been further divided into known quantities to represent sensors measurements and unknown to indicate the quantities to be computed, as in the following:

- ∇: Unknown kinematic information
- $\blacktriangledown$: Known (e.g., measured) kinematic information
- $\diamond$: Unknown dynamic information
- $\blacklozenge$: Known (e.g., measured) dynamic information

In general, kinematic variables can be measured by means of gyroscopes, accelerometers, or simply inertial sensors. When attached on link i^{th}, these sensors provide angular and linear velocities and accelerations $(\omega, \dot{\omega}, \dot{p}, \text{and } \ddot{p})$ at the specific location where the sensor is located. We can represent this measurement in the graph with a *black triangle* ($\blacktriangledown$) and an additional edge from the proper link where the sensor is attached to the triangle. As usual, the edge has an associated reference frame, in this case corresponding to the reference frame of the sensor. An unknown kinematic variable is represented by a *white triangle* (∇) with an associated edge going from the link (where the unknown kinematic variable is attached) to the triangle. Similarly, we introduce two new types of nodes with a rhomboidal shape: *black rhombus* ($\blacklozenge$) to represent known (i.e., measured) wrenches and *white rhombus* ($\diamond$) to represent unknown wrenches which need to be computed. The reference frame associated to the edge will be the location of the applied or unknown wrench. The complete graph for the iCub is shown in Fig. 6.5.

From the graph structure, we can define the update rule that brings information across edges, and by traversing the graph, we therefore compute either dynamical or kinematic unknowns ($\diamond$and ∇, respectively). For kinematic quantities this is

$$\begin{aligned} \omega_{i+1} &= \omega_i + \dot{\theta}_{i+1} z_i, \\ \dot{\omega}_{i+1} &= \dot{\omega}_i + \ddot{\theta}_{i+1} z_i + \dot{\theta}_{i+1} \omega_i \times z_i, \\ \ddot{p}_{i+1} &= \ddot{p}_i + \dot{\omega}_i \times r_{i,i+1} + \omega_{i+1} \times (\omega_{i+1} \times r_{i,i+1}), \end{aligned} \tag{6.8}$$

where z_i is the z-axis of $\langle i \rangle$, i.e., we propagate information from the base to the end-effector visiting all nodes and moving from one node to the next following the edges. The internal dynamics of the manipulator can be studied as well: if the dynamical parameters of the system are known (mass m_i, inertia I_i, center of mass C_i), then we can propagate knowledge of wrenches applied to, e.g., the end-effector (f_{n+1} and μ_{n+1}) to the base frame of the manipulator so as to retrieve forces and moments f_i, μ_i:

$$\begin{aligned} f_i &= f_{i+1} + m_i \ddot{p}_{C_i}, \\ \mu_i &= \mu_{i+1} - f_i \times r_{i-1,C_i} + f_{i+1} \times r_{r_i,C_i} + I_i \dot{\omega}_i + \omega_i \times (I_i \omega_i), \end{aligned} \tag{6.9}$$

where

$$\ddot{p}_{C_i} = \ddot{p}_i + \dot{\omega}_i \times r_{i,C_i} + \omega_i \times (\omega_i \times r_{i,C_i}), \tag{6.10}$$

noting that these are the classical recursive Newton-Euler equations. Knowledge of wrenches enables the computation of w_i as needed in (6.2) or the corresponding joint torques from $\tau_i = \mu_i^{\mathrm{T}} z_{i-1}$.

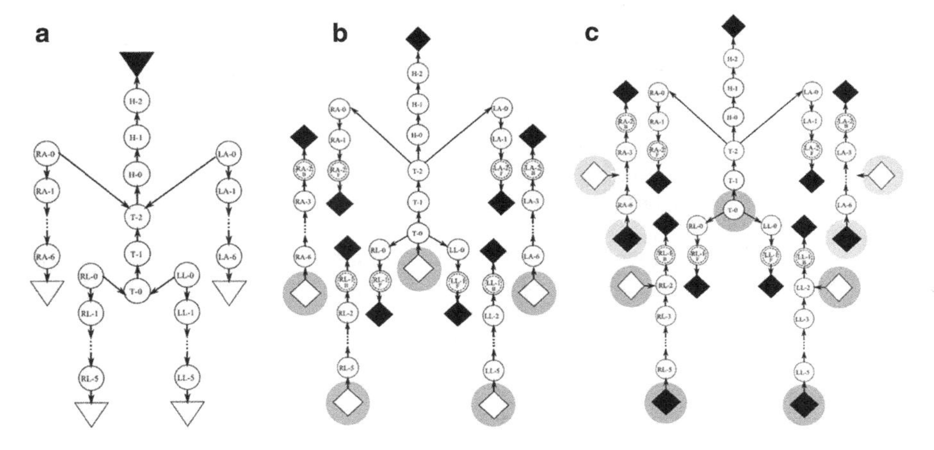

Fig. 6.5 Representation of iCub's kinematic and dynamic graph. In (**a**): iCub's kinematics. The inertial sensor measure (*black traingle*) is the unique source of kinematic information for the whole branched system. (**b**): iCub's dynamics when the robot is standing on the mainstay and moving freely in space. Given the four FTSs, the main graph is cut by the four links hosting the sensors, and a total of five subgraphs are finally generated. The unknowns are the external wrenches at the end-effectors: if the robot does not collide with the environment, they are zero, whereas if a collision happens, then an external wrench arises. The displacement between the expected and the estimated wrenches allows detecting contacts with the environment under the hypothesis that interactions can only occur at the end-effectors. The external wrench on top of the head is assumed to be null. Notice that the mainstay is represented by an unknown wrench *white rhombus*. (**c**): iCub's dynamics when the robot is crawling (four points of contact with the ground). As in the previous case, five subgraphs are generated after the insertion of the four FTSs measurements, but unlike the free-standing case, here the mainstay wrench is removed, being the iCub on the floor. Specific locations for the contacts with the environment are given as part of the task: the unknown external wrenches (*white rhombus*) are placed at wrists and knees, while wrenches at the feet and palms are assumed known and null (*black triangle*). Interestingly, while moving on the floor, the contact with the upper part could be varying (e.g., wrists, palms, elbows), so the unknown wrenches could be placed in different locations than the ones shown in the graph

6.3.2 Validation and Further Improvements

In order to validate computation of the dynamics, we compared measurements from the FTSs with their model-based prediction. The wrenches w_s from the four six-axes FTSs embedded in the limbs are compared with the analogous quantities $\hat{w}_s$ predicted by the dynamical model during unconstrained movements (i.e., null external wrenches). Kinematic and dynamic parameters are retrieved from the CAD model of the robot. Sensor measurements w_s can be predicted assuming known wrenches at the limb extremities (hands or feet) and then propagating forces up to the sensors. In this case, null wrenches are assumed because of the absence of contact with the environment. Table 6.1 summarizes the statistics of the errors $(w_s - \hat{w}_s)$ for each limb during a given, periodic sequence of movements, with the robot supported by a rigid metallic mainstay and with the limbs moving freely

Table 6.1 Error in predicting FT sensor measurement (see text for details)

	ε_{f0}	ε_{f1}	ε_{f2}	$\varepsilon_{\mu 0}$	$\varepsilon_{\mu 1}$	$\varepsilon_{\mu 2}$
$\bar{\varepsilon}$	−0.3157	−0.5209	0.7723	−0.0252	0.0582	0.0197
σ_ε	0.5845	0.7156	0.7550	0.0882	0.0688	0.0364
Right arm: $\varepsilon \equiv \hat{w}_{s,\,RA} - w_{s,\,RA}$						
$\bar{\varepsilon}$	−0.0908	−0.4811	0.8699	0.0436	0.0382	0.0030
σ_ε	0.5742	0.6677	0.7920	0.1048	0.0702	0.0332
Left arm: $\varepsilon \equiv \hat{w}_{s,\,LA} - w_{s,\,LA}$						
$\bar{\varepsilon}$	−1.6678	3.4476	−1.5505	0.4050	−0.7340	0.0171
σ_ε	3.3146	2.7039	1.7996	0.3423	0.7141	0.0771
Right leg: $\varepsilon \equiv \hat{w}_{s,\,RL} - w_{s,\,RL}$						
$\bar{\varepsilon}$	0.2941	−5.1476	−1.9459	−0.3084	−0.8399	0.0270
σ_ε	1.8031	1.8327	2.3490	0.3365	0.8348	0.0498
Left leg: $\varepsilon \equiv \hat{w}_{s,\,LL} - w_{s,\,LL}$						

SI units: f: [N], μ: [Nm]

without self-collision or contact with the environment. Table 6.1 shows the mean and the standard deviation of the errors between measured and predicted sensor wrench during movement. Figure 6.6 shows a comparison between w_s and $\hat{w}_s$ for the left arm (without loss of generality, all limbs show similar results).

Subsequently we investigated methods to improve the estimates of the robot dynamics. In another set of experiments, we thus compared various nonparametric learning methods with the rigid body model just presented. We refer the interested reader to Gijsberts and Metta (2011). We report here only the main findings. The task of learning here is the estimation of the wrenches due to the internal dynamics (w_i) given the FTS readings (w_s) and the robot configuration $(q, \dot{q}, \ddot{q})$; we do not take into account inertial information.

We compared various methods from the literature as, for example, the widely used local weighted projection regression (LWPR), the local Gaussian process (LGP), and Gaussian process regression (GPR) as presented by Nguyen-Tuong et al. (2008) with an incremental version of kernel ridge regression (also known as sparse spectrum Gaussian process) with the aim of maintaining eventually an incremental open-ended learner updating the estimation of the robot dynamics on-line. Our incremental method relies on an approximation of the kernel (see Rahimi and Recht 2008) based on a random sampling of its Fourier spectrum. The more random features, the better the approximation. We considered approximations with 500, 1,000, and 2,000 features. In the following we call KRR the plain kernel ridge regression method and RFRR^D the random feature version for D features. Various datasets (e.g., Barret, Sarcos) were used from the literature [for comparison Nguyen-Tuong et al. (2008)] before applying the method to the iCub.

The results in Fig. 6.7 show that KRR often outperforms GPR by a significant margin, even though both methods have identical formulations for the predictive mean and KRR hyperparameters were optimized using GPR. These deviations indicate that different hyperparameter configurations were used in both experiments. This is a common problem with GPR in comparative studies: the marginal

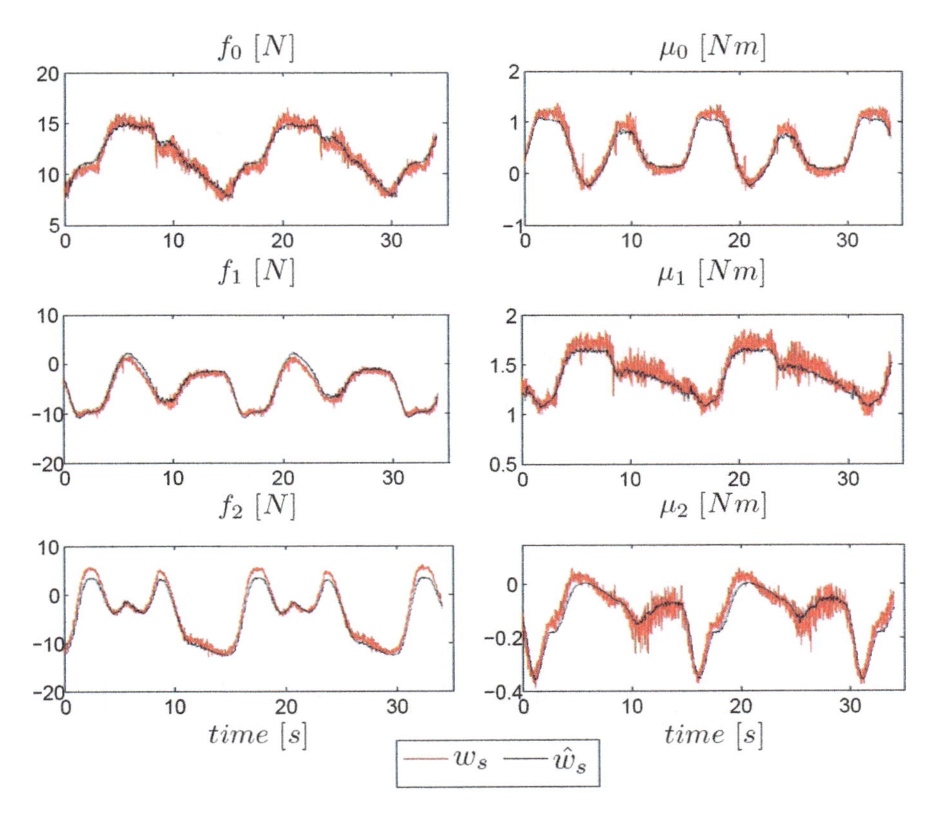

Fig. 6.6 Comparison between the wrench measured by the FT sensor and that predicted by the model, during a generic contact-free movement of the left arm. The three plots on the *left* are forces expressed in [N]; the three *rightmost plots* are the moments in [Nm]

likelihood is non-convex and its optimization often results in a local optimum that depends on the initial configuration. Hence, we have to be cautious when interpreting the comparative results on these datasets with respect to generalization performance. The comparison between KRR and RFRR, trained using identical hyperparameters, remains valid and gives an indication of the approximation quality of RFRR. As expected, the performance of RFRR steadily improves as the number of random features increases. Furthermore, RFRR^{1000} is often sufficient to obtain satisfactory predictions on all datasets. RFRR^{500}, on the other hand, performs poorly on the Barrett dataset, despite using distinct hyperparameter configurations for each degree of freedom. In this case, RFRR^{1000} with a shared hyperparameter configuration is more accurate and requires overall less time for prediction.

Figure 6.8 shows how the average nMSE develops as test samples are predicted in sequential order using either KRR or RFRR. RFRR requires between 5,000 and 10,000 samples to achieve performance comparable to KRR. The performance of

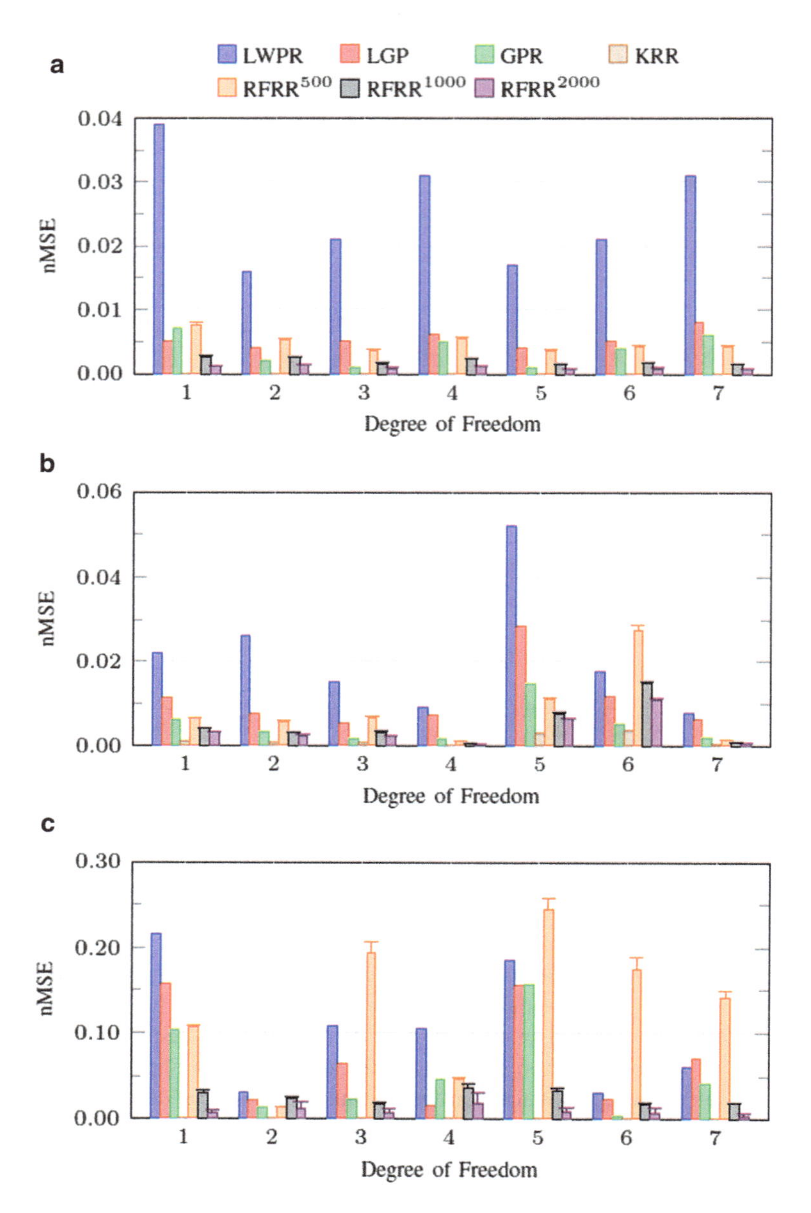

Fig. 6.7 Prediction error per degree of freedom for the (**a**) simulated Sarcos, (**b**) Sarcos, and (**c**) Barrett datasets. The results for LWPR, GPR, and LGP are taken from Nguyen-Tuong et al. (2008). The mean error over 25 runs is reported for RFRR with $D \in 500, 1{,}000, 2{,}000$, whereas error bars mark a distance of one standard deviation. Note that in some cases the prediction errors for KRR are very close to zero and therefore barely noticeable

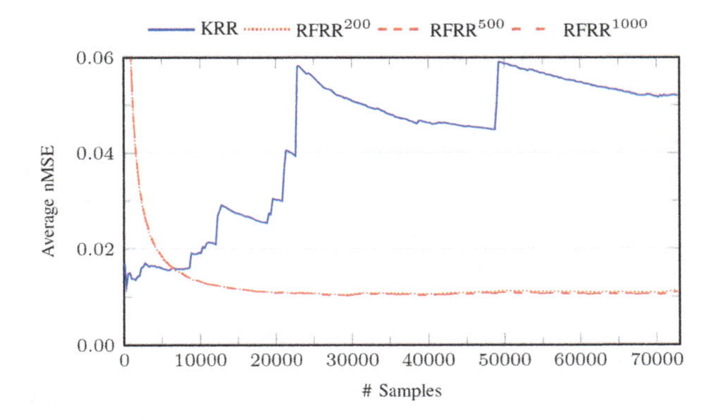

Fig. 6.8 Average prediction error with respect to the number of test samples of KRR and incremental RFRR with $D \in 200, 500, 1{,}000$ on the iCub dataset. The error is measured as the nMSE averaged over the force and torque output components. The standard deviation over 25 runs of RFRR is negligible in all cases; for clarity we report only the mean without error bars

KRR, on the other hand, decreases over time. In particular on the iCub dataset it suffers a number of large errors, causing the average nMSE to show sudden jumps. This is a direct consequence of the unavoidable fact that training and test samples are not guaranteed to be drawn from the same distribution. Incremental RFRR, on the other hand, is largely unaffected by these changes and demonstrates stable predictive performance. This is not surprising, as RFRR is incremental, and thus (1) it is able to adapt to changing conditions, and (2) it eventually has trained on significantly more samples than KRR. Furthermore, Figure 6.8 shows that 200 random features are sufficient to achieve satisfactory performance on either dataset. In this case, model updates of RFRR require only 400 μs, as compared to 2 ms and 7 ms when using 500 or 1,000 random features, respectively. These timing figures make incremental RFRR suitable for high-frequency loops as needed in robot control tasks.

In conclusion, this shows that for a relatively complex robot like the iCub, good estimation of the internal dynamics is possible and that a combination of nonparametric and parametric methods can provide simultaneously good generalization performance and fast and incremental learning. Not surprisingly, lower errors are obtained with learning. In the next section, we see how to build on this controller to generate whole-body movements.

6.4 Prioritized Whole-Body Motion-Force Control

In this section we show how to calculate the motor torques τ_d to achieve a certain set of tasks, sometimes simultaneously. Here we exploit the redundancy of the humanoid body to satisfy multiple tasks by building a hierarchy with prioritization in the task execution. Our goal is to build a control framework that is sound, optimal, and efficient. We are also interested in the method's capabilities, i.e., whether it allows inequality bounds (e.g., to respect joint limits), force, and position control. A control framework is *sound* if the control action of any task does not affect the performance of any higher-priority tasks. A framework is *optimal* if its control action minimizes the error of each task, under the constraint of being sound. The *capabilities* of a framework concern the types of tasks and systems that it can control. Finally, a framework is *efficient* if its computational complexity is minimal, considering its capabilities (typically, the more capable a method, the higher the computational complexity). In this context, efficiency is strictly related to the number of computed (pseudo)inverses, matrix multiplications, and the computation of the inertia matrix.

In the following, we indicate with $\mathbb{S}_+^n$ the set of symmetric positive-definite $n \times n$ matrices. We want to design position tracking control laws for a rigid robot with n degrees of freedom. The equation of motion of the robot in free space may be written as before:

$$M(q)\ddot{q} + h(q, \dot{q}) = \tau \tag{6.11}$$

where $q \in \mathbb{R}^n$ are the joint coordinates, $\tau \in \mathbb{R}^n$ are the joint torques, $M(q) \in \mathbb{S}_+^n$ is the joint space inertia matrix, and $h(q, \dot{q}) \in \mathbb{R}^n$ contains all the nonlinear terms such as Coriolis, centrifugal and gravity terms. A position tracking task for the robot is described as a time-varying constraint $f(q) = x_{\mathrm{r}}(t)$, where $x_{\mathrm{r}}(t) \in \mathbb{R}^m$ is the reference task trajectory and $f : \mathbb{R}^n \rightarrow \mathbb{R}^m$ is a generic function of the joint angles (e.g., the forward kinematics). Since we assume that the control inputs are the joint torques τ, we can only affect instantaneously the joint accelerations $\ddot{q}$. To express the task in terms of $\ddot{q}$, we differentiate the constraint twice with respect to time:

$$J(q)\dot{q} = \dot{x}_r(t), \quad J(q)\ddot{q} + \dot{J}(q)\dot{q} = \ddot{x}_{\mathrm{r}}(t) \tag{6.12}$$

where $J(q) = \frac{\partial}{\partial q} f(q) \in \mathbb{R}^{m \times n}$ is the task Jacobian. In the following, dependency upon t, q, and $\dot{q}$ is no longer shown to simplify notation. Since we use the second derivative of the constraint, in real situations a drift is likely to occur. To prevent deviations from the desired trajectory and to ensure disturbance rejection, we design a proportional-derivative feedback control law:

$$\ddot{x}^* = \ddot{x}_{\mathrm{r}} + K_d(\dot{x}_{\mathrm{r}} - \dot{x}) + K_p(x_{\mathrm{r}} - x) \tag{6.13}$$

where $\ddot{x}^* \in \mathbb{R}^m$ is the desired task acceleration, whereas $K_{\mathrm{d}} \in \mathbb{S}_+^m$ and $K_{\mathrm{p}} \in \mathbb{S}_+^m$ are the derivative and proportional gain matrices, respectively. Following Peters et al. (2007), we formulate the control problem as constrained minimization (this approach is called Unifying Framework—UF in the following):

$$\tau_{\mathrm{d}} = \mathrm{argmin}_{\tau \in \mathbb{R}^n} \left|\left|\ddot{x} - \ddot{x}^*\right|\right|^2, \\ s.t. \begin{cases} M\ddot{q} + h = \tau \\ J\ddot{q} + \dot{J}\dot{q} \end{cases} \tag{6.14}$$

For the typical case $m < n$, this problem has infinite solutions:

$$\tau_d = \left(JM^{-1}\right)_V^\dagger \left(\ddot{x}^* - \dot{J}\dot{q} + JM^{-1}h\right) + \left(I - \left(JM^{-1}\right)_V^\dagger JM^{-1}\right)\tau_0 \tag{6.15}$$

where $\tau_0 \in \mathbb{R}^n$ is an arbitrary vector, $V \in \mathbb{S}^n$ is an arbitrary matrix and $A_V^\dagger = V^{\frac{1}{2}} \left(AV^{\frac{1}{2}}\right)^\dagger = VA^{\mathrm{T}}\left(AVA^{\mathrm{T}}\right)^\dagger$ is the pseudoinverse of the matrix A, weighted by V. If A is full rank, then we can also write $A_V^\dagger = VA^{\mathrm{T}}(AVA^{\mathrm{T}})^{-1}$. By choosing a particular pair of (V, τ_0), we get the solution that minimizes $\left|\left|V^{-\frac{1}{2}}(\tau - \tau_0)\right|\right|^2$ (Bjorck 1996). Setting $\tau_0 = 0$, and varying V, we get different well-known control laws, reported in Table 6.2; the second row reports the operational space control law of Khatib (Sentis and Khatib 2005), which selects the torques generated by a hypothetical force applied at the control point.

Without loss of generality, given that $M \in \mathbb{S}_+^n$, we can set $V = M^2W$, where $W \in \mathbb{S}_+^n$ is another arbitrary matrix, so that Eq. (6.15) simplifies to

$$\tau_{\mathrm{d}} = MJ_W^\dagger \left(\ddot{x}^* - \dot{J}\dot{q} + JM^{-1}h\right) + MN_W M^{-1}\tau_0 \tag{6.16}$$

where $N_W = I - J_W^\dagger J$ is a weighted (nonorthogonal) nullspace projector.

6.4.1 Hierarchical Extension of UF

This approach can manage an arbitrary number of tasks N, each characterized by a desired acceleration $\ddot{x}_i^*$ and Jacobian J_i. To ensure the correct management of task conflicts, the tasks need prioritization: the higher the number i of the task, the higher its priority, i.e.:

$$\tau_{\mathrm{d}} = M\ddot{q}_1, \\ \ddot{q}_i = \ddot{q}_{i+1} + N_{p(i)W} J_{iW}^\dagger \left(\ddot{x}_i^* - \dot{J}_i\dot{q} + J_i M^{-1}h\right), \quad i \in [1, N] \\ N_{p(i)W} = N_{p(i+1)W} - \left(J_{i+1}N_{p(i+1)W}\right)_W^\dagger J_{i+1}N_{p(i+1)W} \tag{6.17}$$

where $N_p i)W$ is a projector into the nullspace of all the tasks $\{j|j > i\}$, computed with the recursive formula proposed in []. The computation is initialized setting $\ddot{q}_{N+1} = 0$ and $N_{p(N)} = I$. If the state of the robot is completely controllable, which is usually the case, then this formulation simplifies to

Table 6.2 Control laws for different values of the weight matrix V

V	Minimize	Control law, τ_d	Reference
I	$\|\tau\|^2$	$M^{-1}J^{\mathrm{T}}\left(JM^{-2}J^{\mathrm{T}}\right)^{\dagger}\left(\ddot{x}^{*}-\dot{J}\dot{q}+JM^{-1}h\right)$	WBCF (Sentis and Khatib 2005)
M	$\tau^{\mathrm{T}}M^{-1}\tau$	$J^{\mathrm{T}}\left(JM^{-1}J^{\mathrm{T}}\right)^{\dagger}\left(\ddot{x}^{*}-\dot{J}\dot{q}+JM^{-1}h\right)$	
M^2	$\|M^{-1}\tau\|^2$	$MJ^{\mathrm{T}}\left(JJ^{\mathrm{T}}\right)^{\dagger}\left(\ddot{x}^{*}-\dot{J}\dot{q}+JM^{-1}h\right)$	

$$
\begin{aligned}
\tau_{\mathrm{d}} &= M\ddot{q}_1 + h, \\
\ddot{q}_i &= \ddot{q}_{i+1} + N_{p(i)W}J_{iW}^{\dagger}\left(\ddot{x}_i^{*} - \dot{J}_i\dot{q}\right), \quad i \in [1, N]
\end{aligned}
\tag{6.18}
$$

The accelerations of each task $\ddot{q}_i$ are projected into the nullspace of the higher priority tasks; this guarantees that the framework is sound. However, this approach is not optimal, because each task is solved independently and then projected into the nullspace of the higher-priority tasks. This does not ensure the minimization of the error of each task. In the case of the WBCF as reported in Sentis and Khatib (2005), the hierarchical extension differs considerably. The reader is referred to the above mentioned paper for a complete presentation of the WBCF.

6.4.2 *Hybrid Control*

Hybrid position/force control can be realized by setting the joint space control torques to

$$
\tau_0 = h - J_c^T f^* \tag{6.19}
$$

where $J_c(q) \in \mathbb{R}^{k \times n}$ is the contact Jacobian, f^* are the desired contact forces, and $k \in \mathbb{R}$ is the number of independent directions in which the robot can apply force. Substituting τ_0 into the desired control torques (6.16), we get

$$
\tau_{\mathrm{d}} = MJ_W^{\dagger}\left(\ddot{x}^{*} - \dot{J}\dot{q}\right) + h - MN_W M^{-1}J_c^{\mathrm{T}}f^{*} \tag{6.20}
$$

where the applied forces act in the nullspace of the tracking task.

6.4.3 *Task Space Inverse Dynamics*

The development of a new method is compelling since none of the existing methods is jointly sound, efficient, and optimal. For example, we would like to shove off the computation of the inertia matrices pseudoinverses which have a cost of $O(N^3)$. On the contrary for specific choices of V and τ_0 in (6.15), the solution takes the form of $\tau_{\mathrm{d}} = M(q)\ddot{}_1 + h$ which we can calculate without explicitly computing M through the $O(n)$ recursive Newton-Euler algorithm (RNEA). Unfortunately this is not optimal since tasks at lower priority may not be performed correctly even in cases where they do not conflict with the higher-priority tasks. Our methods, called task space inverse dynamics (TSID), follows the approach outlined so far with a different hierarchical extension. We minimize the error of each task under the constraint of not affecting any higher-priority task. At each minimization step, we carefully select the weight matrices used in the pseudoinverses, so as to simplify the resulting control laws. This leads to an efficient formulation, while preserving the optimality property. We start considering position tracking control only, and then we introduce force control tasks.

6.4.3.1 Weight Matrix and Joint Space Stabilization

The weight matrix V (or equivalently W) introduced in the resolution of (6.15) can play two different roles. In case there is no secondary task (i.e., $\tau_0 = 0$), V determines the cost to be minimized (e.g., $\|\tau\|^2$, $\|\ddot{q}\|^2$). In case there is a secondary task, V specifies the metric that is used to measure the distance between τ and τ_0. Using the nullspace of a task to minimize some measure of effort is appealing and it is also rooted in some deep principle of human motor control (Flash and Hogan 1985). While this approach may be feasible in simulation, unfortunately in reality it leads to singular configurations and/or hitting of joint limits (Peters et al. 2007). The subspace of joint accelerations that does not affect the task is not controlled, so its behavior is determined by disturbances and errors in the model of the manipulator. Even in simulation, if the initial conditions of the robot have nonzero joint velocities, failing to use a secondary task may result in joint space instability. The reason for this behavior is obvious: the effort of stabilizing in joint space is not task relevant and it would increase the cost (Peters et al. 2007). Peters et al. (2007) suggest to add a joint space motor command for stabilization. A common approach is to design the postural task to attract the robot toward a desired posture q_{p}. We compute the desired joint accelerations as $\ddot{q}_{\mathrm{p}}^* = K_{\mathrm{p}}(q_{\mathrm{p}} - q) - K_{\mathrm{d}}\dot{q}$, where $K_{\mathrm{p}} \in \mathbb{S}_+^n$ and $K_{\mathrm{d}} \in \mathbb{S}_+^n$ are the proportional and damping gain matrices, respectively. In the following we always include the postural task to minimize $\left\|\ddot{q} - \ddot{q}_{\mathrm{p}}^*\right\|^2$, under the constraint of not affecting any other task. This ensures stabilization of the manipulator in joint space.

6.4.3.2 Framework Derivation

In the following we only state the results of our approach and we leave the derivation to further reference papers as, for example, (De Lasa and Hertzmann 2009). Consider a general scenario in which the robot has to perform N position tracking tasks $T_1 \ldots T_N$ and a postural task T_0 (with desired joint accelerations $\ddot{q}_{\mathrm{p}}^*$) to stabilize any redundancy. Taking inspiration from Peters et al. (2007), we formulate the control problem as a sequence of constrained minimizations:

$$\begin{array}{lll}(T_N)\ r_N = \min_{\tau\in\mathbb{R}^n} g_N(\tau) & s.t.\ M\ddot{q}+h=\tau & \\ (T_i)\ r_i = \min_{\tau\in\mathbb{R}^n} g_i(\tau) & s.t.\ M\ddot{q}+h=\tau, & g_j(\tau)=r_j \forall j>i \\ (T_0)\ \tau_{\mathrm{d}} = \mathrm{argmin}_{\tau\in\mathbb{R}^n}\left\|\ddot{q}-\ddot{q}_{\mathrm{p}}^*\right\|^2 & s.t.\ M\ddot{q}+h=\tau, & g_j(\tau)=r_j \forall j>0\end{array} \tag{6.21}$$

where $g_i(\tau) = ||J_i\ddot{q} + \dot{J}\dot{q} - \ddot{x}_i^*||^2$ is the cost associated to the task T_i. The solution of 21 is given by

$$\begin{array}{l}\tau_{\mathrm{d}} = M\ddot{q}_0 + h \\ \ddot{q}_i = \ddot{q}_{i+1} + N_{p(i)W}\left(J_i N_{p(i)W}\right)_W^{\dagger}\left(\ddot{x}_i^* - \dot{J}_i\dot{q} - J_i\ddot{q}_{i+1}\right) \quad i\in[0,N]\end{array} \tag{6.22}$$

where $J_0 = I$ and $\ddot{x}_0^* = \ddot{q}_{\mathrm{p}}^*$. The computation is initialized setting $\ddot{q}_{N+1} = 0$ and $N_{p(N)} = I$. Once again, by selecting the weight matrix W, we can vary the form of the control law. Interestingly enough though, the solution τ_{d} is independent of W. This is because the only role of W is to weight the cost in the nullspace of all the tasks, but here the postural task ensures that there is no nullspace left (because any control action affects the postural task). It is then reasonable to choose W so as to simplify the computation. If we set $W = I$, then all the nullspace projectors $N_{pi)}$ become orthogonal, so they are equal to their pseudoinverses, i.e., $N_{pi)}^{\dagger} = N_{pi)}$. This simplifies the formulation (6.22) to

$$\begin{array}{l}\tau_{\mathrm{d}} = M\left(\ddot{q}_1 + N_{p(0)\ddot{q}_{\mathrm{p}}^*}\right) + h \\ \ddot{q}_i = \ddot{q}_{i+1} + \left(J_i N_{p(i)}\right)^{\dagger}\left(\ddot{x}_i^* - \dot{J}_i\dot{q} - J_i\ddot{q}_{i+1}\right) \quad i\in[1,N]\end{array} \tag{6.23}$$

In this form, kinematics and dynamics are completely decoupled: we solve first the multitask prioritization at the kinematic level computing $\ddot{q}_1$, and then we compute the torques to get the desired joint accelerations. This formulation does not require the computation of a pseudoinverse for the postural task, because it exploits the property of orthogonal projectors of being equal to their pseudoinverses. Moreover, it can be efficiently computed with the RNEA, without explicitly calculating M.

6.4.3.3 Force Control

If the robot is in contact with the environment, its equations of motion become:

$$M(q)\ddot{q} + h(q,\dot{q}) - J_{\mathrm{c}}(q)^{\mathrm{T}} f = \tau \tag{6.24}$$

where $J_{\mathrm{c}}(q) = \frac{\partial x_{\mathrm{c}}}{\partial q} \in \mathbb{R}^{k\times n}$ is the contact Jacobian (or constraint Jacobian), $x_{\mathrm{c}} \in \mathbb{R}^k$

is the robot contact point, and $f \in \mathbb{R}^k$ are the contact forces (or constraint forces). To control the contact forces, we need a model of the contact dynamics. The most common choices are the linear spring contact model and the rigid contact model. The first model assumes that the environment at the contact point behaves like a linear spring, i.e., $k_s(x_c - x_e) = f$, where k_s is the contact stiffness and $x_e \in \mathbb{R}^k$ is the environment contact point. Assuming k_s to be known, force is a known function of position, and therefore the force control problems can be translated into position control problems. The rigid contact model is more interesting, since it introduces constraints into the problem formulation. When the manipulator is in rigid contact with the environment, its motion is subject to k nonlinear constraints. In general we can consider these constraints as nonlinear functions of the joint angles, velocities, and time: $c(q, \dot{q}, t) = 0$. To include these constraints into the control problem, we express them as $J_c(q)\ddot{q} = b(q, \dot{q}, t)$. We write then the optimization problem as

$$\begin{aligned} \tau_d &= \operatorname{argmin}_{\tau \in \mathbb{R}^n} \|f - f^*\|^2, \\ s.t. &\begin{cases} M\ddot{q} + h - J_c^T f = \tau \\ J_c \ddot{q} = b \end{cases} \end{aligned} \tag{6.25}$$

where $f^* \in \mathbb{R}^k$ are the desired contact forces. We can express the infinite solutions of the problem as

$$\tau_d = M\left(J_c^\dagger b + N_c \ddot{q}_0\right) + h - J_c^T f^* \tag{6.26}$$

where $\ddot{q}_0 \in \mathbb{R}^n$ is an arbitrary vector. This control law is one of our main contributions to this type of control problems, since it allows implementing force control without computing matrix M, while characterizing the redundancy of the task through $\ddot{q}_0$.

6.4.3.4 Hierarchical Framework

We finally extend our multitask formulation to include force control. The rigid force control task, if any, has to take the highest priority because it is an actual physical constraint that cannot be violated by definition. We assume that the robot has to perform $N - 1$ position control tasks. On top of those, we place a rigid force control task (for the sake of simplicity, here we assume holonomic constraints, i.e., $b(q, \dot{q}, t) = -\dot{J}_c \dot{q}$, with reference force f^* and Jacobian $J_N = J_c$:

$$\begin{aligned} \tau_d &= M\left(\ddot{q}_1 + N_{p(0)} \ddot{q}_p^*\right) + h - J_c^T f^*, \\ \ddot{q}_i &= \ddot{q}_{i+1} + \left(J_i N_{p(i)}\right)^\dagger \left(\ddot{x}_i^* - \dot{J}_i \dot{q} - J_i \ddot{q}_{i+1}\right) \quad i \in [1, N] \end{aligned} \tag{6.27}$$

where $\ddot{x}_N^* = \ddot{x}_c = 0$, $\ddot{q}_{N+1} = 0$, and $N_{p(N)} = I$. In summary, after the extension to force control, we can notice that kinematics and dynamics are still decoupled, so the computational complexity has not increased and τ_d can be efficiently computed with the RNEA.

6.4.4 Validation and Experiment

We tested the TSID against the Unifying Framework (UF) (Peters et al. 2007) and the Whole-Body Control Framework (WBCF) (Sentis and Khatib 2005) on a customized version of the Compliant huManoid (Coman) simulator (Dallali et al. 2013). The robot has 23 DoFs: 4 in each arm, 3 in the torso and 6 in each leg. We adapted the simulator to make the robot rigid and fully-actuated (we fixed the robot base and we removed the joint passive compliance). Direct and inverse dynamics, both in simulation and control, were efficiently computed using C language functions, generated with the Robotran (2012) symbolic engine. Contact forces were simulated using linear spring-damper models [stiffness 2×10^5 N/m and damping 10^3 Ns/m, as proposed in Dallali et al. (2013)] with realistic friction. To integrate the equations of motion, we used the Simulink variable step integrator *ode23t*, with relative and absolute tolerance of 10^3 and 10^6, respectively. The tests were executed on a computer with a 2.83 GHz CPU and 4 GB of RAM.

6.4.4.1 Trajectory Generation

To generate reference position-velocity-acceleration trajectories, we used the approach presented in Pattacini et al. (2010) (see also Sect. 6.5, which provides approximately minimum-jerk trajectories). The trajectory generator is a third order dynamical system that takes as input the desired trajectory $x_d(t)$ and outputs the three position-velocity-acceleration reference trajectories $x_r(t)$, $\dot{x}_r(t)$, $\ddot{x}_r(t)$. The reference position trajectory follows the desired position trajectory with a velocity that depends on the parameter "trajectory time" (always set to 1.0 s in our tests). We set all proportional gains $K_p = 10$ s^{-2} and all derivative gains $K_d = 5$ s^{-1}. The pseudoinverse calculations are all performed using the "damped pseudoinverse" technique to guarantee stability near singularities.

6.4.4.2 Test 1: Feasible Task Hierarchy

In this test the robot performs four tasks (see also Fig. 6.9):

- F: 3 DoFs, apply a normal force of 20 N on a wall with the right hand
- T2: 3 DoFs, track a circular trajectory with the left hand
- T1: 1 DoF (x coordinate), track a sinusoidal reference with the neck base
- T0: 23 DoFs, maintain the initial joint posture

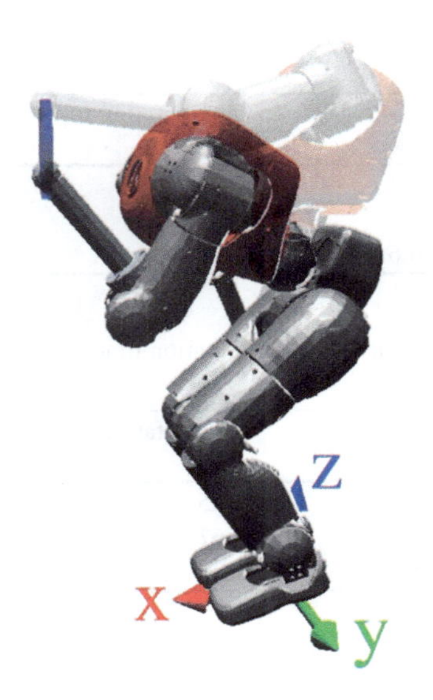

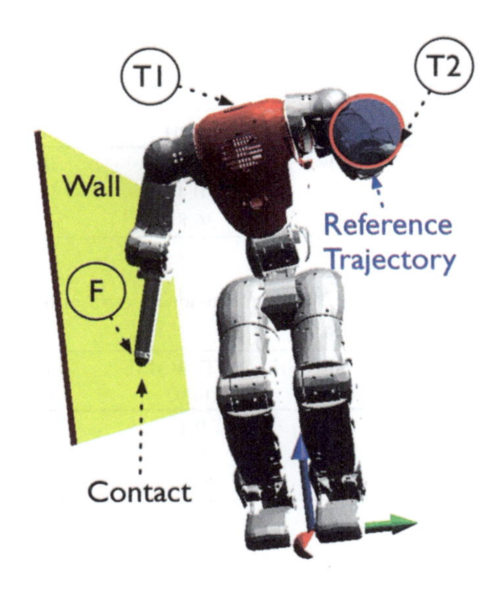

Fig. 6.9 Coman executing Test 1. Task F controls the force exerted by the right hand against the wall. Task T2 moves the left hand along the circular reference trajectory depicted as a red circumference. Task T1 moves the neck base back and forth along the x-axis

The first three tasks are always compatible, so the robot should be able to perform them with negligible errors. Table 6.3 reports the root-mean-square error (RMSE) for each task and the mean computation time of the control loop. We compute the RMSE as $\sqrt{\frac{1}{N_t}\sum_{t=0}^{T}||x(t) - x_r(t)||^2}$, where N_t is the number of samples used in the summation. The evaluation criteria proposed in Sect. 6.4 are strictly connected to the data of Table 6.3: the error of the primary task F concerns the *soundness*, the errors of the nonprimary tasks (T2, T1, T0) concern the *optimality*, and the computation time concerns the *efficiency*. As expected, the UF performs poorly on the nonprimary tasks, because it is not optimal. Both WBCF and TSID achieve good tracking on all tasks, but the computation time of WBCF is $\approx 2.6\times$ the computation time of our method.

6.4.4.3 Test 2: Unfeasible Task Hierarchy

In this test the robot performs the same four tasks of the previous test with one modification: task T1 controls the 3D Cartesian position of the neck base (rather than the x coordinate only). This modification makes the simultaneous satisfaction of all tasks impossible, i.e., the desired trajectory is not reachable. We thus expect a significant error for task T1 and task F and T2 with negligible errors. Table 6.4 shows that, as for test 1, UF performs poorly on the nonprimary tasks, whereas WBCF has higher computational demand than the other two methods. The small

Table 6.3 Test 1: Root-mean-square error of the four tasks and average computation time of the controller

Controller	F-RMSE (N)	T2-RMSE (mm)	T1-RMSE (mm)	T0-RMSE (mm)	Computation time (deg) (ms)
TSID	0.1	0.4	0.1	7.1	0.24
WBCF	0.1	0.4	0.1	7.1	0.64
UF	0.1	36.8	30.1	6.6	0.25

Table 6.4 Test 2: Root-mean-square error of the four tasks and average computation time of the controller

Controller	F-RMSE (N)	T2-RMSE (mm)	T1-RMSE (mm)	T0-RMSE (mm)	Computation time (deg) (ms)
TSID	0.0	0.1	21.5	5.5	0.25
WBCF	0.0	0.3	21.5	5.5	0.67
UF	0.0	23.8	62.4	5.1	0.26

difference between TSID and WBCF in the RMSE of task T2 is due to the behavior of the damped pseudoinverses when close to the singularity.

In summary, we have shown that it is possible to build efficient controllers for the movement of complex humanoid robots even when multiple tasks are requested. We have shown that certain nice properties can be maintained simultaneously, i.e.:

1. *Optimality*: TSID minimizes the error of each task under the constraint of not affecting any higher-priority task (it is thus also *sound*).
2. *Capabilities*: TSID allows for position/velocity/acceleration control and soft/rigid contact force control.
3. *Efficiency*: TSID computes the desired joint torques in $O(n)$ using the Recursive Newton-Euler algorithm because it needs neither the joint space inertia matrix M nor the task space inertia matrices Λ's.

Additional work in this direction can certainly improve the flexibility of the method as, for example, by including the ability to deal with inequality constraints (e.g., joint limits or torque bounds), the capability of high-level planning to keep the robot away from singularities, and more importantly, the ability of controlling a floating base robot that moves autonomously in the environment. In the following we concentrate on a specific—but important—subproblem, i.e., reaching and pointing.

6.5 Reaching and Pointing

We consider the general problem of computing the value of joint angles q_{d} in order to reach a given position in space $x_{\mathrm{d}} \in \mathbb{R}^3$ and orientation $\alpha_{\mathrm{d}} \in \mathbb{R}^4$ of the end-effector (where α_{d} is a representation of rotation in axis/angle notation). Note that q_{d} can be directly connected to the input of the impedance controller described in Sect. 6.3. It is desired that the computed solution satisfies a set of additional constraints expressed as generic inequalities—we see later the reason for constraining the solution of the optimization problem. This can be stated as follows:

$$\begin{aligned} q_{\mathrm{d}} &= \operatorname{argmin}_{q \in \mathbb{R}^n}\left(\left|\left|\alpha_{\mathrm{d}} - K_\alpha(q)\right|\right|^2 + \beta\left(q_{\mathrm{rest}} - q\right)^T W\left(q_{\mathrm{rest}} - q\right)\right), \\ s.t. &\begin{cases} \left|\left|x_{\mathrm{d}} - K_x(q)\right|\right|^2 < \varepsilon \\ q_{\mathrm{L}} < q < q_{\mathrm{U}} \end{cases} \end{aligned} \tag{6.28}$$

where K_x and K_α are the forward kinematic functions for the position and orientation of the end-effector for a given configuration q, q_{rest} is a preferred joint configuration, W is a diagonal weighting matrix, β a positive scalar weighting the influence of the terms in the optimization, and ε a parameter for tuning the precision of the movement. Typically $\beta < 1$ and $\varepsilon \in [10^{-5}, 10^{-4}]$. The solution to (6.28) has to satisfy the set of additional constraints of joint limits $q_{\mathrm{L}} < q < q_{\mathrm{U}}$ with q_{L}, q_{U} as the lower and upper bounds, respectively. In the case of the iCub, we solved this problem for ten DoFs—seven of the arm and three of the waist—and we determined the value of q_{rest} so that the waist is as upright as possible. The left and right arm can be both controlled by switching from one or the other kinematic chain (e.g., as a function of the distance to the target).

We used an interior point optimization technique to solve the problem in (6.28). In particular we used IpOpt (Wätcher and Biegler 2006), a public domain software package designed for large-scale nonlinear optimization. This approach has the following advantages:

1. Quick convergence. IpOpt is reliable and fast enough to be employed in control loops at reasonable rates (tens of milliseconds), as, e.g., compared to more traditional iterative methods such as the cyclic coordinate descent (CCD) adopted in Hersch and Billard (2008).
2. Scalability. The intrinsic capability of the optimizer to treat nonlinear problems in any arbitrary number of variables is exploited to make the controller structure easily scalable with the size of the joint space. For example, it is possible to change at run time from the control of the 7-DoF iCub arm to the complete 10-DoF structure inclusive of the waist or to any combination of the joints depending on the task.
3. Automatic handling of singularities and joint limits. This technique automatically deals with singularities in the arm Jacobian and joint limits and can find solutions in virtually any working conditions.
4. Tasks hierarchy. The task is split in two subtasks: the control of the orientation and the control of the position of the end-effector. Different priorities can be assigned to the subtasks. In our case the control of position has higher priority with respect to orientation (the former is handled as a nonlinear constraint and thus is evaluated before the cost).

5. Description of complex constraints. It is easy to add new constraints as linear and/or nonlinear inequalities either in task or joint space. In the case of the iCub, for instance, we added a set of constraints that avoid reaching the limits of the tendons that actuate the three joints of the shoulder.

Once q_{d} is determined as described above, there is still the problem of generating a trajectory from the current robot configuration q to q_{d}. Simultaneously, we would like to impose suitable smoothness constraints to the trajectory. This has been obtained by using the Multi-Referential Dynamical Systems approach (Hersch and Billard 2008), whereby two dynamical controllers, one in joint space and another in task space, evolve concurrently (Fig. 6.10). The coherence constraint, that is, $\dot{x} = J\dot{q}$, with J the Jacobian of the kinematics map, guarantees that at each instant of time, the trajectory is meaningful. This is enforced by using the Lagrangian multipliers method and can be tuned to modulate the relative influence of each controller (i.e., to avoid joint angle limits). The advantage of such a redundant representation includes the management of the singularities while maintaining a quasi-straight trajectory profile of the end-effector in the task space—reproducing a humanlike behavior (Abend et al. 1982).

Differently from the work of Hersch and Billard, we designed a feedback trajectory generator instead of the VITE (Vector-Integration-To-Endpoint) method used in open loop. A complete discussion of the rationale of the modifications to the trajectory generation is outside the scope of this paper; the interested reader is referred to Pattacini et al. (2010). Reasons to prefer a feedback formulation include the possibility of smoothly connecting multiple pieces of trajectories and correcting on-line for accumulation of errors due to the enforcement of the constraints of the multi-referential method.

6.5.1 Validation and Further Improvements

As earlier for the dynamics, we compared our method with other methods from the literature. The comparison with the method of Hersch and Billard (2008) was almost immediate since the work was developed on the iCub. This provides the multi-referential approach together with the VITE trajectory generation at no cost. Additionally, we included in the assessment another controller representing a more conventional strategy that uses the damped least-squares (DLS) rule (Deo and Walker 1992) coupled with a secondary task that comprises the joint angle limits by means of the gradient projection method (Lee et al. 2007). This solution employs the third-party package Orocos (http://www.orocos.org/kdl), a tool for robot control that implements the DLS approach and whose public availability and compliance with real-time constraints justified its adoption as one of the reference controllers.

In the first experiment, we put to test the three selected schemes in a point-to-point motion task wherein the iCub arm was actuated in the "7-DoF mode" and where the end-effector was controlled both in position and orientation. Results

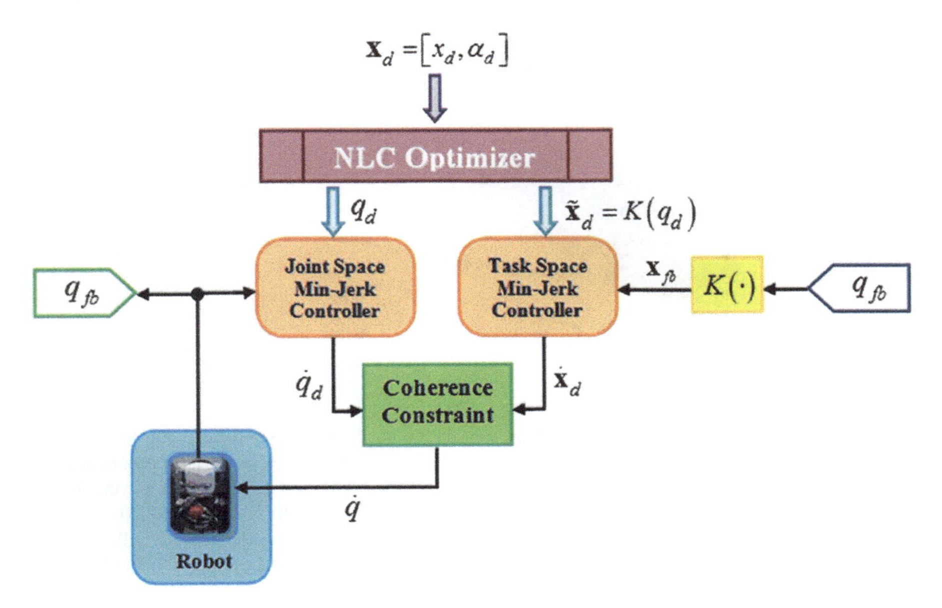

Fig. 6.10 The multi-referential scheme for trajectory generation. K is the forward kinematics map; q_{fb} is the vector of encoder signals

show that paths produced by our controller and by the DLS-based system are well restricted in narrow tubes of confidence intervals and are quite repeatable; conversely the VITE is affected by a much higher variability. Figure 6.11 highlights results for a set of ten trials of a typical reaching task where the right hand is moved from a rest position to a location in front of the iCub with the palm directed downward.

Table 6.5 summarizes the measured in-target errors for the three cases: all the controllers behave satisfactorily, but the DLS achieves lower errors because it operates continuously on the current distance from the target x_{d}, being virtually capable of canceling it at infinite time. On the contrary, strategies based on the interaction with an external solver bind the controller module to close the loop on an approximation $\tilde{x}_{\mathrm{d}}$ of the real target that is determined by the optimization tolerances as in (6.28).

Additional experiments tend to favor our method. For example, measuring the jerk of the resulting trajectory shows a gain of our method by 43 % from the VITE and of about 69 % from DLS. This turns out to be crucial for more complicated trajectories when speed factors make the minimum jerk controller even more advantageous.

Further improvements can be made on the quality of the inverse kinematic results by means of machine learning. As for the dynamics, we initially estimated the function K from the CAD models of the iCub. This is a good initial guess in need of refinement. The goal here is therefore to design a procedure that allows enforcing eye-hand coordination such that, whenever the robot reliably localizes a target in

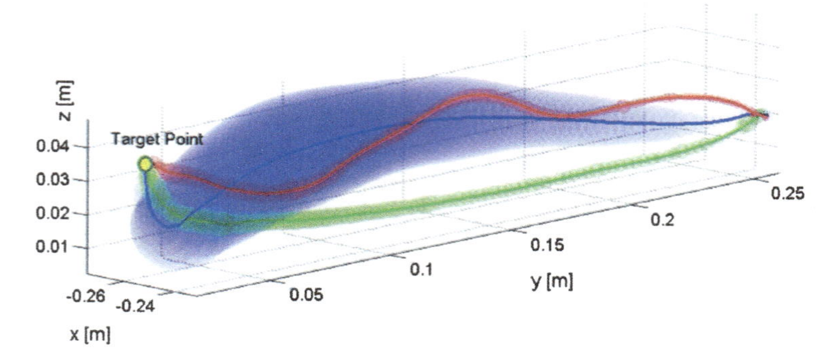

Fig. 6.11 Point-to-point Cartesian trajectories executed by the three controllers: the VITE-based method produces on average the blue line, the minimum-jerk controller result is in green, and the DLS system using Orocos in red. Bands containing all the measured paths within a confidential interval of 95 % are drawn in corresponding colors. Controller settings are $T = 2.0$ s for the minimum-jerk system; $\alpha = 0.008, \beta = 0.002, K_P = 3$ for the VITE (see Hersch and Billard 2008) for the meaning of the parameters); and $\mu = 10^{-5}$ for the damping factor of the DLS algorithm

Table 6.5 Mean errors along with the confidence levels at 95 % computed when the target is attained. An average measure of the variability of executed path is also given for the three controllers

Controller	Position error	Orientation error	Mean radius of the trajectory band
VITE	$1.3 \pm 1.4 \times 10^{-3}$ mm	0.041 ± 0.05 rad	10 ± 10.8 mm
Min-jerk	$3.0 \pm 1.3 \times 10^{-3}$ mm	0.048 ± 0.008 rad	2.5 ± 1.5 mm
DLS	$1.3 \pm 1.4 \times 10^{-3}$ mm	0.016 ± 0.028 rad	2.0 ± 1.36 mm

both cameras, it can also reach it. Here we further simplified the problem (from the visual point of view) and decided to learn only the position of the end-effector (x, y, z) since the orientation of the hand in the image is difficult to detect reliably. For this problem, the input space is defined by the position of the hand (or the target) in the two cameras (u_l, v_l) and (u_r, v_r) with respect to the current head configuration.

To sum up, having defined the input and the output space, the map M that is to be learned is

$$(x, y, z)_{\mathrm{H}} = M\big(u_l, v_l, u_r, v_r, T, V_s, V_g\big), \tag{6.29}$$

where $(u_l, v_l, u_r, v_r) \in \mathbb{R}^4$ represent the visual input of the position of the hand in the iCub cameras, whereas $(T, V_s, V_g) \in \mathbb{R}^3$ accounts for the proprioceptive part of the input designating the tilt, the pan, and the vergence of the eyes; finally, $(x, y, z)_{\mathrm{H}} \in \mathbb{R}^3$ is the Cartesian position of the hand expressed in the head-centered frame.

This map can be learned by a regression method if enough training samples are available and these can be in turn collected if we can measure (u_l, v_l, u_r, v_r) by

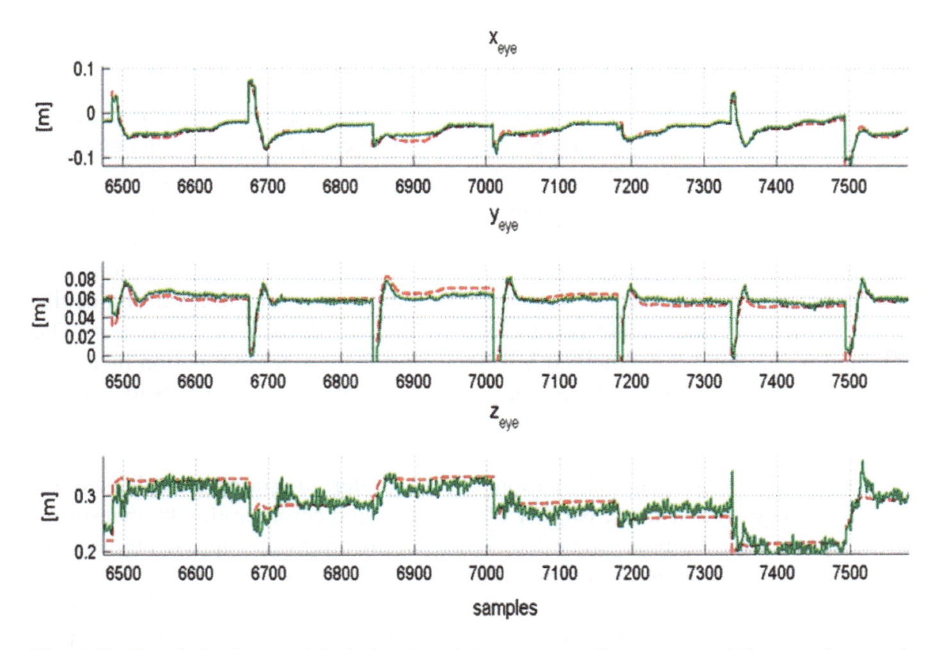

Fig. 6.12 The desired target (*dashed red*) and the corresponding outputs of the neural network (*green*) for the three Cartesian coordinates in the head-centered frame

means of vision (see Sect. 6.7). Some preliminary results by using a sigmoidal neural network from Matlab (Neural Network Toolbox) trained with backpropagation can be seen in Fig. 6.12. The training phase is carried out off-line. The neural network consists of 7 nodes in the linear input layer, 50 nodes for the hidden layer implemented with the ordinary hyperbolic tangent function, and 3 nodes in the linear output layer: an overall number of 15,000 samples has been employed for training and validation, whereas 5,000 samples have been used for testing. The neural network provides a very good estimation of M as demonstrated by the testing phase. Notably, as expected, the z component estimation is the most affected by noise since it accounts principally for the distance of the hand from the head, a value that is not directly measured by the cameras but only indirectly from binocular disparity. The inspection of the mean and standard deviation supports this claim, i.e., mean error 0.00031 m and standard deviation of 0.0055 m for the x and y components and about twice as big for z.

In summary, it is relevant to outline here that an upcoming activity has been planned with the purpose to replace the off-line training phase with a fully online version that resorts to random features as in Gijsberts and Metta (2011) and will eventually make the robot learn the eye-hand coordination completely autonomously.

6.6 Grasping

Once the hand is suitably close to an object, the robot can certainly plan to act on it. Eventually, grasping is the end goal of moving a complex body in the environment, to act and change the "state" of objects to achieve a number of possible goals as e.g., fetch an object, move it, bring it somewhere else, etc. Here we focus on power grasp, which is characterized by large areas of contact between the object and the surfaces of the palm and fingers. Our method seeks object regions that match the curvature of the robots palm. The entire procedure relies on binocular vision, which provides a 3D point cloud of the visible part of the object. The obtained point cloud is segmented in smooth surfaces. A score function measures the quality of the graspable points on the basis of the surface they belong to. A component of the score function is learned from experience and it is used to map the curvature of the object surfaces to the curvature of the robot's hand. The user can further provide top-down information on the preferred grasping regions (e.g., handles). We guarantee the feasibility of a chosen hand configuration by measuring its manipulability. We prove the effectiveness of the proposed approach by tasking a humanoid robot to grasp a number of unknown real objects.

Before deciding how to grasp an object, we need to define where to grasp it. Usually the answer to this problem is not unique; in fact, if one has to lift an object, he can put his hand in several different positions. If we limit our analysis to power grasp, then the number of possible locations gets smaller, but still, there is no a universally accepted rule on where to take an object. Several factors influence how a person performs a grasp (Cutkosky and Howe 1990); some of them regard the object shape and dimension, while others regard the weight of the object and its surface roughness as well as the task at hand.

In our implementation we take into account some of these factors in the process of extracting a set of significant points on the object surface. We first create a 3D point cloud of the visible part of the object (from a single viewpoint), using the stereo vision system of the iCub. We subsequently compute a minimum bounding box enclosing the point cloud, estimating the approximate dimension and orientation of the object with respect to the robot's root frame. Unsupervised learning techniques are employed to segment the reconstructed cloud in smooth regions. We finally look for the regions that best approximate the robotic palms curvature. As shown in Roa et al. (2012) and Chalon et al. (2010), spreading the fingers and enclosing the object against the palm significantly helps in obtaining a stable grasp. Hence we limit our search to the most compatible surfaces under the criterion that they have to match the palm size and curvature. Firstly, we guarantee that the hand lies in a visible region; therefore we select, among the obtained smooth regions, those large enough as compared to the size of the palm. We then apply a uniform sampling on the selected clusters of points, retrieving a smaller number of points along with their normals. Each point here represents the center of a planar region computed on the point's neighborhood with an area similar to the area of the robots palm. This set of points is ranked with the help of a score function, which takes into

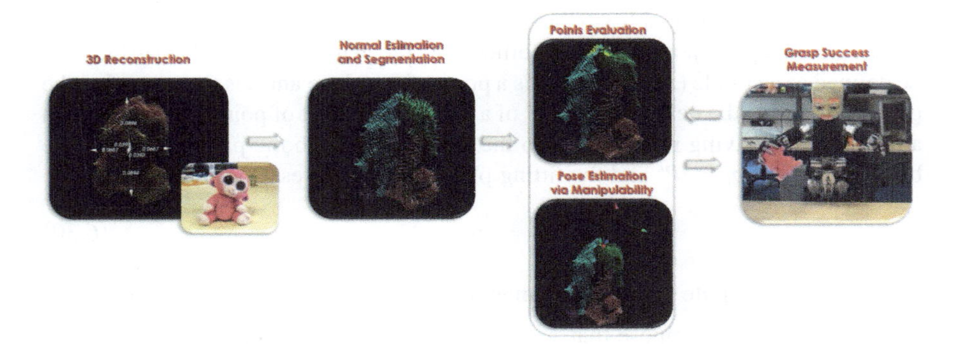

Fig. 6.13 The grasping pipeline: we start by reconstruct the object's shape in 3D resulting in a point cloud representation, which is then segmented. We extract surface normals and isolate connected smooth regions. We then rank the best points on the basis of a composite score function taking into account the object shape and size, and eventually including top-down information. Subsequently the best end-effector position and pose are estimated on the basis of the robot manipulability measure. If the grasp is successful, the score function is adjusted by updating the coefficients of an incremental least-square support vector machine

account the local shape properties around the points, as well as simple heuristics on the object dimension. This defines the best regions from where to extract grasping points. The user can also provide top-down information to bias the point selection process. Since vision is not enough to ensure a stable grasp, we select a set of N points that got the highest scores, and finally we pick a feasible hand configuration on the basis of the robot manipulability. The complete pipeline is schematized in Fig. 6.13.

6.6.1 Reconstructing and Segmenting the Point Cloud

Three-dimensional information can significantly improve the quality of robotic grasps, as it enables a more precise estimation of cues such as surface curvatures and normals. We rely on stereo vision algorithms in order to retrieve 3D information. We use the Hirschmuller algorithm (2008) to estimate the depth map, and we project each pixel of the object in the 3D space. We then estimate a minimum bounding box enclosing the point cloud, in order to obtain the approximate dimension of the object. We employ a technique based on the convex hull of the point cloud, which is analyzed using rotating calipers algorithms (Barequet and Har-Peled 2001). The next step selects where to place the end-effector. Here we would like to guarantee that the hand lies in a region that is large enough with curvature similar to that of the palm. We employ the region growing segmentation (Rabbani et al. 2006) that segments the object point cloud into a set of smooth connected regions. This method starts with the computation of surface normals as an estimation of the normal of a plane tangent to the surface passing by each point.

This is obtained through a least-square fitting on each point's neighborhood (Radu 2009). Given a point p and its neighborhood P^k, the plane tangent to the surface can be defined as a couple $(x, \overline{n})$, where x is a point of the plane and $\overline{n}$ is the normal to the plane. We define the neighborhood P^k of a point p as the set of points that lies within a circular area having radius equal to the radius of the robotic palm. The distance between a point $p_i \in P^k$ and the fitting plane can be expressed as

$$\text{dist}_i = (p_i - x)\overline{n}. \tag{6.30}$$

In order to compute the plane parameters, we need to minimize the distance dist_i for each point. If we impose that x is the centroid of the neighborhood (i.e., $x = \frac{1}{k} \sum_{i=1}^{k} p_i$), then the solution for $\overline{n}$ can be calculated by analyzing the eigenvectors and eigenvalues of the covariance matrix:

$$C = \frac{1}{k}\sum_{i=1}^{k}(x - p_i)(x - p_i)^{\mathrm{T}} \tag{6.31}$$

Once the normals of all points have been computed, a seed point p is chosen and every point $p_i \in P^k$ is evaluated; p_i will be added to the current cluster only if it is locally connected to the seed p and if the angle between the normals of p and p_i is smaller than a specified threshold; otherwise it is added to the list of potential seeds. The point cloud is thus subdivided into several regions having similar curvatures. Later in order to assure grasp stability, we select only the regions that contain a sufficient number of points. We effectively impose the condition that the hand is placed on a smooth and large enough surface of the object.

6.6.2 Points Evaluation

Appropriate end-effector positions are ranked by means of a score function which biases those with specific characteristics. We choose the N points with the highest score as returned by a function that weighs the object shape and dimension:

$$s(p) = w_1 \cdot v(p) + w_2 \cdot m(p) \tag{6.32}$$

where $v(p)$ is an auto-adaptive function representing the evaluation of visual properties at the point p and $m(p)$ is a fixed component that depends on the object dimension. $m(p)$ can integrate a user-defined task component. w_1 and w_2 are relative weights which can be chosen empirically to balance the contribution of the two components:

1. *Visual component*: The first part of the score function takes into account the shape of the object. In particular, we would like to grasp the object on a point

which lies on a surface having a curvature similar to the curvature of the robots palm, so that the hand can adapt on the object. Since good curvature values are not immediately computable, we use machine learning to approximate a relation between the robot's hand curvature and the curvature of a surface centered in a point p. In order to ensure that the hand will adapt on the object, the neighborhood of the evaluated point p will have the same area as the robot's hand. We relate the local curvature of the surface to a grasp success measure g, which is evaluated on the basis of the robot's own exploration. In particular, the grasp success measurement is a binary value (0 or 1), and it is provided by a grasp detector mechanism. To achieve such detection, we exploit the intrinsic elasticity of the iCub fingers; in particular we employ a technique that retrieves a measure of contact occurring on the distal phalanxes by comparing the actual joint position θ_j with the prediction $\hat{\theta}_j$ provided by a linear model of the joint actuation, given as input the motor position $\theta_{m(j)}$. High discrepancy between the feedback and the prediction corresponds to increasing external pressures; in this case we assign $g = 1$, otherwise $g = 0$. The map is trained from a set of input–output pairs acquired during free movements of the fingers (contactless). It is also possible to update the robot's experience continuously by learning the map between the curvature c computed on the surface centered at the point p and the grasp success/failure g. We use the same least-square support vector machine algorithm described in Sect. 6.3.2.

2. *Modality component*: The location of the grasp point on the object is an important element in choosing the grasping location. For example, if the object has one dimension much larger than the others, then selecting a point along the larger dimension increases the chances of a stable grasp. The rationale is that grasping an object that is too large for the hand is doomed to fail. On the contrary, if the object is too small, then it would be better to place the hand on the top of it. Following these considerations, we define three modality-specific biases, which thus assign higher scores to the points that, respectively, lie in the top, right, or left regions with respect to the robot's root frame. Objects have also specific affordances; hence it is reasonable to assume that the grasping mode depends on the task at hand. Since we are dealing with power grasp of unknown objects, we cannot define complex object-specific affordances. We have to content ourselves with generic task biases as, for instance, taking an object to give it to a person or taking the object to explore it as for learning tactile classification. To this aim, we can simply analyze the position of the point with respect to the rest of the object. For instance, if the task is to pass an object to a person waiting with her hand open, palm up, we can assume that the end-effector position is better located on the top part of the object. We leave this choice to a user-tunable parameter in our score function. In addition, we would like the hand to reach far from the border of the visible portion of the object since the computation of the surface normals tends to be noisier at the borders. This condition is easily satisfied by privileging points that lie far from the corner points of the minimum bounding box. In summary, given π_j,

$j = 1,\ldots,nc = 8$ corner points of the minimum enclosing bounding box, the preference for points on the top part of the object can be formulated as follows:

$$t(p) = \sqrt{|p_z - c_z|/\text{dim}_z} + \sum_{j=1}^{nc} \frac{||p - \pi_j||}{nc} \tag{6.33}$$

where p_z is the z component of the point p, c_z is the z component of the center of the object, and dim_z is the dimension of the object along the z-axis with respect to the robot's root frame.

6.6.3 Grasp Parameters Estimation

Once a number of suitable candidate points has been computed as illustrated above, we have to determine the best grasping point and the corresponding pose of the robots end-effector. This last step has to take into account the robot kinematics in order to ensure a feasible grasp. For each candidate point, we evaluate a set of possible orientations in terms of their manipulability index; given this measure, the most suitable point and orientation of the end-effector is selected.

We would like the hand to be parallel to the surface at the contact point, and thus we ask that the z-axis of the end-effector be parallel and opposite to the surface normal computed at the point under evaluation. We then sample the plane determined by the z-axis and passing through the point p by identifying n possible orientations for the x- and y-axes. We make use of Ipopt (Wätcher and Biegler 2006) as before to solve the inverse kinematics resulting in the joint configuration that satisfies the desired position and orientation of the hand using 10 degrees of freedom of the robot (7 for the arm and 3 for the torso). Notably, we find a reliable solution in only about 0.04[s], and we can consequently explore hundreds of possible robot configurations in a handful of seconds. Each resulting joint configuration is evaluated using the standard manipulability measure (Yoshikawa 1985):

$$w(\theta) = \sqrt{\det\left(J(\theta)J(\theta)^{\mathrm{T}}\right)} \tag{6.34}$$

where θ is the current joint configuration and J is the Jacobian matrix of the robot. Manipulability is further augmented with a penalty term that considers the distance from the joint limits:

$$P(\theta) = 1 - \exp - k \prod_{j=1}^{nj} \frac{\left(\theta_j - l_j^-\right)\left(l_j^+ - \theta_j\right)}{\left(l_j^+ - l_j^-\right)^2} \tag{6.35}$$

where θ_j is the current position of the jth joint, l_j^+ is the jth joint upper limit, l_j^- is the jth joint lower limit, and k is a scaling factor that weights the behavior of the measure near joint limits. Summarizing, we aim at finding a suitable position and orientation of the end-effector, such that the associated joint configuration θ optimizes the following:

$$\underset{\theta}{\operatorname{argmax}} \left(w(\theta) + P(\theta)\right) \tag{6.36}$$

The manipulability measure, combined with the direction of the normal, also defines the most suitable hand that should be used for a given grasp.

6.6.4 Experimental Validation

We validate grasping by conducting three different experiments. We start with a qualitative experiment, where we show that the same object, rotated by different amounts, can still be grasped reliably. Then we demonstrate that we can learn the relation between the curvature of an object region and its influence on a successful grasp. We finally perform a large number of grasp actions on several objects lying in different positions with respect to the robot, and we show that the robot can grasp them with a high success rate. In the context of these experiments, we used 19 of the 53 degrees of freedom (DOF) of the iCub, considering the 3 DOFs of the torso along with the 7 DOFs of the arm and 9 DOFs of the hand.

6.6.4.1 Rotating Object

To demonstrate that the system is robust against object rotations, we run a qualitative test using an elongated cylindrical container as shown in Fig. 6.14, placed at four different orientations with respect to upright direction: 0°, –45°, 45°, and 90°. It turns out that the modality component of the score function correctly rewards points that are lateral to the cylinder principal axis in the tested cases. As a result, the iCub adapts the grasp action accordingly (Fig. 6.14).

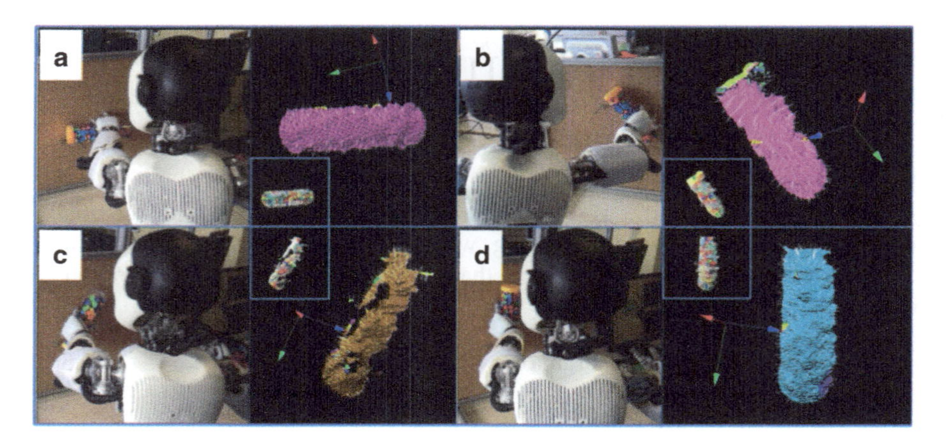

Fig. 6.14 Four different experiments with the same object. A cylinder is rotated respectively, by 0° (**a**), –45° (**b**), 45° (**c**), and 90° (**d**). The *rightmost plot* on each panel (**a–d**) shows the segmented object. The color coding shows that a single region is detected. Grasping is successful in all cases

6.6.4.2 Mapping Evaluation

The validation of the learning procedure and the resulting map between local surface curvature and the grasp success rate is carried out on a training set of 100 data points. These points are collected on the objects shown in Fig. 6.15. The 100 trials are performed imposing $w_2 = 0$; therefore only the curvature component is taken into account to evaluate the grasp success. Trials are carried out choosing points with random curvature values in order to explore the entire function domain. Figure 6.15 (bottom left) shows the results of learning. Abscissa and ordinates represent the curvature normalized between 0 and 1 and the grasp success rate, respectively. We can infer that surfaces with curvature values between 0.03 and 0.2 are suitable for the iCub's palm, and they usually lead to successful grasps. Conversely, surfaces too flat or with higher curvature rates tend to yield unsuccessful grasps. To verify whether the maximum of the function identifies a critical curvature, we designed a dedicated experiment with two grasping sessions on the cylindrical container (Fig. 6.15, see bottom-center image), which presents both flat and curved surfaces. In the first session, we let the robot perform 30 grasps by choosing points with curvature close to the limits of unsuccessful grasp ($c > 0.3$). In the second session, an additional set of 30 grasps is collected by rewarding points with curvature close to the maximum. We report a grasp success rate of 60 % on the first session, and a significantly higher rate (90 %) on the second session, proving that grasping performance considerably changes as a function of the curvature of the chosen point. Notably, a relatively small set of 100 samples is sufficient to learn the curvature map.

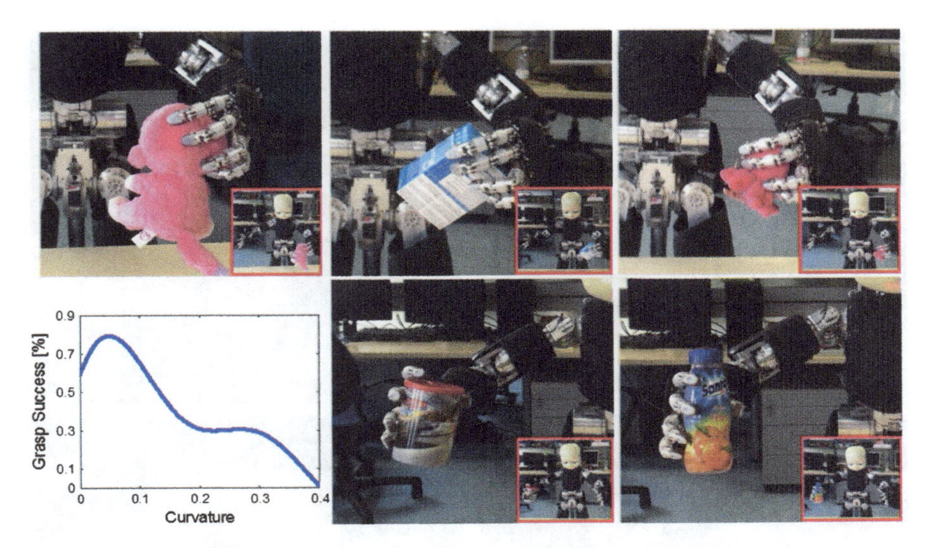

Fig. 6.15 *Bottom left*: the learned map between object curvatures and successful grasps. Curvature is normalized between 0 and 1. Points with curvatures in the range of 0.1 and 0.2 are preferable as they are likely to bring about successful grasps

6.6.4.3 Complete Pipeline

To evaluate the complete system, we define a performance indicator as follows: a grasp is successful if the robot can hold it firmly without dropping it. The experiment we present here also demonstrates that the curvature map (learned earlier) generalizes to novel objects. We execute 20 trials on each object in the test set (Fig. 6.16), i.e., 80 trials in total, achieving an overall success rate of 91.25 %. Such accuracy makes these algorithms suitable to be employed in robust manipulation tasks. As grasping lacks a standardized benchmark, we compare our approach with a simple top grasp (grasping the object always from the top), which has been widely used in the past. We tested this more stereotyped grasp on the same objects showed in Fig. 6.16 carrying out 20 trials per object as before. The success rate for the cylinder and the bottle was significantly lower (15 % for both) quite obviously because of their elongated shape that makes the top grasp unsuitable. We also achieved 65 % for the stuffed dog and 80 % for the cube. These results confirm the considerable performance gain of the complete grasping pipeline.

6.7 Vision

The remaining element in this journey through the structure of the iCub controllers is certainly vision. We strive to provide reliable estimates of the position and shape of objects in space since this enables the control of action as presented earlier

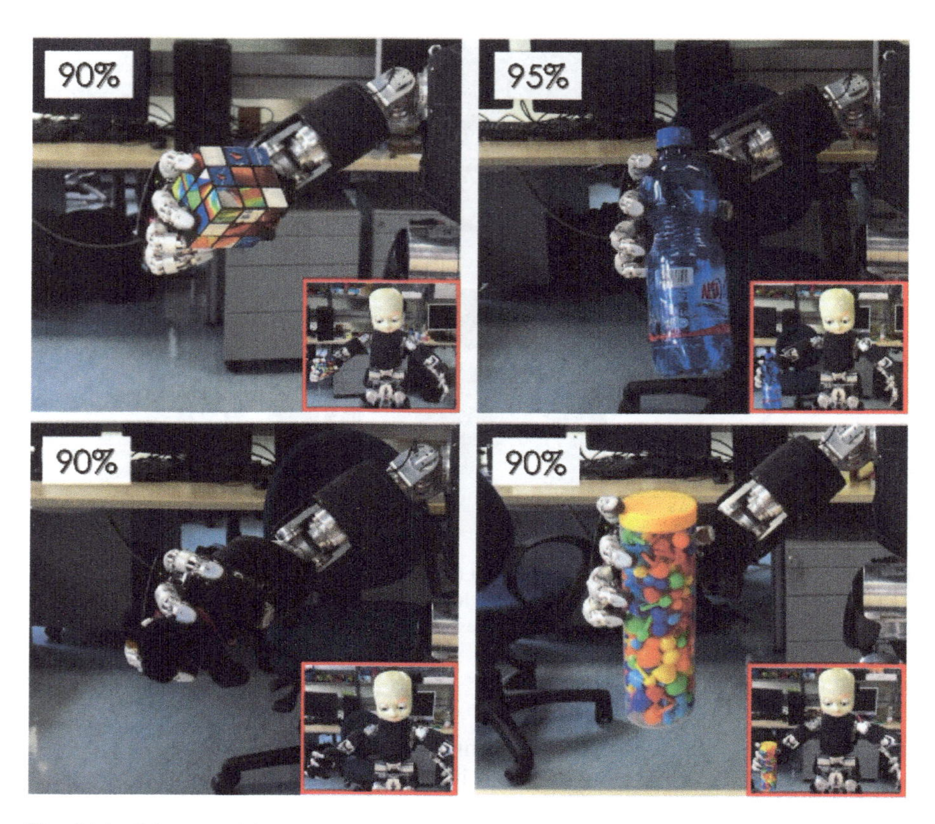

Fig. 6.16 Objects used for testing with their respective success rates over 20 trials

(reaching and grasping). One appealing visual cue is motion and we have been recently able to devise a method which provides motion segmentation independent from the movement of the cameras. Another important source of information is 3D vision which enables the extraction of partial object shape which in turn is useful for the control of grasping. For 3D vision we used a standard method and we refer the reader to the paper by Hirschmuller (2008). The estimation of visual motion is instead described next.

6.7.1 Optical Flow

Our method is based on the analysis of failures of the standard Lucas–Kanade algorithm (1981). As a general rule, in order to verify that the instant velocity v of a point p has been correctly estimated, the patch W around that point in the image I_t is compared to the patch of the same size at $p + v$ in the new image I_{t+1} (where the original point is supposed to have moved). Given a suitable threshold Θ_M, the discrepancy measure

$$M(p) = \sum_{q \in W} (I_t(p + q) - I_{t+1}(p + v + q))^2 \tag{6.37}$$

is then used to evaluate whether tracking was correctly performed ($M(p) < \Theta_M$) or not ($M(p) \geq \Theta_M$). It is thus interesting to analyze empirically when the Lucas–Kanade algorithm tends to fail and why. Conclusions from this investigation will lead directly to a method to perform independent motion detection. The main empirical circumstances in which errors in the evaluation process of the optical flow arise are three:

- Speed. The instantaneous velocity of the point is too large with respect to the window where motion is being considered. Hence, the computation of temporal derivatives is difficult.
- Rotations. The motion around the point has a strong rotational component and thus, even locally, the assumption regarding the similarity of velocities fails.
- Occlusions. The point is occluded by another entity and obviously it is impossible to track it in the subsequent frame.

Tracking failures caused by high punctual speed depend exclusively on the scale of the neighborhood where optical flow is computed. This issue is usually solved by the so-called pyramidal approach which applies the Lucas–Kanade method at multiple image scales. This allows evaluating iteratively larger velocities first and then smaller ones. Instead we determined empirically that when rotations cause failures in the tracking process, this is often a consequence of a movement independent from that of the observer. The third situation in which Lucas–Kanade fails, is caused by occlusions. In this context the main role in determining whether optical flow has been successfully computed is played by the speed at which such occlusion takes place.

We therefore look for points where tracking is likely to fail as soon as one of the conditions discussed is met, i.e., flow inconsistencies due to rotations or occlusions. In detail, we run Lucas–Kanade over a uniform grid on the image, perform the comparison indicated in (6.37), and then filter for false positives (isolated failures). The results are a set of independent moving blobs.

We tested the method both in controlled situations (a small robotic device moving linearly in front of the iCub) and, more generally, in tracking people and other moving objects in the laboratory. Figure 6.17 shows results of tracking with both stationary and moving cameras (therefore without and with ego-motion, respectively). In the configuration considered, a linear speed of 10 cm/s corresponds to one pixel per frame in a 30 frames-per-second (fps) acquisition. Experiments were conducted up to 100 cm/s and with the iCub head adding movement up to 40 deg/s.

The sequence of images in Fig. 6.18 is an example of a more naturalistic tracking. In spite of the complexity of the background, it is evident from the images

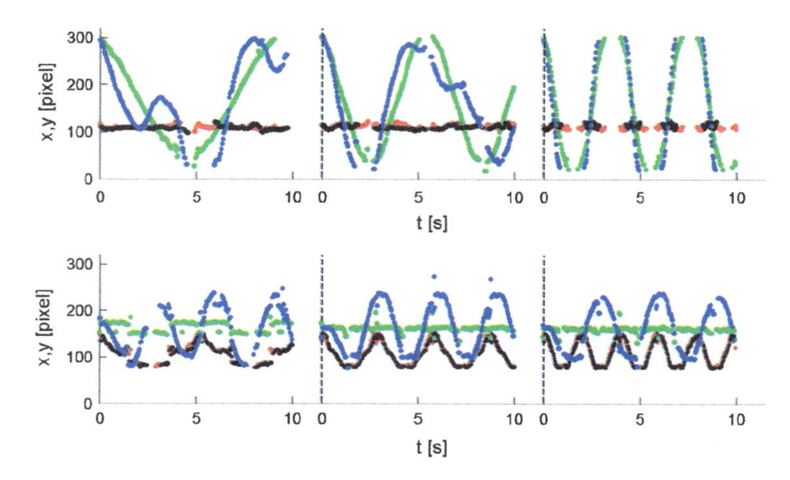

Fig. 6.17 Trajectories of the x, y coordinates of the center of mass of the areas detected as moving independently. The cart is moving parallel (*up*) or orthogonal (*down*) with respect to the image plane. The plots are reported for the following cart speeds: from *left* to *right* 20, 40, 100 cm/s. Colors legend: (1) *green* for x and *red* for y in the case of a static head; (2) *blue* for x and *black* for y in the case of a head rotating at 20 deg/s

that our method produces robust detection of the moving target with a behavior that varies smoothly in time and is consistent with respect to the two different views acquired from the left and right cameras of the robot. In particular, the movement of the target is effectively tracked both when the person is far from the robot (frames 1 and 6) as well as when he gets closer to it (frames 2–5). Furthermore a substantial modification to light conditions exists with a maximum of brightness reached approximately at frame 4. The algorithm is robust to occlusions: this is visible at the frames in which pillars and posters cover the person. Notably, at frame 3 another person sitting at the table produces a secondary blob with his hand. This distractor is of limited size and it does not interfere with the task since the tracker is instructed to follow the largest blob in the sequence.

These are the data that at the moment the iCub uses for attention and for tracking and which are eventually passed to the reaching controller described earlier. We favored robustness to accuracy here in order to be able to run learning methods and exploration of the environment for considerable periods of time (e.g., as for collecting the 20,000 samples mentioned in Sect. 6.5.1). Our experiments show that this goal has been fully achieved.

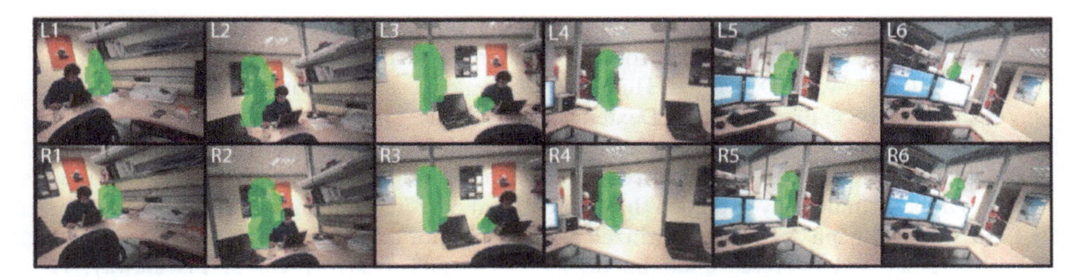

Fig. 6.18 A sequence of images recorded during the real time stereo tracking of a person walking in front of the iCub: six images are shown in temporal order from L1 to L6 (*left camera*) and R1 to R6 (*right camera*). The walking person is highlighted with a *green blob* using the result of proposed algorithm

6.8 Conclusions

This chapter deals with the problem of building a reliable architecture to control movement by relying on sensory data in a humanoid robot where many degrees of freedom need to be coordinated. We have shown original solutions to vision (using motion), to kinematics (using robust optimization and a multi-referential trajectory formulation), and to dynamics (by enabling impedance control from a set of FTSs and tactile sensors). Although certain aspects of these methods are somewhat traditional, their specific application and combination is novel. We took particular care in testing all methods rigorously and comparing them with other methods in the literature.

Furthermore, the entire implementation of this software is available, following the iCub policies, as open source (GPL) from the iCub repository. These libraries and modules, besides running on the iCub, are available to the research community at large. The algorithms are almost always embedded in static libraries ready to be picked up by others.

The iCub repository can be found at http://www.icub.org and browsed on Source-Forge (http://www.sourceforge.net). Several videos of the iCub showing the methods described in this paper are available on the Internet and in particular at this site: http://www.youtube.com/robotcub.

References

Abend W, Bizzi E, Morasso P (1982) Human arm trajectory formation. Brain 105:331–348

Arbib MA (1981) Perceptual structures and distributed motor control. In: Brooks VB (ed) Handbook of physiology, vol. II, motor control. American Physiological Society, Bethesda, MD, pp 1449–1480

Barequet G, Har-Peled S (2001) Efficiently approximating the minimum-volume bounding box of a point set in three dimensions. J Algorithm 38:91–109

Bjorck A (1996) Numerical methods for least squares problems. Society for Industrial Mathematics, Philadelphia, PA

Chalon M, Grebenstein M, Wimboeck T, Hirzinger G (2010) The thumb: guidelines for a robotic design. In: IEEE/RSJ international conference on intelligent robots and systems
Cutkosky MR, Howe RD (1990) Human grasp choice and robotic grasp analysis. In: Venkataraman ST, Iberall T (eds) Dexterous robot hands. Springer, New York, NY
Dallali H, Mosadeghzad M, Medrano-CerdaGA, Docquier N, Kormushev P, Tsagarakis N, Li Z, Caldwell D (2013) Development of a dynamic simulator for a compliant humanoid robot based on a symbolic multibody approach. In: International conference on mechatronics, Vicenza
De Lasa M, Hertzmann A (2009) Prioritized optimization for task-space control. In: 2009 IEEE/RSJ international conference on intelligent robots and systems, vol 3, Piscataway, NJ, pp 5755–5762
Deo AS, Walker ID (1992) Robot subtask performance with singularity robustness using optimal damped least-squares. In: IEEE international conference on robotics and automation
Eljaik J, Li Z, Randazzo M, Parmiggiani A, Metta G, Tsagarakis N, Nori F (2013) Quantitative evaluation of standing stabilization using stiff and compliant actuators. In: Robotics: science and systems 2013, Berlin, 24–28 June
Featherstone R, Orin DE (2008) Dynamics—chapter 2. In: Siciliano B, Khatib O (eds) Springer handbook of robotics. Springer, Berlin
Fitzpatrick P, Metta G, Natale L (2008) Towards long-lived robot genes. Robot Auton Syst 56(1): 29–45
Flash T, Hogan N (1985) The coordination of arm movements: an experimentally confirmed mathematical model. J Neurosci 5:1688–1703
Gallese V, Fadiga L, Fogassi L, Rizzolatti G (1996) Action recognition in the premotor cortex. Brain 119:593–609
Gibson JJ (1977) The theory of affordances. In: Shaw R, Bransford J (eds) Perceiving, acting and knowing: toward an ecological psychology. Lawrence Erlbaum, Hillsdale, NJ, pp 67–82
Gijsberts A, Metta G (2011) Incremental learning of robot dynamics using random features. In: IEEE international conference on robotics and automation, Shanghai, 9–13 May
Hersch M, Billard AG (2008) Reaching with multi-referential dynamical systems. Auton Robot 25 (1–2):71–83
Hirschmuller H (2008) Stereo processing by semiglobal matching and mutual information, TPAMI
Ihrke CA, Parsons AH, Mehling JS, Griffith BK. Planar torsion spring. Patent, June 2010
Lallee S, Yoshida E, Nori F, Natale L, Metta G, Warneken F, Dominey PF (2010) Human-robot cooperation based on interaction learning. In: Sigaud O, Peters J (eds) From motor learning to interaction learning in robots, vol 264. Springer, Heidelberg
Lee HY, Yi BJ, Choi Y (2007) A realistic joint limit algorithm for kinematically redundant manipulators. In: IEEE international conference on control, automation and systems
Lucas BD, Kanade T (1981) An iterative image registration technique with an application to stereo vision. In: Proceedings of IJCAI, pp 674–679
Metta G (2010) The iCub website. http://www.iCub.org
Metta G, Vernon D, Sandini G (2005) The RobotCub approach to the development of cognition: implications of emergent systems for a common research agenda in epigenetic robotics. In: 5th epigenetic robotics workshop, Nara, July 2005
Metta G, Natale L, Nori F et al (2010) The iCub humanoid robot: an open-systems platform for research in cognitive development. Neural Netw 23:1125–1134
Miyamoto H, Schaal S, Gandolfo F, Gomi H, Koike Y, Osu R, Nakano E, Wada Y, Kawato M (1996) A kendama learning robot based on bi-directional theory. Neural Netw 9:1281–1302
Nguyen-Tuong D, Peters J, Seeger M (2008) Computed torque control with nonparametric regression models. In: American control conference (ACC 2008), 2008 June, pp 212–217
Parmiggiani A, Maggiali M, Natale L, Nori F, Schmitz A, Tsagarakis N, Santos-Victor J, Becchi F, Sandini G, Metta G (2012a) The design of the iCub humanoid robot. Int J HR 9(4):1–24

Parmiggiani A, Metta G, Tsagarakis N (2012b) The mechatronic design of the new legs of the iCub robot. In: IEEE-RAS international conference on humanoid robots (HU-MANOIDS2012), Osaka, Japan, 29 November–1 December

Pattacini U, Nori F, Natale L, Metta G, Sandini G (2010) An experimental evaluation of a novel minimum-jerk cartesian controller for humanoid robots. In: IEEE/RSJ international conference on intelligent robots and systems, Taipei, 18–22 October, pp 1668–1674

Peters J, Mistry M, Udwadia FE, Nakanishi J, Schaal S (2007) A unifying framework for robot control with redundant DOFs. Auton Robot 24:1–12

Rabbani T, van den Heuvel F, Vosselmann G (2006) Segmentation of point clouds using smoothness constraint. In: ISPRS commission V symposium 'Image Engineering and Vision Metrology'

Radu BR (2009) Semantic 3d object maps for everyday manipulation in human living environments, Ph.D. dissertation, Computer Science department, Technische Universität München, Germany

Rahimi A, Recht B (2008) Random features for large-scale kernel machines. Adv Neural Inf Process Syst 20:1177–1184

Roa M, Argus M, Leidner D, Borst C, Hirzinger G (2012) Power grasp planning for anthropomorphic robot hands. In: IEEE international conference on robotics and automation

Robotran webpage (2012) http://www.robotran.be

Sciavicco L, Siciliano B (2005) Modelling and control of robot manipulators, 2nd edn, Advanced text-books in control and signal processing. Springer, London

Sentis L, Khatib O (2005) Synthesis of whole-body behaviors through hierarchical control of behavioral primitives. Int J HR 2:505–518

The Orocos website. http://www.orocos.org/kdl

Tilley AR (2002) The measure of man & woman: human factors in design. Wiley Interscience, New York, NY

Tsagarakis NG, Metta G, Sandini G et al (2007) iCub: the design and realization of an open humanoid platform for cognitive and neuroscience research. Adv Robot 21(10):1151–1175

Tsagarakis N, Li Z, Saglia J, Caldwell D (2011) The design of the lower body of the compliant humanoid robot cCub. In: Proceedings of the IEEE international conference on robotics and automation (ICRA), May, pp 2035–2040

Vernon D, Metta G, Sandini G (2007) A survey of cognition and cognitive architectures: implications for the autonomous development of mental capabilities in computational systems. IEEE transactions on evolutionary computation, special issue on AMD, vol 11, April

Villani L, De Shutteer J (2008) Force control—chapter 7. In: Sicilian B, Khatib O (eds) Springer handbook of robotics. Springer, Berlin

von Hofsten C (2004) An action perspective on motor development. Trends Cogn Sci 8:266–272

Wätcher A, Biegler LT (2006) On the implementation of a primal-dual interior point filter line search algorithm for large-scale nonlinear programming. Math Program 106(1):25–57

Yoshikawa T (1985) Manipulability of robotic mechanisms. Int J Robotics Res 4(2):3–9

Chapter 7
Towards a "Brain-Guided" Cognitive Architecture

Vishwanathan Mohan, Pietro Morasso, and Giulio Sandini

7.1 Introduction

Motor control and motor cognition have been under intensive scrutiny for over a century with a growing number of experimental and theoretical tools of increasing complexity. Still we are far away from a real understanding which can allow us, for example, to integrate what we know in large-scale projects like VPH (Virtual Physiological Human). In a sense, the abundance of new behavioral, neurophysiological, and computational approaches may worsen the situation, by "flooding" researchers with frequently incompatible evidence, losing view of the overall picture. An aspect of this tendency is to quickly dismiss earlier "old-fashioned" ideas on the basis of specific but narrow new evidence. This chapter argues in the opposite direction, revisiting old-fashioned notions, like synergy formation, equilibrium point hypothesis (EPH), and body schema, in order to *reuse* them in a larger context, focused on whole-body actions: this context, typical of humanoid robotics, stresses the need of efficient computational architectures, capable to defeat the curse of dimensionality determined by the frightening "trinity": complex body + complex brain + complex (partly unknown) environment. The idea is to organize the computational process in a local to global manner, grounding it on emerging studies in different areas of neuroscience, while keeping in mind that motor cognition and motor control are inseparable twins, linked through a common body/body schema. The long-term goal is to make a humanoid robot like iCub capable of "cumulative learning." A humanoid robot should mirror both the complexity of the human form and the brain that drives it to exhibit equally complex and often creative behaviors! This requires to emulate the gradual process of infant "cognitive development" in order to investigate the underlying interplay among multiple sensory, motor, and cognitive processes in the framework of an integrated system: a coherent,

V. Mohan (✉) • P. Morasso • G. Sandini
Central Research Laboratory, Istituto Italiano di Tecnologia, Genova, Italy
e-mail: vishwanathan.mohan@iit.it

R. Cingolani (ed.), *Bioinspired Approaches for Human-Centric Technologies*,
DOI 10.1007/978-3-319-04924-3_7, © Springer International Publishing Switzerland 2014

purposive system that emerges from a persistent flux of fragmented, partially inconsistent episodes in which the human/humanoid perceives, acts, learns, remembers, forgets, reasons, makes mistakes, introspects, etc. We aim at linking such a model building approach with emerging trends in neuroscience, taking into account that one of the fundamental challenges today is to "causally and computationally" correlate the incredibly complex behavior of animals to the equally complex activity in their brains. This requires to build a shared computational/neural basis for "execution, imagination, and understanding" of action, while taking into account recent findings from the field of "connectomics," which addresses the large-scale organization of the cerebral cortex, and the discovery of the "default mode network" of the brain. We will particularly focus, in the near future, on the organization of memory instead of "learning" per se because this helps understanding development from a more "holistic" viewpoint that is not restricted to "isolated tasks" or "experiments." Computationally the proposed architecture should lead towards novel nonlinear, non-Turing computational machinery based on quasi-physical, non-digital interactions grounded in the biology of the brain.

7.2 Background Concepts on Body and Embodiment

7.2.1 Embodiment

Robotics has long been disputed between approaches that are fully dependent on the exploitation of the affordances provided by the specific features/structure of the robot "body" and approaches, based on artificial intelligence (AI) principles, that neglect "embodiment" and operate in a completely abstract domain. The "vehicles" proposed by Valentino Braitenberg (1986) are examples of the former approach: in spite of the fact that the control hardware is simply a reactive system, which directly links the sensors to the actuators, vehicles' behaviors can be surprisingly adaptive and exhibit remarkable features that are commonly attributed to some kind of "intelligence." There are also many biological counterparts of Braitenberg's vehicles, such as the Aplysia depilans (Kandel and Tauc 1965), which emphasize the fact that adaptive behavior does not require a central nervous system but can emerge in very simple networks of biological neurons as well. However, it is quite clear that purely reactive systems (or reflexes, in the neurophysiological jargon) can only work effectively with very simple bodies.

Nevertheless, a very influential theory proposed by Charles Sherrington (1904) that dominated the understanding of human neurophysiology for over half a century is based on a simple generalization of the reactive architecture, by positing that reflexes are the basic modules of the integrative action of the nervous system, thus enabling the entire body to function towards one definite goal at a time. A similar point of view was defended by Rodney Brooks in robotics (Brooks 1991), as a drastic alternative to GOFAI (Good Old-Fashioned Artificial Intelligence), by proposing a bottom-up design, named *Subsumption Architecture*, that is supposed to achieve "intelligence without representation": this architecture is organized in layers, decomposing complicated intelligent behavior into many "simple" behavioral modules, which in turn are organized into layers of simpler behaviors, down to reflex-like mechanisms. Each layer implements a particular goal of the agent, and higher layers are increasingly general and abstract. However, this kind of layered bottom-up architecture scales up badly when one attempts to deal with complex bodies and complex behaviors in a complex environment.

In contrast with the Sherringtonian view, Hugo Liepmann (1905) was the first one to suggest that actions are generated from within, requiring the existence of an *internal state* where they would be encoded, stored, and ultimately performed independently of the stimuli coming from the external environment. To account for the implementation of action plans, he proposed that the elementary chunks of action are assembled according to an internal representation: he called *movement formula* the result of this process, i.e., an anticipatory hierarchical structure where all the aspects of an action are represented, before it is enfolded in time. Liepmann's legacy is still quite influential in motor neuroscience, although the term *movement formula* was later replaced by several others, like *engram*, *schema*, or *internal model*. In the same vein, Nikolai Bernstein (1935) had an interesting analogy for explaining this mode of organization: he suggested that the representation of an action must contain, "like an embryo in an egg or a track on a gramophone record," the entire scheme of the movement as it is expanded in time and it must also guarantee the order and the rhythm of the realization of this scheme.

In the field of human motor cognition, only recently advanced brain imaging techniques allowed to gain direct access to cognitive/mental states in the absence of overt behavior, thus making clear that actions involve a covert stage. It is now accepted that the covert stage is a representation of the future that includes

- The goal of the action
- The means/tools to reach it
- The consequences on the body
- The effects on the external world

Covert and overt stages thus represent a continuum, such that every overtly executed action implies the existence of a covert stage, whereas a covert action does not necessarily turns out into an overt action. Jeannerod (2001) provided a very important contribution by formulating the Mental Simulation Theory, which posits that cognitive motor processes such as motor imagery, movement observation, action planning, and verbalization share the same representations with motor execution. Jeannerod interpreted this brain activity as an internal simulation of a detailed representation of action and used the term *S-state* for describing the corresponding time-varying mental states. The crucial point is that since S-states occurring during covert actions are, to a great extent, quite similar to the states occurring during overt actions, then it is not unreasonable to posit that also real, overt actions are the results of the same internal simulation process. Running such internal simulations on an interconnected set of neuronal networks is, in our view, the main function of what is known as *body schema*.

7.2.2 Synergies

Synergy is a compound noun of Greek origin that implies the interaction and cooperation of two or more elements for carrying out some function or work which is difficult or impossible to achieve with isolated elements. Bernstein (1935) was among the first ones to use this term for describing the complexity of the motor system, recognizing that the central problem in the neural control of movement is *motor redundancy*, namely the imbalance between (a small number of) task-related variables and the (extremely large number of) muscles and mechanical degrees of freedom (DoF). He suggested that the brain uses synergies to solve this problem, giving this term a strongly *cybernetic* meaning, indeed years before Norbert Wiener invented the term cybernetics: the idea, although not developed in a mathematical model, was that synergies allow the brain to get rid of task-irrelevant degrees of freedom, thus focusing on the simpler problem of mastering a smaller number of task-relevant variables. In this sense, a synergy can be conceived as a "dimensionality-reduction device," and as such it has been criticized by some (e.g., Diedrichsen and Classen 2012) considering that deterministic constraints on the evolution of DoFs would imply the inability to achieve large subsets of physically possible postures, an inability which is contradicted by a number of experimental findings in speech motor control, whole-body reaching, brain–machine interfaces, etc. However, this criticism can be overcome by supposing that the computational mechanism, responsible for constraining DoFs and muscle activation patterns in such a way to allow a small number of command variables to coordinate them in a purposive manner, is not hardwired but is sensitive to task requirements, imposing task-related constraints in the preparation time of an action. In this view, biologically plausible synergy formation mechanisms must be multireferential, in the sense of allowing task-modulated bidirectional dynamic interactions among different spaces: end-effector space, joint and muscles space, and possibly spaces related to the DoFs of manipulated tools. If such dynamic interactions are acquired by the brain of a subject via training in the real world, they will incorporate implicitly causality constraints, thus allowing a synergy formation mechanism to bind together high-dimensionality and low-dimensionality computational processes. This means that dimensionality reduction can coexist with full dimensionality representation also in a deterministic framework, provided that suitable dynamic processes link the different spaces. Later on we describe a mathematical model, based on Passive Motion Paradigm (PMP), that can achieve this goal.

In recent years a lot of effort has been focused on *muscle synergies* (D'Avella et al. 2003). It has been found that, for a wide variety of motor tasks, muscle activation patterns evolve in low-dimensional manifolds and thus can be approximated by the linear composition of a small set of predefined/primitive patterns or modules, i.e., the basis vectors of such low-dimensional subspace. However, from this empirical evidence, can we conclude that muscle synergies are explicitly encoded or stored in the brain, thus becoming the building blocks of the synergy formation mechanism? It is possible indeed that the observed correlations and regularities are not determined by the immediate readout of hypothetic modules, for which there is no concrete evidence, but the effects of a multireferential neural dynamics that does not need to explicitly store or encode a number of high-dimensional patterns. It has been shown, for example, by Kutch and Valero-Cuevas (2012), that biomechanical constraints can explain the low-dimensionality of muscle synergies, without the need of an explicit neural coding, and it is conceivable that the specific dynamic modules incorporate such constraints in the production of synergistic patterns. A recent study with frog leg muscles before and after transection at different levels of the neuraxis (Roh et al. 2011) shows that muscle synergies are organized within the brain stem and spinal cord and are activated by descending commands. Moreover, microstimulation of cortical areas (Overduin et al 2012) is capable of evoking muscle synergies that match those extracted from natural movements. But again, this does not imply that muscle synergies are explicitly coded in the corticospinal motor system, although it is compatible with the neural origin of such synergies (Bizzi and Cheung 2013).

It is also worth mentioning that the idea of storing muscle synergies, as basic motor primitives, is similar to the rationale of the model proposed years before by Rosenbaum et al. (1995), which defends the idea that motor planning is based on "goal postures," selected from a "database" of stored postures. "Goal postures" take the place of "muscle synergies," but the underlying idea is the same: using a limited, but sufficiently rich, number of high-dimensional patterns to be combined by a synergy formation process. The underlying issue, in our opinion, is *memory vs. computation trade-off*: is it better to find the solution of a problem by storing a database of predefined solutions or by simulating an internal, generic, computational model? The answer is not unique and probably the brain can switch between one method and the other in different situations. However, in the case of whole-body motor control, the curse of dimensionality, namely, the exponential growth of computational complexity when the number of recruited degrees of freedom increases, is likely to hit the memory solution earlier than the computational solution.

7.2.3 Motor Synergies and Motor Imagery

Recent discoveries about motor imagery are slowly revolutionizing our grasp of motor control and motor cognition. Motor imagery, which can be defined as the set of mental processes occurring when a movement is imagined or practiced without performing it in an overt way, shares many features with brain activities in real actions, as made explicit by means of brain imaging techniques (Decety 1996). The practical relevance of this empirical finding comes from the effectiveness of mental practice for improving performance in athletic skills (Suinn 1972) and the fact that stroke patients can use mental practice to regain motor function (Sharma et al. 2006). We should also take into account that, in spite of similarities, there is also evidence that motor imagery and neural processes during overt motor behavior are not exactly the same (Coelho et al. 2012). Nevertheless, the same existence of motor imagery indicates that muscle synergies are unlike as basic building blocks of the synergy formation circuitry and suggests that what occurs in the brain, during mental rehearsal or mental training, reflects an endogenous dynamics, not a dynamics related to the neuromuscular system, as involved in overt movements. In other words, "muscleless" motor synergies, occurring in covert movements, might be the hidden building blocks which stand behind the recorded muscle synergies.

In any case, there is mounting evidence accumulated from different directions such as brain imaging studies (Frey and Gerry 2006; Grafton 2009), mirror neuron systems (Rizzolatti et al. 1996; Rizzolatti and Luppino 2001; Rizzolatti and Sinigaglia 2010), and embodied cognition (Gallese and Sinigaglia 2011; Gallese and Lakoff 2005) that generally supports the idea that action "generation, observation, imagination, and understanding" share similar underlying functional networks in the brain: distributed, multicenter neural activities occur not only during imagination of movement but also during observation and imitation of other's actions (Buccino et al. 2001; Anderson 2003; Frey and Gerry 2006; Grafton 2009; Iacoboni 2009) and comprehension of language, namely action-related verbs and nouns (Pulvermüller and Fadiga 2010; Glenberg and Gallese 2012). Such neural activation patterns include premotor and motor areas as well as areas of the cerebellum and the basal ganglia. During the observation of movements of others, an entire network of cortical areas, called "action observation network," is activated in a highly reproducible fashion (Grafton 2009). The central hypothesis that emerges out of these results is that motor imagery and motor execution draw on a shared set of cortical and subcortical mechanisms underlying motor cognition.

On the other hand, single-cell recordings of motor cortical neurons have provided an apparently different picture, showing that those neurons are characterized by rather broad tuning functions and suggesting the theory of population coding of some kind of population parameter. However, after the early seminal study by Georgopoulos et al. (1986), who proposed that movement direction might be the coded parameter, alternative interpretations were proposed also on theoretical ground (Mussa-Ivaldi 1988), by showing that the same experimental findings can be correlated indeed with different movement-related parameters. Other experimental studies have also shown that the activity of motor cortical neurons correlates with a broad range of parameters of motor performance from spatial target location to hand or joint motion, joint torque, muscle activation patterns, etc. In other words, the correlation between an internal variable, such as the discharge frequency of a motor neuron, and a specific aspect of an empirically measured movement is a very weak form of explanation of the organization of the motor system.

This kind of indeterminacy is also found in a related area of motor control study: the attempt to explain motor invariants, such as the speed–accuracy trade-off (Woodworth 1899), the bell-shaped speed profile of aiming movements

(Morasso 1981), or the power law relating the speed and curvature profiles of continuous drawing movements (Lacquaniti et al. 1983), by means of optimization processes to be associated with the main synergy formation process. Also in this case the empirically characterized smoothness of natural movements is compatible with different optimization criteria, but fails to identify in a strong manner a single organizing principle. Thus, the quest for the prevailing motor parameter directly encoded by neuron firing and the optimization criterion specifically employed in the neural control of movements both appear to be an elusive "holy grail." The crucial point, in our opinion, is that the direct encoding/storage of specific features or criteria is basically a static concept: it may be appropriate, at least as a first-order approximation, for describing sensory/perceptual processing but fails to capture the essence of "ergonomics" (in the wide sense of the word's etymology), namely, the capability of human beings to generate extremely complex spatiotemporal patterns, required for performing purposive actions, while interacting with external systems and environments. Another essential feature of "ergonomics" is flexibility, in the sense that each action can potentially recruit all the DoFs of the whole body, with the requirement of a rapid reorganization of the specifically recruited body parts as a function of task and environmental requirements. This makes the static encoding of movement parameters impossible or at least nonfunctional.

The alternative to static encoding is endogenous dynamics of brain circuitry which indirectly supplies the outflow of motor commands and, in turn, is sensitive to the inflow of reafferent signals. This is an idea supported by Churchland et al. (2012) who recently proposed that the evolution over time of the state vector of a cortical map (namely, the instantaneous distribution of firing rates for all the neurons of a map) can be better characterized by a nonlinear differential equation, driven by some external input vector, rather than by a direct static encoding of movement parameters. In this framework, the tuning properties of individual neurons are unintended consequences of the fact that the state vector (or population code) is causally determining the motor outflow, although in an indirect way. We agree with this idea, but we should also consider that it has been around for at least two decades, although as the opinion of a small minority: we welcome its resurrection in the context of new evidence and renewed thinking.

7.2.4 Motor Synergies and the Equilibrium Point Hypothesis

The concept of synergy, as a "dimensionality-reduction device," was accompanied in early studies by the attempt to assign a regulatory role to the "springlike" behavior of muscles (Bernstein 1935) when such springness was indeed suggested by several experimental studies in the 1960s and 1970s (Asatryan and Feldman 1965; Bizzi and Polit 1978, among others). The central idea was that there is no chance in trying to explain biological movement in terms of engineering servomechanism theory, an approach supported, for example, by Marsden et al. (1972), first of all because muscles are not force/torque generators like electrical motors but mainly because the propagation delays in the feedback loop are a severe, potential source of instability. In contrast, intrinsic muscle stiffness has two strong beneficial effects: (1) it provides, locally (i.e., in a muscle-wise manner), an instantaneous disturbance compensation action, and (2) it induces, globally (i.e., in a total body-wise manner), a multidimensional force field with attractor dynamics. This allows to achieve complex body postures "for free," without a complex, high-dimensional computational process, but simply by allowing the intrinsic dynamics of the neuromuscular system to seek its equilibrium state.

In this framework, movement becomes the transition from an equilibrium state to another, with the remarkable property of "equifinality" (Kelso and Holt 1980), namely, the fact that movement endpoints should be scarcely affected either by small, transient perturbations or by variations in the starting position of the body. Such attractor properties of motor control were confirmed by several studies of electrical stimulation of different parts of the nervous system, such as interneurons in the spinal cord of the frog (Giszter et al. 1993) or pyramidal neurons in the precentral cortex of the monkey (Graziano et al. 2002).

In reality, the picture is more complicated, in the sense that detailed experimental investigations show, for example, that muscles can only be approximated by ideal springs and that equifinality can be somehow violated by small, impulsive force disturbances (Popescu and Rymer 2000) or specific environmental conditions. In spite of this, we believe that EPH can explain a lot of the overall rationale underlying synergy formation, although it cannot cover the whole range of situations. Consider, for example, the stability of the upright standing body and the coordination in whole-body aiming movements: in this case, muscle stiffness alone is insufficient to achieve stability (Loram and Lakie 2002) and requires a parallel intermittent control action (Asai et al. 2009); on the other hand, the appropriate synchronization of ankle and hip strategies, which is essential for whole-body aiming, is nicely explained by means of an extended force field-based coordination model (Morasso et al. 2010), based on the Passive Motion Paradigm (see below).

Motor imagery is quite important, again, for framing the discourse in the right perspective. Since in humans and other species in the high stages of phylogenetic development, actions can be goal oriented, not necessarily stimulus oriented, and can occur in anticipation of events/stimuli or in learned cycles, real/overt actions can alternate with covert/mental actions in order to optimize the chance of success in a game or during social interaction. Therefore, overt actions are just the tip of an iceberg: under the surface it is hidden a vast territory of actions without movements (covert actions) which are at the core of *motor cognition*. This has two main consequences: (1) the format of spatiotemporal patterns of purposive actions, namely, the organization of the synergy formation process, must be shared by covert and overt actions; (2) this format cannot be strictly dependent upon the physics of the body and the neuromuscular system, because in covert actions there is no motion of body masses or contraction of the muscles. We may then derive the hypothesis that the endogenous dynamics of cortical maps is basically the same in overt movements, when it drives the formation of neuromuscular activation patterns, and in covert movements, when it carries out mental simulations of the same movements. This concept is implicit in the Mental Simulation Theory (Jeannerod 2001), and in a similar line of reasoning, we may quote recent experiments on motor planning in tasks that require the careful coordination of rotation and translation of objects (Cohen and Rosenbaum 2011): these experimental results support theories of synergy formation as a process that generates holistic body changes between successive goal postures (Rosenbaum et al. 1995, 2001) or the Ideomotor Theory, which claims that actions are triggered by the anticipation of intended effects (Herbort and Butz 2012).

7.2.5 Motor Synergies and the Body Schema

That humans have an integrated, internal representation of their body (the body image or body schema[1]) is strongly suggested by the variety of pathological conditions which can only be explained by a deficient internal representation (Head and Holmes 1911). More recent studies (for reviews see Graziano and Botvinick 2002; Haggard and Wolpert 2005) have identified the different cortical areas that may contribute to this function (area 5 in the superior parietal lobe and possibly premotor and motor areas) and the multimodal integration of proprioceptive, visual, tactile, and motor feedback signals that is necessary for maintaining a coherent spatiotemporal organization. It has also been suggested that such continuous body experience may be one of the key elements for allowing the emergence of individual self-consciousness. However, the role of the body schema in synergy formation needs to be investigated more in depth. We believe indeed that running internal simulations on an interconnected set of neuronal networks is perhaps one of the main functions of the body schema. Therefore, the body schema must not be considered as a static structure, like the Penfield's homunculus, but a dynamical system that generates goal-oriented, spatiotemporal, sensorimotor patterns.

This view of the body schema is clearly multireferential and resonates well with many ideas investigated in the framework of embodied cognition: (1) *cognition is situated*, in the sense that it is an online process which takes place in the context of task-relevant sensorimotor information; (2) *cognition is time pressured*, i.e., it is constrained by the requirements of real-time interaction with the environment, what is also known as "representational bottleneck" (Brooks 1991; Pfeifer and Scheier 1998, among others); (3) the *environment is part of the cognitive system*, including both the physical and social environment; (4) *cognition is intrinsically action oriented* and even "off-line cognition," namely, cognition without overt action, is body based as argued by Lakoff and Johnson (1999), who remarked that in most

[1] The difference between body image and body schema is disputed and is somehow fuzzy. For our purpose we assume that they are two sides of the same coin: the former one stresses the static component, mainly based on proprioceptive information, whereas the latter is related to the dynamic synergy formation function.

occasions abstract concepts are based on metaphors grounded in bodily experience/activity.

We agree with Brooks (1991) that "the world is its own best model," but we also believe that a human being, as well as a humanoid robot, needs an internal model or representation of its own body or body schema, extended with an internal representation of the environment and the mastered tools that allow him/her/it to succeed in physical/social interaction. Such body schema does not need to be a faithful biomechanical model, including the finest details of flesh and bones. It is just a skeleton or middleware representation where it is possible to play plausible spatio-temporal games, required at the same time and formulated in the same language by *motor cognition* and *motor control*. The power of the concept is that a well-trained agent can use it to interpret/anticipate the actions of other agents or also imagine actions that are physically impossible but crucially important for figuring out the solution of a difficult task (Fig. 7.1).

The introduction of the body schema as a middleware implies two important concepts in the analysis of the organization of action: one concept is the necessity and the convenience to separate motor cognition from motor control, in a multireferential framework; the other concept is the identification of different time frames. The first concept is related to flexibility and the necessity of degrees of abstraction in the acquisition of skills. Mental reasoning and mental training can be powerful and effective only if it is possible to abstract from specific environmental conditions that can require different control strategies. The capability of abstraction is made possible by a body schema that allows to formulate real and imagined actions in the same format. This logic separation of motor cognition and motor control implies the identification of three different time frames: (1) *learning time*, for acquiring an approximate representation of the model modules; (2) *preparation time*, for recruiting the necessary body parts, configuring the networks, and setting up the specific task-dependent components; and (3) *real time*, for running the internal simulation of the body model and thus generating control patterns either for covert or overt actions.

7.2.6 Implementing the Body Schema by Means of the Passive Motion Paradigm

The PMP (Mussa Ivaldi et al. 1988) was conceived as an extension of the EPH from motor control to motor cognition. The idea is to think that there are two attractor dynamics, nested one inside the other, which cooperate for action generation: the more internal one expresses an endogenous brain activity, related to an internal model or body schema, and is the one that is responsible for covert movements (as such, it does not involve body masses, muscle stiffness, and muscle synergies); the latter attractor dynamics, related to the conventional EPH, exploits the physical equilibrium states determined by the biomechanics of the body. Our hypothesis is

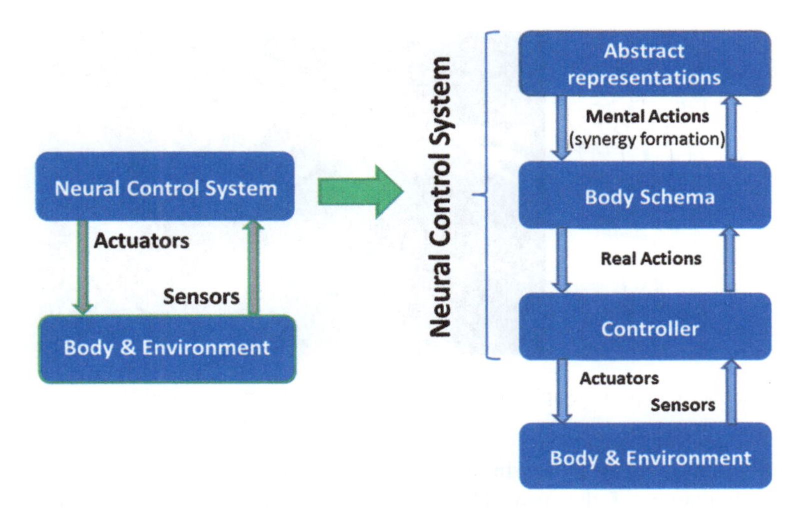

Fig. 7.1 Purely reactive system (*left panel*) vs. cognitive system (*right panel*)

that the two dynamical regimes are compatible and integrated in the same structure, allowing subjects to shift effortlessly from mental simulations of actions to real actions and back, in agreement with the evidence coming from brain imaging.

The Passive Motion Paradigm is a force field-based mechanism of synergy formation that allows to coordinate the motion of a redundant set of articulations while carrying out a task, like reaching or tracking an object. Originally, it was formulated in order to demonstrate that, when carrying out inverse kinematics with a highly redundant system, it is not necessary to introduce an explicit optimization process. The idea can be expressed, in qualitative terms, by means of the animated puppet metaphor (Fig. 7.2 left panel) or the "flying hand metaphor" (Fig. 7.2 right panel), suggested by Marc Jeannerod. The key point, in both cases, is that in reaching movements, it is not the proximal part of the body which is *pushing* the end effector to the target but the other way around: the end effector is *pulled* towards the target by the force field and in turn pulls the rest of the body.

In mathematical terms, let us represent the intention to reach a target $\vec{p}_{\mathrm{T}}$ by means of a force field $\vec{F}_{\mathrm{H}}$, aimed at the target and attached to the hand $\vec{p}_{\mathrm{H}}$.[2] $\vec{F}_{\mathrm{H}}$ is mapped into an equivalent torque field $\vec{T}_{\mathrm{A}}$, acting on all the joints of the arm (vector $\vec{q}$), by means of the transpose Jacobian matrix J_{B} [3]: it is worth mentioning that the

[2] In the simplest case of a linear model, this field is elastic and is characterized by a stiffness matrix K: $\vec{F}_{\mathrm{H}} = K\left(\vec{p}_{\mathrm{T}} - \vec{p}_{\mathrm{H}}\right)$.

[3] The Jacobian matrix of the arm is defined as follows: $J_{\mathrm{B}} = \frac{\partial \vec{p}_{\mathrm{H}}}{\partial \vec{q}}$. It maps motion and effort in opposite directions: $\frac{d\vec{p}_{\mathrm{H}}}{dt} = J_{\mathrm{B}} \frac{d\vec{q}}{dt}$ and $\vec{T}_{\mathrm{A}} = J_{\mathrm{B}}{}^{\mathrm{T}} \vec{F}_{\mathrm{H}}$.

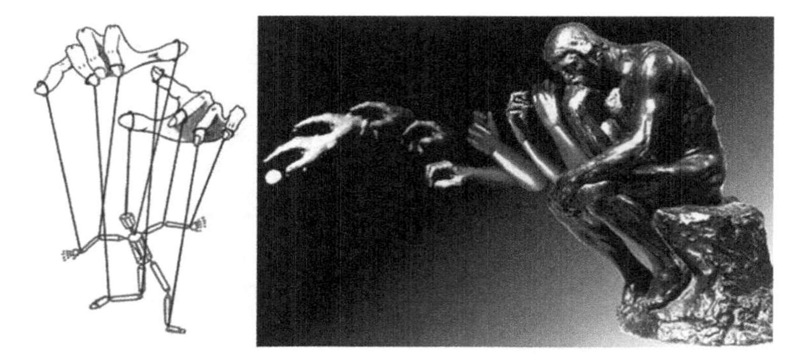

Fig. 7.2 Animated puppet metaphor (*left panel*). Flying hand metaphor (*right panel*)

torque field has a much higher dimensionality than the force field as a consequence of the redundancy of the arm. The torque field induces in the body schema a distribution of incremental joint rotations, modulated by the admittance matrix A. In turn, the joint rotation pattern is mapped into the corresponding hand motion pattern, thus updating the attractor force field and closing the computational loop:

$$\underbrace{\begin{cases} \dfrac{d\vec{p}_{\mathrm{H}}}{dt} = J_{\mathrm{B}}\dfrac{d\vec{q}}{dt} \\ \vec{F}_{\mathrm{H}} = K\left(\vec{p}_{\mathrm{T}} - \vec{p}_{\mathrm{H}}\right) \cdot \Gamma(t) \end{cases}}_{\text{Hand space}} \quad \begin{matrix} \leftarrow J_{\mathrm{B}} \leftarrow \\ \rightarrow {J_{\mathrm{B}}}^{\mathrm{T}} \rightarrow \end{matrix} \quad \underbrace{\begin{cases} \dfrac{d\vec{q}}{dt} = A\vec{T}_{\mathrm{A}} \\ \vec{T}_{\mathrm{A}} = {J_{\mathrm{B}}}^{\mathrm{T}}\vec{F}_{\mathrm{H}} \end{cases}}_{\text{Arm joint space}} \tag{7.1}$$

The mathematical description of the PMP summarized by (7.1) can be expressed graphically by means of the bock diagram of Fig. 7.3. The transient induced by the activation of the force field is terminated when the target is reached, if it is reachable. If the target is not reachable, for example, if it is outside the workspace, the final posture is the one that minimizes the final positioning error. It should be noted that all the computations in the loop are "well posed" and thus this computational model is robust and cannot fail. In any case, if the force field remains stationary during the movement, the acquisition of the new equilibrium state occurs in an asymptotic manner, and thus reaching time is not controlled. Such time can be controlled by means of a technique proposed by the group of Michael Zak (1988), called terminal attractor dynamics, which consists of a suitable nonlinear modulation of the force field, which tends to diverge to infinity when time approaches the intended deadline. The $\Gamma(t)$ function or nonlinear time-base generator implements such modulation. The function can be considered as a kind of "neural pacemaker" (Barhen et al. 1989), and a biologically plausible representation can be identified in the cortico-basal ganglia–thalamocortical loop and the well-established role of the basal ganglia in the initiation and speed control of voluntary movements. In other words, *synergy* formation requires a *symphonic* director, not a mere metronome, namely, a coordination entity that, in addition to giving the tempo, recruits the

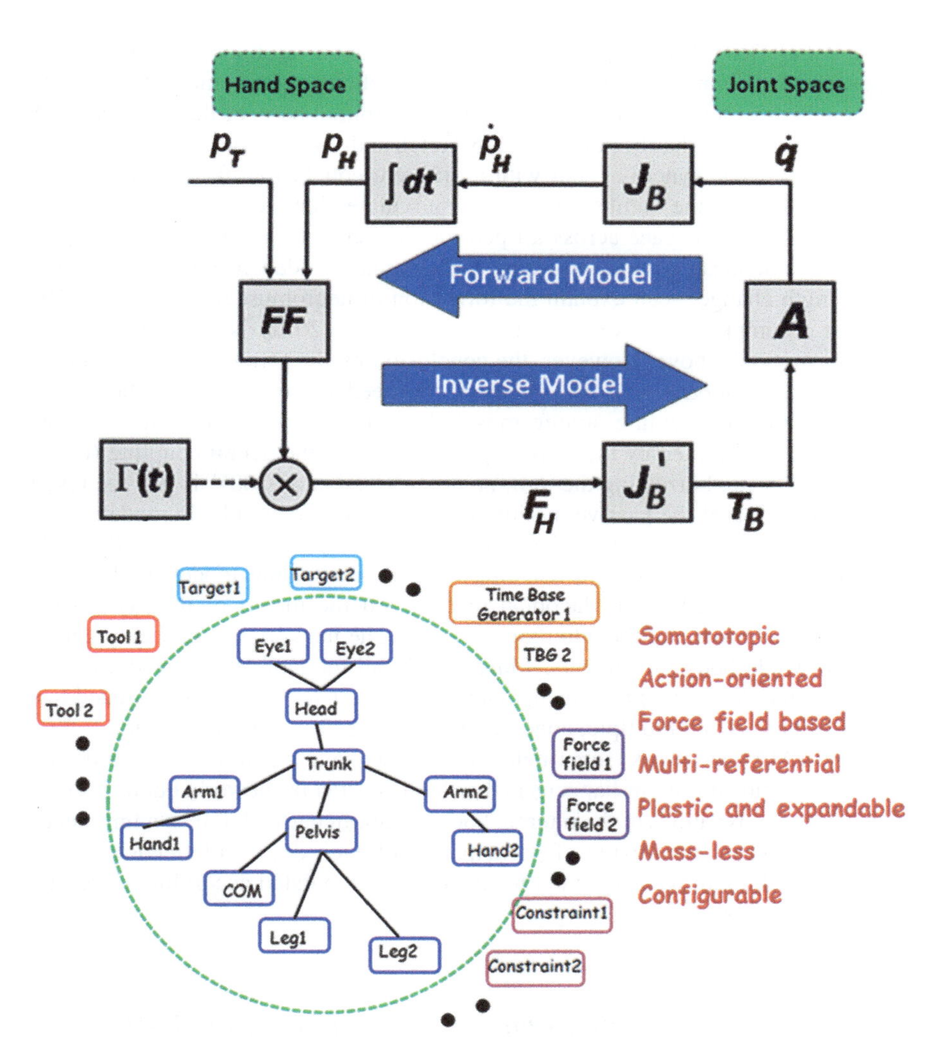

Fig. 7.3 *Top panel*: PMP network. The basic kinematic constraint that links the hand and joint spaces is represented by the Jacobian matrix. Additional constraints, in the hand and joint spaces, can be represented by means of corresponding force or torque fields. *Bottom panel*: Articulated body schema within the PMP framework, to be configured in the preparation time of an action with a selection of tools, targets, time-base generators, and specific constraints

different sections of the orchestra, modulates the emphasis of the different melodic pieces, etc.: the gating action of the function is the key element of this symphonic action.

The $\Gamma(t)$ function was not present in the original PMP model, and it was added later on (Mohan and Morasso 2011; Mohan et al. 2009, 2011a, b) when the model was applied to the iCub robot (Metta et al. 2010). The movements determined by the model are described as "passive" in the sense that the animation of a marionette is passive: the joint rotation patterns are not explicitly programmed but are the consequences of applying a set of forces to the terminal parts of the marionette. A similar point of view has been followed by Kutch and Valero-Cuevas (2012) in their analysis of muscle synergies, but with a different conclusion: they show that the biomechanics of the limbs constrain musculotendon length changes to a low-dimensional subspace across all possible movement directions and then propose that "a modest assumption"—that each muscle is independently instructed to resist length change—can explain the formation of neuromuscular synergies. The "modest assumption" of Kutch and Valero-Cuevas (2012) is equivalent to the "passive motion" above. However, the conclusion by the former authors (namely, that "muscle synergies will arise without the need to conclude that they are a product of neural coupling among muscles") is not the only possible one. The alternative, exemplified by the PMP hypothesis, is that the neural coupling (or the organized S-state, borrowing the terminology of Jeannerod 2001) is just the result of the simulation of the passive motion induced by the internal body model.

The simple PMP network of Fig. 7.3 (top panel) is just an example of the body schema employed in a simple reaching task. Basically, the model of the body schema is embedded in the Jacobian matrix, and the model of the task in the force field generator and the admittance matrix. The network can be easily generalized to whole-body movements, which recruit all the DoFs of the body, can be expanded in order to integrate manipulated tools, and can be easily specialized to a variety of tasks, even multiple, concurrent tasks (Fig. 7.3, bottom panel).

In the PMP framework, force fields, admittance, and stiffness matrices do not refer to physical entities, as happens in the classical EPH framework, but to features of the attractor dynamics of the internal body model. In particular, the "admittance" matrix A specifies the degree of participation of each degree of freedom to the common reaching movement, and thus it can be manipulated according to specific task requirements.

7.2.7 A Biologically Plausible Implementation of the PMP

A biologically plausible neural architecture that is consistent with the PMP dynamics described by (7.1) or the model of Fig. 7.3 is described in Morasso et al. (1998). It is formulated in terms of collection of macro-neurons, each of which summarizes the activity level of a cortical column, and characterized by a nonlinear ordinary differential equation ODE, gated by the same $\Gamma(t)$ function defined above. These neural ensembles can be considered "maps" because the lateral connections correspond to a semi-regular grid. The rate of change of the activity of each macro-neuron is modulated by three elements: (1) a local inhibitory input; (2) a recurrent neighboring excitatory input, due to lateral connections inside the map; and (3) another excitatory input originating from external sources. The model is consistent with what is known about the cytoarchitecture of motor cortical areas.

In fact, the majority of synapses in the mammalian neocortex originate from cortical neurons. In particular, lateral connections from superficial pyramids tend to be characterized by recurrent excitation with other pyramids (about 80 % of the total), while only about 20 % of the synaptic connections are with inhibitory intra-columnar interneurons (Nicoll and Blakemore 1993). It is well known that recurrent excitation in neural networks can implement many interesting functions, like finite-state automata, associative memories, or spatiotemporal pattern formation (McCulloch and Pitts 1943; Cohen and Grossberg 1983; Hopfield 1984; Morasso et al. 1998). On the other hand, inhibitory synaptic connections are an important part of the intrinsic circuitry of the neocortex, serving to modulate the propagation of sensory information.

More specifically, the inhibitory local field is expressed by a simple "leaky integrator." The recurrent lateral connections are excitatory and approximately symmetric, as in Hopfield networks, thus making sure that the map is stable, i.e., has an attractor dynamics. We also assume that the pattern of lateral connectivity is acquired through a process of babbling and self-organization, thus encoding the dimensionality and topology of the sensorimotor space represented by the map. The distribution of activity throughout the map via the lateral connections is normalized by a mechanism of gating inhibition that takes into account, for each macro-neuron, the average activity of its neighbors (Reggia et al. 1992; Morasso et al. 1998). Finally, the input field, broadcasted to the map by another map or by thalamo-cortical projections, is channeled to a limited population of macro-neurons via a mechanism of shunting interaction that induces a cluster of activity in the neural population around the neuron that resonates with the input field.

The equilibrium states of this network architecture are characterized by clusters of activation in register with the peak of the external field, i.e., a population code matching the external input field. After a shift of the input field, corresponding to the selection of a new target, the combination of symmetric recurrent excitation, gating inhibition, and shunting interaction induces in the map an attractor dynamics characterized as follows: first, a diffusion process (which initially flattens the population code, spreading the activity pattern over a large part of the network) and, then, a re-sharpening process around the target. The combination of the two processes can be described as a moving hill, namely, the propagation of the population code towards the new target.

Suppose now to instantiate two cortical maps, with the same network dynamics but with different dimensionality and connectivity: for example, a map for representing hand position and the other for representing arm configuration (in the case of arm motor control) or a map for representing speech sounds and the other for representing configurations of the vocal tract (in the case of speech motor control). Both cases are characterized by a high degree of redundancy, and thus the latter map will have a larger number of units and a more complex connectivity than the former one. We may suppose that during a process of self-supervising learning or Piagetian circular reaction (Kuperstein 1991), it was possible to acquire two sets of topology-representing intra-connections for the two maps and, at the same time, a set of interconnection between the maps. As a consequence of the redundancy of the system, we may expect that interconnectivity will be "many to one," i.e., each neuron of the hand map will be connected to many neurons of the arm map, thus representing in a distributed manner the "null-space" of the kinematic transformation between the two spaces.

The external field acting on each map is a combination of a bottom-up external input and an input coming from the cross-connection of the two maps. If no external input is provided, the two maps excite each other, via the two corresponding population codes, representing, for example, the current configuration of the arm and the corresponding position of the hand. Starting from this equilibrium state, if an external input is activated in the hand map, identifying a target position, then an overall dynamics will be induced in both maps by spreading activation via inter- and intra-connections until the population code of the hand settles in the target positions and the population code of the arm in one of the many corresponding arm configurations. In principle, this distributed architecture can be extended, up to a full-body representation, by including cortical maps of different body parts as well as cortical representations of manipulated tools (Maravita and Iriki 2004).

The "universal" gating action of the $\Gamma(t)$ function is critical for making sure that the multiple population codes in a whole-body cortical architecture remain consistent throughout the overall transient from one equilibrium condition to a new one. It can be considered as a deadline enforcing mechanism, and it has been conceived originally for attributing terminal attractor dynamics to associative memories of large size, namely, for assuring that the equilibrium state is achieved in a finite time, independent of the network size and topology. This kind of nonlinear, broadcasted gating action is generally appropriate for coordinating the timing in large-scale, distributed systems, such as different cortical maps. Moreover, the computational necessity of guaranteeing ordinal and temporal structure in complex biological or artificial organisms is supported by recent behavioral experiments (Kornysheva et al. 2013) that suggest the existence of independent ordinal and temporal structures and advocate a nonlinear multiplicative neural interaction of temporal and ordinal signals in the production of motor patterns.

7.2.8 *Separating Motor Control from Motor Cognition and Integrating Them via the Body Schema*

Figure 7.1 (right panel) illustrates the concept that the body schema can be considered as an internal model which serves as a middleware between the covert virtual movements generated by a motor cognitive machinery and the overt movements generated by the motor controller. In the simplest case (typically used by iCub as a default control mode), the covert movements provide reference trajectories for all the DoFs which are then controlled as a bunch of independent PD-controlled servomechanisms. However, this may not be appropriate in a number of significant situations, in particular in the case of unstable tasks.

An example is whole-body reaching while standing. A biomimetic approach, based on PMP, for synergy formation of whole-body movements in humanoid robots is described by Morasso et al. (2010). It is supposed to combine a double task: (1) a focal task (reaching or approaching as much as possible a target in 3D space) and (2) a postural task (keeping the vertical projection of the center of mass inside the support base of the standing body). The synergy formation mechanism uses two force fields applied to the body schema: one linked to the hands for the focal part and the other linked to the pelvis for the postural part, thus implementing a hip strategy of stabilization. Remarkably, the simulated patterns generated by the model are consistent with distinctive aspects of human behavior for this kind of task, namely, the synchronized velocity peaks of the reaching hand and the forward shift of the center of mass. However, this PMP-based mechanism is massless and is not yet a control system because it does not provide specific stabilization signals of the inverted pendulum which, at least approximately, represents the standing body. The intrinsic instability of the inverted pendulum model is due to the fact that the rate of growth of the gravity-related toppling torque is greater than the stiffness of the critical joint involved in the stabilization of the standing body, namely, the ankle. Therefore, a controller is needed for providing ankle torque control signals that stabilize the inverted pendulum. A continuous-time PD feedback controller applied to the ankle does not work because the delay of the feedback signals (sway angle and sway speed) becomes itself a source of instability. However, such delay-induced instability can be avoided by means of an intermittent controller (Asai et al. 2009), which closes the loop according to a decision mechanism based on the analysis of the trajectories of the inverted pendulum in the phase space: this mechanism achieves bounded stability, consistent with the recorded sway movements of the standing body, in a robust way. A recent paper (Morasso et al. 2013) demonstrates the feasibility of extending the intermittent controller from quiet standing to dynamic standing. It integrates in a bidirectional manner the PMP synergy formation mechanism, which generates time-varying reference joint rotations, with the intermittent controller which switches on/off the feedback control law according to the current state of the pendulum. In other situations, as in grabbing/pushing in which there is a physical interaction, the control part of the synergy might be more concerned with a modulation of the end-effector stiffness, in order to take into account task-dependent features like fragility of the manipulated objects. In any case, stiffness modulation requires, as a prerequisite, the selection and real-time adjustment of appropriate body postures that can be naturally provided by the animated body schema.

7.3 Beyond Embodiment: Building a Brain to Understand the Brain

In the first part of this chapter, we summarized some concepts about the necessity and usefulness of embodiment and body schema as basic building blocks in the process of building a cognitive architecture of a humanoid robot like iCub. However this is only a kind of preliminary groundwork, and the actual construction is an exciting work in progress. As a matter of fact, our ongoing adventure to build a cognitive architecture for iCub in many ways is linked to the three apparently disparate citations above, namely, the power of understanding fundamental principles through a model building approach, which is essentially decentralized, local to global, nonlinear, non-digital: smooth flow through time and space. All of this relates to cumulative learning and organization of memories in our brain as well as in iCub cognitive system. Indeed our own individual experiences play a fundamental role in leading us to exhibit numerous instances of creativity, rationality, and irrationality in our behaviors. Use of "experience" to go "beyond experience" is important simply because we all inhabit a continuously changing world where neither everything can be known nor can everything be experienced. In order to succeed and ultimately survive, diverse "chunks of knowledge" emerging from one's past experiences have to be integrated and exploited flexibly in the context of the present state of affairs to ensure smooth realization of goals. How the brain achieves such diversity in control is a central challenge facing both neuroscience and cognitive robotics today.

Simply put, beyond a point a software programmer cannot travel the journey of a cognitive robot. Instead, like natural cognitive agents, cognitive robots must also be endowed with mechanisms that enable them to efficiently organize their sensorimotor experiences into their memories, remember and exploit them effectively when needed to realize their goals, and, at the same time, keep learning new things. Enabling them to do so presents a unique opportunity to emulate the gradual process of infant development and investigate the underlying interplay between multiple sensory, motor, and cognitive processes from the perspective of an integrated system that perceives, acts, learns, remembers, forgets, reasons, makes mistakes, introspects, etc. To this effect, even simple experiments with a humanoid like iCub offer us an exciting medium to "build a brain to understand the brain" and contemplate numerous open questions related to the emergence of embodied cognition: how do structures of bodily experience gradually "work their way up" to form abstract patterns of inferences? How do playful interactions between the body and the world sculpt the memories of a cumulative learning robot? When and how do mechanisms related to abstraction, consolidation, and forgetting play a role in shaping cumulative learning and sensorimotor development? What is the role of the teacher in minimizing "blind" trial and error exploration and motivating and influencing the developmental curve? How do all these questions, phrased in the context of a gradually learning and developing humanoid, relate to emerging trends in neuroscience? And finally, to which extent this kind of "cognitive biomimetism" is effective in shaping humanlike capabilities in a humanoid robot? We are currently investigating these fundamental issues with the help of numerous playful experiments with iCub that attempt to achieve cumulative development of procedural, semantic, and episodic memories and the parallel development of a brain-guided computational framework to organize and creatively exploit such learned knowledge for the realization of goals.

In general, after the tryst with GOFAI, most current research in the field of cognitive developmental robotics appreciates the fact that "sensorimotor experience precedes representation" and cognition is gradually bootstrapped through a cumulative process of learning by interaction (physical and social) within the zone of proximal development (Vygotsky 1978) of the agent. This approach indeed has roots in Wiener's cybernetics (1948), Varela and Maturana's autopoiesis (1974), Chiel and Beer's neuroethology (1997), Clark's situatedness (1997), Hesslow's simulation hypothesis (Hesslow 2002; Hesslow and Jirenhed 2007), and Thompson's enactive cognition (2007). The obvious reason to pursue this path is because it is impossible to predict and program at design time every possible situation in every time instance to which an artifact may be subjected to in the future. Straight robot programming approaches work for simple machines performing targeted functions but certainly not for general-purpose robotic companions envisaged to interact with humans in unstructured environments. Complementing the extrinsic application of specific value, the embodied/enactive approach is also relevant from an intrinsic viewpoint of understanding our own selves—understanding how interactions between body and the brain shape the mind and shape action and reason. This is because in addition to the range of direct problems typical of conventional physics, which involve computing effects of forces on objects, brains of animals have also to deal with inverse, typically ill-posed, problems of learning, reasoning, and choosing actions that would enable realization of one's goals and hence ultimately survive. Strikingly, many of the inverse problems faced by the brain to learn, reason, and generate goal-directed behavior, together with the ability to make predictions inherent with the solution of direct problems, are indeed analogous to the ones roboticists must solve to make their robots act cognitively in the real world. At the same time, it is only fair to say that in spite of extensive research scattered across multiple scientific disciplines and prevalence of numerous machine learning techniques, the present artificial agents still lack much of the resourcefulness, purposefulness, flexibility, and adaptability that biological agents so effortlessly exhibit. Certainly, this points towards the need to develop novel computational frameworks that go beyond the state of the art and endow cognitive agents with the capability to learn cumulatively and use past experience effectively "to connect the dots" when faced with novel situations.

Looking at the incessant loop of gaining experience and using experience, typical of biological species that exhibit some form of cognition, learning and reasoning can be seen as foreground and background alternating each other as intricately depicted in the artistic creations of Escher. In an intriguing work during the early days of embodied/enactive cognition, Mark Johnson (1987) playfully remarked that "we are animals but we are also rational animals," emphasizing the fact that, like learning, the structure of reasoning and inference also does not transcend the structure of bodily experience. The centrality of embodiment directly influences "what" and "how" things can be meaningful to us, the ways in which our understanding of the world is gradually bootstrapped by experience and the ways in which we reason about them. In this essence, we believe that for cognitive robots foreseen to operate in open-ended unstructured environments, learning and reasoning must cumulatively drive each other in a closed loop: more learning leading to better reasoning and inconsistencies in reasoning driving new learning. In neural computation, this implies that part of the cortical substrates activated during perceptual and motor learning (i.e., when an agent gains experience) are also activated when an agent reasons and simulates the causal consequences of its actions. While resonance between top-down and bottom-up information flows is a measure of the quality of learning, dissonance is the stepping stone to novelty detection for gaining more experience and learning further. Such neural reuse also makes sense considering the fact that brain is a product of evolution, meant to support the survival of a species in its natural environments, and importantly operates under constraints of space, time, and energy. A wealth of emerging evidence from neuroscience substantiates this fact (see Gallese and Sinigaglia 2011; Grafton 2009; Martin 2009; Bressler and Menon 2010; Hesslow and Jirenhed 2007 for recent reviews). We believe that this aspect must be an essential design feature in future cognitive robots that have any chance to survive, cooperate, and assist humans in the real world. While emerging results from functional imaging and behavioral studies may serve as a guiding light, there is still an urgent need to also focus on "cognitive computation" and look deeper into the underlying computational principles in order to create artificial cognitive systems that can both be "practically useful" and in turn shed deeper insights into the ongoing "neural computation" in the brain. In this context, building up on an intriguing review a decade back by Germund Hesslow (2002), we believe that computational architectures driving cognitive robots must include the three following basic building blocks that form the core of the embodied simulation hypothesis:

1. **Simulation of action through animation of the PMP-based body schema** This building block was discussed in detail in the Background section. In general one may ask why does a cognitive robot like iCub need a body schema. Simply put, for the same reason a human or a chimp needs it: without one, it would be unable to use its "complex body," take advantage of it, and ultimately survive. In general, for an organism with a complex body inhabiting an unstructured world, the purpose of "action" is not just restricted to shaping motor output to generate movement but also to provide the self with information on the feasibility, consequence, and understanding of "potential actions" (which could lead to realization of "goals"). We already suggested the "iceberg metaphor" to explain this state of affairs; by adding to it, we should say that there must be continuity between what is above and what is below the surface: the "link or the middleware," we suggest, is the body schema mechanism. We note here that until recently the issue of body schema has not been very popular in cognitive

robotics in comparison to the concept of embodiment. These are not the same things. If you have a body schema, you also have embodiment but not the other way around. Vernon et al. (2010) in their discussion on a roadmap for cognitive development in humanoid robots present a catalogue of cognitive architectures, but in none of them the concept of body schema is a key element. However, emerging trends in neuroscience act as a motivating force to revisit old ideas like synergy formation, EPH, and body schema and reuse them in a larger context to arrive at a shared computational/neural basis for "execution, imagination, and understanding" of action in humans and humanoids.

2. **Simulation of perception and distributed organization of semantic memory** Imagining to perceive something is similar to actually perceive it, only difference being that the perceptual activity is generated top-down rather than by environmental stimuli. While this perspective has been emphasized in the reviews of Hesslow (2002, 2007) and Grush (2004), among others, more recent developments on the organization of semantic knowledge in the brain (see Patterson et al. 2007; Martin 2007, 2009; Martin et al. 2011; Damasio 2010) provide further insights that help to constrain computational architectures for cognitive agents. The main finding from these studies is that conceptual information is grounded in a distributed fashion in "property-specific" cortical networks that directly support perception and action. It is also established that "retrieval" or reactivation of the neural representation can be triggered from partial cues coming from multiple modalities: for example, the sound of a hammer retro-activates its shape representation (Meyer and Damasio 2009), and presentation of a real object or a 2D picture of it can both activate the complete network associated with the object. The results indicate that while there is a fine level of "functional segregation" in the higher-level cortical areas processing sensorimotor information, there is also an underlying cortical dynamics that facilitates cross-modal, top-down, and bottom-up activation of these areas. "Higher level" needs to be emphasized because there is reason to believe that both early stages of perception and late stages of action should not be involved in embodied simulation of action and perception, in order to keep a distinction between overt and covert actions, which we deem important for purposive reasoning: there is evidence of this distinction both from motor (Desmurget and Sirigu 2009) and perceptual studies (Martin 2009).
3. **Global integration through small world organization** From a computational perspective, in a large-scale complex system like the brain, efficient integrative mechanisms require a number of organizational properties, such as minimization of the number of processing steps, efficient wiring for minimizing brain volumes and metabolic cost in the transmission of information, and synchronization of neural processes in order to achieve pattern completion and conflict resolution. Recent developments in the fields of network theory (Barabási 2012, 2003) and connectomics (Sporns 2013) provide useful insights in this direction. The point of intersection is the property of "small worldness" now found to be prevalent in many large-scale networks. In simple terms, "small worlds" are complex systems where individual members form tightly knit local communities,

characterized by dense clustering and very short connection lengths. Since the seminal works of Watts and Strogatz (1998) and Barabási and Albert (1999), it is now established that several complex systems like social networks, transportation networks, power grids, connectivity of the Internet, gene networks, food webs, and patterns in sexually transmitted diseases, among several others, exhibit the "small world" property. Emerging evidence from the analysis of large-scale architecture of the cerebral cortex (Hagmann et al. 2008; Sporns et al. 2002; Sporns 2011, 2013) using techniques like Diffusion Tensor Imaging substantiates the fact that cortical networks of the brain exhibit such small world property. These studies suggest existence of a small set of "hubs" (highly connected cortical patches) that closely interact to facilitate swift cross-modal, top-down, and bottom-up interactions between subnetworks involved in learning, simulating, and representing various sensorimotor information.

It is also worth to highlight that the studies mentioned above, about the simulation of perception and action, also point towards existence of few set of hubs that facilitate both "integration and differentiation" (Patterson et al 2007; Martin 2009; Damasio 2010). Further, with the recent discovery of the default mode network (DMN) in the brain (Buckner and Carroll 2007; Suddendorf et al. 2009; Buckner et al 2008; Bressler and Menon 2010; Addis and Schacter 2012; Addis et al 2009; Hassabis and Maguire 2011; Welberg 2012), it is now also known that a core network of "highly connected" areas is consistently activated when subjects perform diverse cognitive functions like recalling past experiences, simulating possible future events (or prospection) and planning possible actions, and interpreting thoughts and perspectives of other individuals. Recently a homologous network for DMN was also discovered in rats (Lu et al. 2012) further supporting the hypothesis that the structure of DMN was both retained and further enhanced during evolution. In addition to natural systems, these findings provide crucial insights towards creating brain-guided computational architectures that can enhance the survival and productivity of artificial systems beyond the state of the art (e.g., robotic assistants supporting humans in numerous application domains). Figure 7.4 presents a schematic illustration of the recent developments in the fields of neuroscience that we plan to integrate in the cognitive architecture of the iCub.

7.3.1 Organization of a Procedural Memory from "Fast, Green, Embodied, Cumulative Learning"

We believe that central to the issue of procedural memory is the capability of humans and cognitive animals to master the use of tools. In general, the essence of "tool use" lies in our gradual progression from learning to act "on" objects to learning to act "with" objects in ways to counteract limitations of "perceptions, actions, and movements" imposed by our bodies. At the same time, to learn both "cumulatively" and "swiftly," a cognitive agent must be able to efficiently integrate

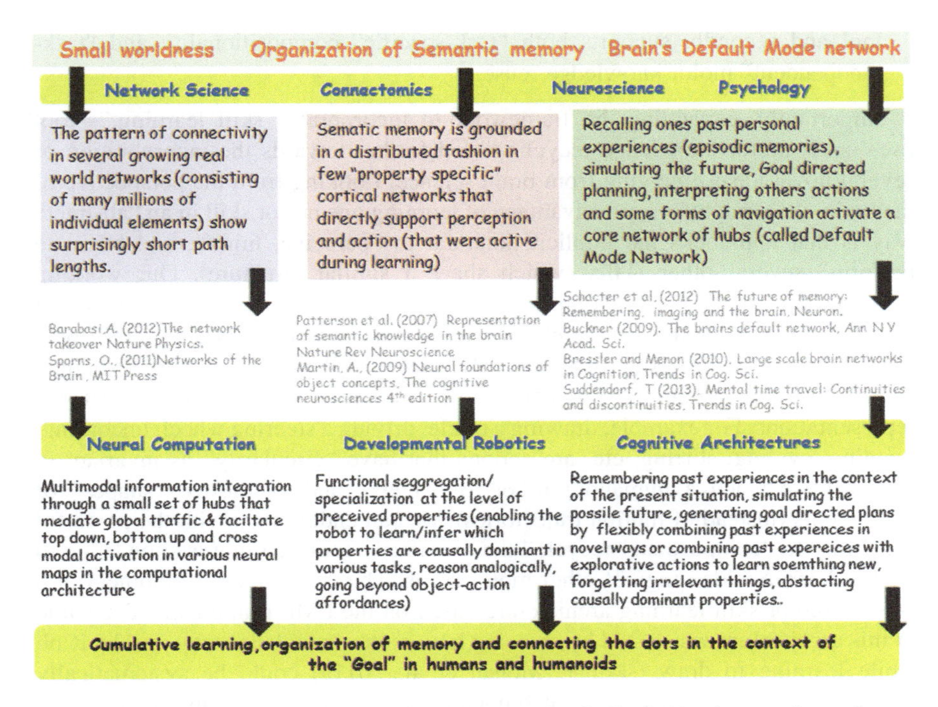

Fig. 7.4 Schematic illustration of the recent developments in the fields of neuroscience that we plan to integrate in the cognitive architecture for iCub

multiple streams of information that aid the learning process itself. Most important among them are social interaction (e.g., imitating a teacher's demonstration), physical interaction (or practice), and "recycling" previously acquired motor knowledge (experience). On the other hand, from the neuroscience perspective, there has been resounding evidence substantiating the fact that action "generation and observation" share underlying functional networks in the brain, and experiments related to "tool use" learning in animals clearly indicate the fact that the a learned "tool" during coordination becomes a part of the acting "body schema" and is coded in the motor system as if it were an artificial hand able to interact with the external objects, exactly as the natural hand is able to do.

For the development of a "motor vocabulary" and a "procedural memory" for iCub, we took into account the following main requirements:

1. The need to learn "fast" and "green," by combining multiple learning streams (social interaction, exploration, recycling of past motor experience);
2. The need to arrive at a shared computational basis for "execution, perception, imagination, and understanding" of action;
3. The need to arrive at general representational framework for motor action generation and skill learning that firstly blurs the distinction between body and

tool and secondly supports both “task-specific” compositionality and “task-independent” motor knowledge reuse.

Importantly, expanding the framework to incorporate “skill learning,” “tool use,” and “motor knowledge recycling” led further towards the incorporation of several novel ideas emerging from brain science. Looking from the perspective of the brain, the straightforward advantage of learning one motor skill in an “abstract” way is that it unlocks the implicit potential to “perceive, mimic, and begin to perform” several other skills (which share a similar structure). Our working hypothesis was that “shape of movement” could be the abstract feature using which motor vocabulary can be efficiently composed and inversely “stored” as a component of the procedural memory. We observed that a wide range of human actions result in formation of trajectories that ultimately result in similar “shape” representations. For example, drawing a circle, driving a steering wheel, uncorking, winding, cycling, stirring, etc. are actions that have “circularity” as invariant in them. If we teach a humanoid robot to perceive and synthesize “shapes” of movements (instead of motion trajectories), we can endow then with the powerful capability to “compose and recycle” the previously acquired motor knowledge to swiftly learn a wide range of other motor skills. This led to the development of a general motor skill learning architecture based on the PMP framework. The value of this architecture was tested by showing how motor knowledge acquired by iCub while learning to draw (skill 1: Mohan et al. 2011a) could be systematically recycled in a task of learning the bimanual control of a toy crane as a tool to “pick up” otherwise unreachable objects in the environment (skill 2: Mohan and Morasso 2012). The underlying mechanism is indeed quite general and can be applied to acquire a wide range of skilled actions in a similar manner.

Figure 7.5 summarizes the central building blocks and high-level information flows that are crucial for constructing a “reusable” and “growing” motor vocabulary and procedural memory in cumulatively learning robots. Three streams of learning are integrated into the architecture: (1) learning through teacher’s demonstration (information flow in black arrow), (2) learning through physical interaction (blue arrow), and (3) learning through motor imagery (loop 1–5). The imitation loop initiates with the teacher’s demonstration and ends with iCub reproducing the observed action. The motor imagery loop is a subpart of the imitation loop, the only difference being that the motor commands synthesized by the PMP-based forward/inverse model are not transmitted to the actuators. This loop hence allows iCub to internally simulate a range of motor actions and only execute the ones that are promising, given the task and the context.

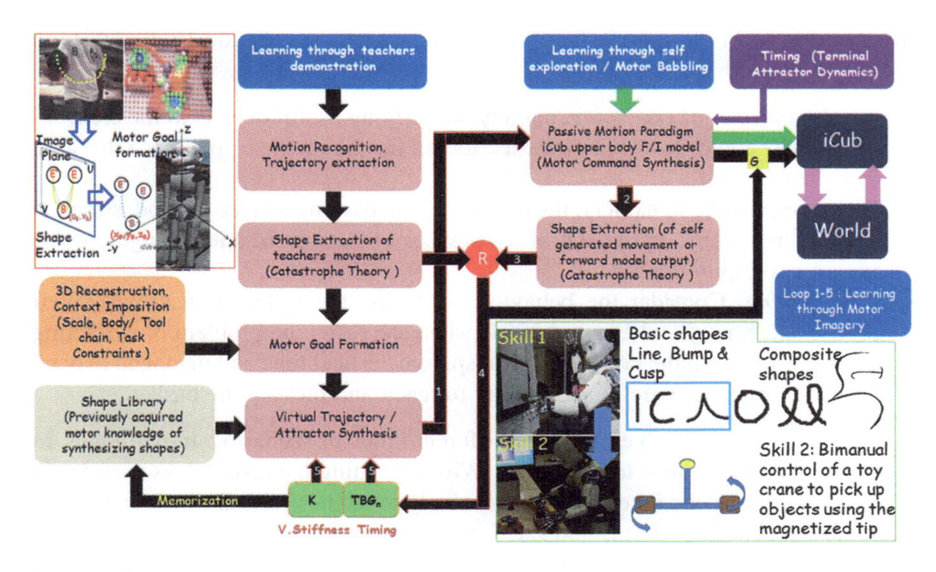

Fig. 7.5 Motor skill learning and action generation architecture for iCub: building blocks and information flows

7.4 Work in Progress: Playful Experiments with iCub for Organizing Episodic and Semantic Memory

If we focus only on learning specific tasks, *embodied procedural memory* is sufficient to drive learning and action generation. However, many questions remain unanswered if we stick to this framework. Let us list a few of them, for summarizing the range of relevant issues:

- How do structures of bodily experience gradually “work their way up” to form abstract patterns of inferences?
- How do we bridge the gap from task-specific “sense” to task-independent “common sense”?
- How do playful interactions between the body and the world sculpt the memories of a cumulatively learning agent?
- When and how do mechanisms related to abstraction, consolidation, and forgetting play a role in cumulative learning?
- What is the specific influence of a teacher in minimizing exploration, motivating, and shaping the developmental curve?

In addition to procedural memory, what we need is semantic and episodic memory (Tulving 1972, 2002) in order to feed in an integrated and bidirectional manner the twin processes of reasoning and learning: more learning driving better reasoning and inconsistencies in reasoning driving new learning. In order to address these problems in the robotic field, it is useful to take inspiration from studies in animal cognition:

- *Causal and spatial reasoning*, namely, identifying useful objects in the environment that could be exploited, as tools, in the context of the otherwise unrealizable goal.
- *Trap tube paradigm*, namely, the problem of recovering a piece of food, stored in a transparent tube, by means of a sticklike object of sufficient length, while avoiding a trap in the tube.
- *Tool making*: Consider the behavior of "Betty, the Caledonian crow" (Weir et al. 2002; Emery and Clayton 2004) when she faced the problem of extracting a food basket from the bottom of a transparent vertical tube and managed to bend a piece of metallic wire in such a way to reach and pick up the basket.

Figure 7.6 shows iCub engaged in different kinds of scenarios. In particular, in these scenarios iCub must learn to push. Why is pushing interesting? As a matter of fact, this skill has been investigated extensively in studies related to understanding of "physical causality" in primates and infants (Visalberghi and Tomasello 1997; Whiten et al 2009; Addessi et al. 2008). It is also known from these studies on animal behavior that different species are different levels of understanding of the causality related to this task. In addition to the multiple utilities of the "push/pull" action itself in the context of assembly operations, what makes it significant is the sheer range of physical concepts that have to be "learned" and "abstracted" in order to execute this action successfully in diverse environmental conditions. For example, it has to be learned that contact is necessary to push, that object properties influence "pushability" (balls roll faster than cubes and it does not matter what is the color of the ball or the cube), that pushing objects gives rise to path of motion in specific directions (the inverse applies for goal-directed pushing), that pushing can be used to support grasping and bring objects to proximity (while working on assembly tasks), and that there can be counterforces that block the pushed object (similar to a goal keeper in football). The requirement to capture/learn such a wide range of physical concepts through "playful interactions" of the baby humanoid with different objects makes this task both interesting and challenging.

Other paradigmatic scenarios can be envisaged, in order to engage iCub in significant goal-directed activities. One of them is *assembling the tallest possible stack* from a set of available objects/toys. This scenario is useful for exploring the computational architecture necessary to enable the robot to efficiently organize and use its own episodic memories related to its various experiences of interacting with different objects, all channelized towards achieving the goal of building the tallest possible stack. Learning takes place cumulatively with the robot playing with different combinations of objects (some previously experienced, some novel) and it goes on in an open-ended fashion. By incrementally exploring and building stacks with various objects, the robot has to learn about their physical properties and relations among different objects in the context of creating the tallest stack. Since the solution itself depends on what objects are available in the "now," to be successful multiple episodes of past experiences have to be remembered and

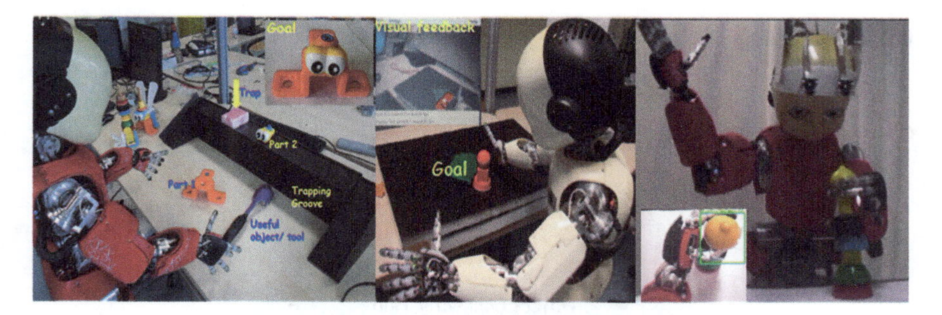

Fig. 7.6 Playful scenarios for iCub to learn and reason

integrated in the context of the present. Hence, the robot is continuously pushed to both exploit "what it knows" from its past experiences in the novel situations and at the same time learn by exploring novel objects, remember its own mistakes, and perform better next time.

7.4.1 The Darwin Perception–Action Loop

Darwin is an EU project whose principal goal is the development and validation of a cognitive architecture to control action in the generation of assembly tasks. Figure 7.7 shows a block diagram of how the lower-level perception–action-related information is organized. At the bottom is the Darwin sensory layer that includes the sensors, associated communication protocols, and algorithms to analyze properties of the objects, such as color, shape, and size. Word information is an additional input coming from the teacher either to issue user goals or interact with the robot. Results of perceptual analysis activate various neural maps (property-specific SOM's in layer 1, provincial hubs) ultimately leading to a distributed representation of the perceived object in the connector hub (top-level object map). These self-organizing maps are trained using standard techniques (Kohonen 1995; Fritzke 1995), and more details with experimental results can be found in Mohan et al. (2013). An interesting aspect of such kind of organization is that as we move upwards in the hierarchy, information becomes more and more integrated and multimodal, and as we move downwards, information is more and more differentiated to the level of perceived properties. The connectivity between hubs and property-specific maps is essentially bidirectional, hence allowing information to move "top-down, bottom-up, or in cross-modal fashion." For example, as illustrated in Mohan et al. (2013), when the robot is issued the goal "grasp a red container" (a new combination of known words describing an object the robot has not encountered before), bottom-up activity in the word map starts spreading through the provincial hub leading to anticipatory top-down activations in the neural maps processing color and shape information. If such top-down activation

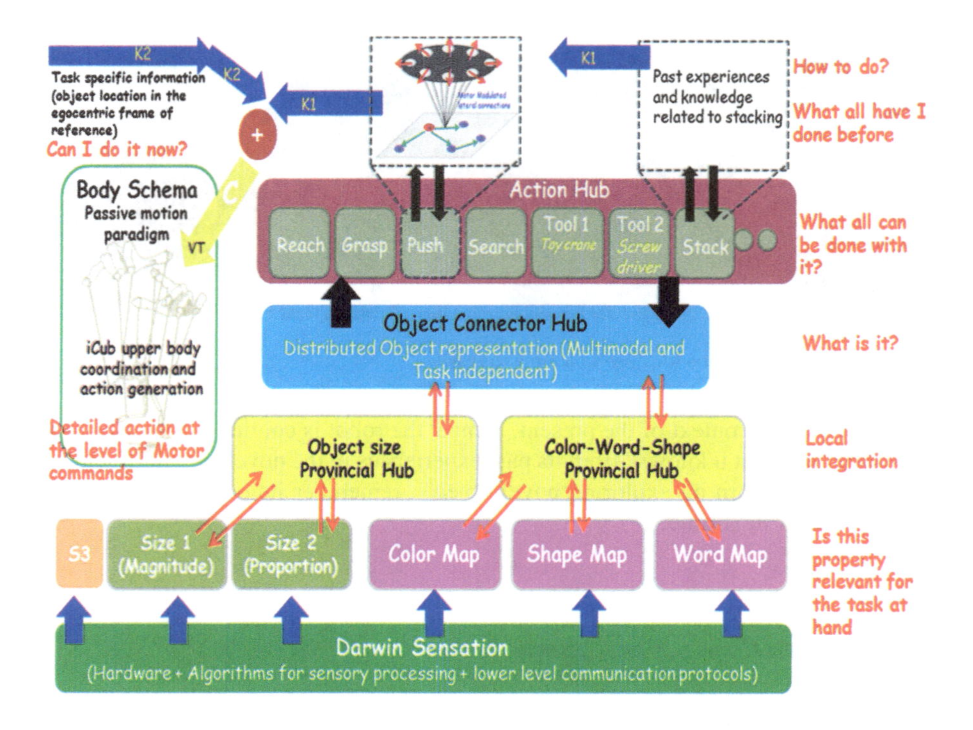

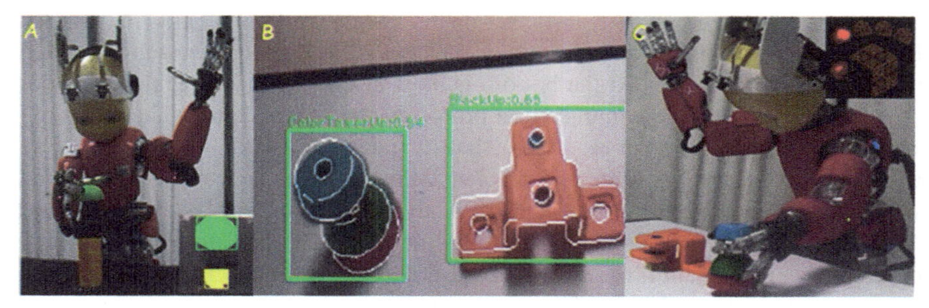

Fig. 7.7 Action–perception loop. *Top panel*: Shows how lower-level sensorimotor information is organized and the main subsystems involved in the "identify–localize–reach–grasp" loop used to generate primitive actions, in the context of creating the tallest possible stack. At the bottom is the sensory layer that includes the sensors, early visual processing, and associated lower-level communication protocols. Results of perceptual analysis activate various property-specific neural maps (property-specific SOM's in layer 1, provincial hubs) ultimately leading to a distributed representation of the perceived object in the connector hub. Hubs perform the role of integration between modalities and enable "top-down, bottom-up, and cross-modal" flow of neural activity. The abstract layer forms the "connector hub" in the action space and consists of single neurons coding for different actions at an abstract level. Note that these single neurons do not code for the action itself but instead have the capability to trigger the complete network responsible for generating the plan to execute the action in the context of the present environment. Finally all plans have to be executed by coordinating the body. This is accomplished by iCub action generation system that decomposes the plans to the level of motor commands to be transmitted to the actuators. *Bottom panel*: Some snapshots of the working loop

resonates with the concurrent bottom-up activation (through the perceptual stream), this is sufficient to lead to the inference that the novel object being perceived is most probably the one the user is requested to grab (Mohan et al. 2013).

This kind of property-specific organization and global integration through hubs is in line with emerging results from neuroscience (van den Heuvel and Sporns 2013; Martin 2009; Meyer and Damasio 2009) as depicted in Fig. 7.3. It is also worth remarking that two important features are made possible by this kind of architecture:

1. The bottom-up processing leads to a distributed representation of the perceived objects (in relation to its perceptual properties color, shape, size) in the object connector hub that identifies the object (in other words coding for "what is it").
2. Due to reciprocal connectivity between the hubs and property-specific maps, it becomes possible to go beyond "object–action" and learn things at the level of "property–action" too: in our embodied framework, "actions" are mediated through the "body" and directed towards "objects" in the environment, according to "tasks."

Playful interactions with objects give rise to sensorimotor experience, learning, and ability to reason in the future. Thus there is the need to connect "object," "action," and the "body." Note that there is a subtle separation between representation of actions at an abstract level ("what all can be done with an object/tool") and the memories related to the action and its consequences ("how to do"). While the former relates to the "affordances" of an object, the latter relates to memories of motor skills, sensorimotor consequences, and anticipated rewards in relation to the goal. The abstract layer forms the "connector hub" and consists of single neurons coding for different action goals like reach, grasp, push, stack, use of different tools, etc. and grows with time as new skills are learned. Single neurons in the connector hub in turn have the capability to trigger the subsystems that hold (procedural, semantic, and episodic) knowledge related to the action (and other actions that may participate as subcomponents). In this sense neurons in the top-level "action connector hub" are similar to "canonical neurons" found in the premotor cortex (Murata et al 1997) that are activated at the sight of objects to which specific actions are applicable. At the same time the detailed knowledge itself is learned/represented in distributed cortical networks which are activated by the action goal (may also involve other sub-actions and sensorimotor memories related to them).

7.4.2 Learning to Build the Tallest Stack Given a Random Set of Objects to Play with

While building the tallest stack, the robot is allowed to explore gradually with a limited set of objects (two at a time, then add a new object, further add another new object, present them in different combinations). The role of the teacher is important as he/she gradually helps the developmental curve, without directly suggesting the solution, but creating situations that can aid new learning, contradictions, and abstractions. At the same time, this scenario is used to explore the organization and flexible use of episodic memory of the robot. The main contents of the episodic memory for this scenario were identified as the temporal order of the robot's "action" on objects and the final reward received by the user. At the same time, the activations in the neurons directly correspond to activations in the "object hubs" and "action hubs" that were active also during explorative learning. For the stacking scenario (depicted in Fig. 7.8), let us consider a very small patch of a simulated neocortex, consisting of 1,000 pyramidal cells. For simplicity in visualization, the 1,000 neurons are organized in a sheetlike structure with 20 rows each containing 50 neurons. Every row may be thought as an event in time (related to object, action, or reward) and the complete memory as an episode of experience (e.g., picking a cylinder and placing it on a mushroom and getting a null reward from the user and vice versa).

This neural network consisting of a sheet of 1,000 pyramidal cells acts as an auto-associative memory that builds up on a recent excitatory–inhibitory neural network proposed by Hopfield (2008). So next time the robot perceives a mushroom (through activations in the color and shape maps), the partial cue is sufficient to recall its past experiences with mushroom (e.g., placing a cylinder on top of it and getting a reward of 0 or placing it on top of the cylinder that was more rewarding). The right panel shows what is "remembered" when these objects are encountered in the future. The neural map (shown in green) depicts the activations in the object connector hub due to the result of bottom-up perception (case 1 only green mushroom and case 2 both mushroom and cylinder). Note that, under such circumstances, the anticipated reward can be used to trigger competition between "remembered episodic experiences" in a way that all memories "compete to survive": survival based on their capability to reenact their plans once again through the body.

7.4.2.1 Interplay Between Episodic Memory and Abstraction

Colors of objects do not affect the way they move when they are used to create the tallest stack. Can this information be abstracted through playful explorative learning and recall of such past experiences? Suppose that we started with the robot playing with green sphere and a yellow cylinder; the teacher now presents the robot with a blue cylinder and orange sphere. Since activity in object hubs reflects activity in property-specific maps that drive them, there is partial similarity in the neural activation of the object hubs; the objects are of different colors but same shapes. Approximate similarity is enough to generate the partial cue and reconstruct the related past experiences. When presented with a blue cylinder and orange sphere, still the past memories of playing with green sphere and a yellow cylinder can be retrieved successfully. Also note that the partial cue is different and contains less information as compared to the partial cues. This is because the objects in the world

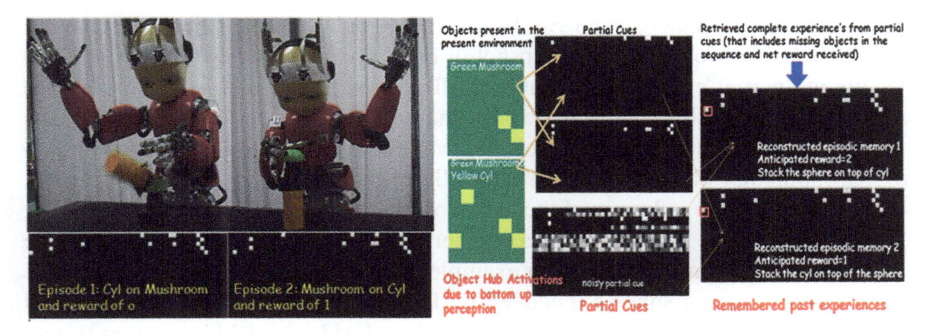

Fig. 7.8 *Left panel* shows explorative attempts to build the tallest stack using a mushroomlike object and a regular cylinder. The formed memories related to object and action (rows 1–4) reflect activation in the neural maps related to object and action; row 5 is the end user reward given to the robot for its performance. *Right panel*: shows what is remembered when the robot encounters objects already explored in the past. The green table depicts the activations in the object connector hub due to the result of bottom-up perception in two cases: (1) only green mushroom and (2) both mushroom and cylinder are shown. In both cases, partial cues generated by bottom-up perception enable the robot to remember its past experiences. In such a computational organization, the anticipated reward (from past explorative experiences) can be used to trigger competition between multiple “remembered episodic experiences”

that are responsible for the generation of partial cues are also different yet share some similarity in “shape” but not “color.” Partial cue leads to the retrieval of the most related and valuable past memory. Even though the robot knows nothing about stacking blue cylinders and orange spheres, it knows something about yellow cylinders and green spheres and anticipates full reward. Thus, the most valuable action sequence from the past is once again executed (now on new objects), and it turns out that the consequence (in terms of reward received) is the anticipated one. In summary, the robot can pin down “causally dominant” properties while experiencing, learning, and remembering in a dynamic “cumulative” fashion.

7.4.2.2 Interplay Between Memory, Prospection, and Creativity

Let us focus again on the task of assembling the tallest possible stack in order to exemplify the creative use of experiences, showing how novel “action sequences” emerge out of “multiple” past experiences, without any need of “blind” exploration. The teacher puts all the objects (cube, small cylinder, large box, and sphere) in front of the robot, to assemble the tallest stack. Let us suppose that iCub only has isolated past experiences with any of them. This is interesting because none of the “past experiences” of the robot has enough information to deal with all these objects at the same time. The challenge is to “combine” knowledge from multiple experiences to come up with a “novel action sequence.”

Let us suppose that four episodic memories have been assimilated and stored in the past: EM1 (cylinder on top of sphere), EM2 (sphere on top of cylinder), EM3 (cube—cylinder—sphere), and EM4 (large box—cube). iCub is then presented to the full set of four objects (first snapshot of Fig. 7.9). The activity in the object hub results in "partial cues" that reconstruct all the four EMs: this is because all the memories (EM1–EM4) have some information related to a "subset" of objects present in the world. However, not all EMs may participate to the construction system, although they compete for controlling the hub (either fully or partially), exerting a top-down influence of the hub. Note that EM1 and EM2 can be wiped out in the competition because there are other competitors that know more (in the context of the present situation). For example, EM3 encodes information related not just to cylinders and spheres (encoded by EM1 and EM2) but also to cubes and hence is a stronger competitor. But in addition to EM3, also EM4 manages to stay alive (it knows something about large objects that none of the other EMs knows anything about). Further, since EM3 and EM4 know something in common (i.e., cubes), they must inhibit each other in order to get control. In this specific example, it happens that the sum of the activities imposed top-down on the hub by EM3 and EM4 is equal to the bottom-up activities. This implies that "the complete action sequence to solve the problem is already available in the isolated past experiences that won the competition" and this applies always independent of how many past experiences claim their control over the hub. Either the most valuable action sequence is directly available (in a single episodic memory), or multiple past experiences may have to be combined in a novel fashion to generate a new behavior. In any case, if the net top-down hub activity is equivalent to the bottom-up hub activity, then even if the environment is "novel," the robot can conclude that its past experiences contain enough information to realize the goal, by optimally combining these past memories into a novel sequence. In summary, action sequence chunks encoded by EM3 and EM4 enter the construction system, by singling out the overlapping object cube highlighted in the red box.

Overlap in knowledge between different remembered experiences is advantageous, because it helps to connect them together. The construction system just employs one simple rule to achieve this: if there are overlaps in knowledge encoded by different "winning" past experiences, bring them as close as possible. In this sense, the overlapping element is similar to an intermediate subgoal (a point of intersection between two different past experiences). After the initial bootstrap explained above, the construction process goes on as illustrated in Fig. 7.9, by combining isolated memories of past experiences, in such a way that a novel sequence emerges: stack the large box at the bottom, then the cube, the small cylinder on top of the cube, and the sphere on top of the small cylinder and anticipate full reward for this! Indeed full reward was given!

More advanced scenarios, such as the one depicted in Fig. 7.10, are being investigated, while following the same *fil rouge* in order to test and improve the cognitive architecture.

Reaching cube with the desired hand pose
First micro sequence of pick and place
Cylinder lifted successfully
Placing cylinder
Cylinder placed, Mushroom lifted
Softly releasing fingers from the mushroom
With drawing the arm, from the stack
Initializing, Tallest stack created

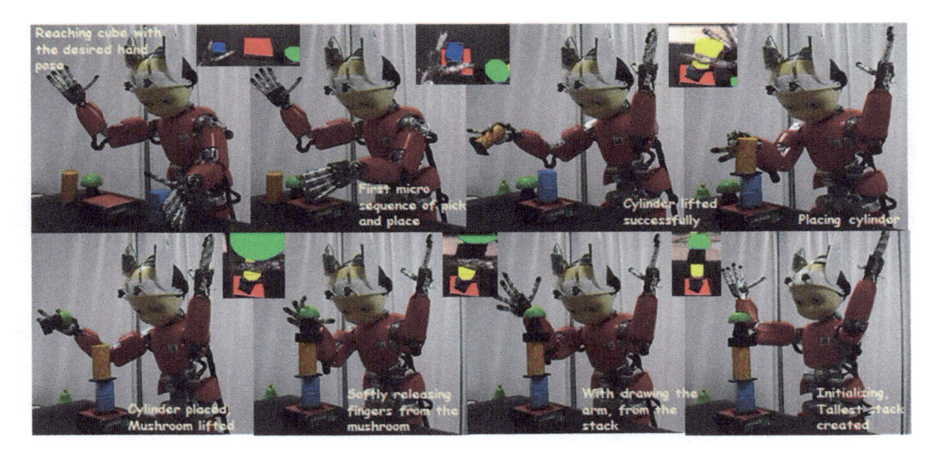

Fig. 7.9 Snapshots of the process of building the tallest stack from an available set of objects by combining past memories without any trial and error exploration

7.5 Concluding Remarks

The world we inhabit is an amalgamation of structure and chaos. There are regularities that could be exploited. Biological or artificial agents, which do this best, have the greatest chances of survival. Often this attempt to survive involves a complex interplay between fundamental mechanisms associated with perception, action learning, memory, abstraction, and prospection that can be investigated in greater detail even through simple "playful" experiments using an integrated system like a baby humanoid (incorporated with basic vision, touch, proprioception, force control, and whole-body coordination). Several experiments related to motor control, skill learning, and organization of procedural, semantic, and episodic memory were presented in this chapter to describe the cross talk between these fundamental processes operating in a "cumulatively" developing cognitive robot. All of this is organized in multiple interacting subsystems that synergistically come together in the context of the "goal" executed in the present (sometimes combined with new explorative interactions). Such interplay plays a fundamental role in ensuring that not everything needs to be learned and explored and not everything needs to be memorized (even memories compete to survive in the neural substrate and get their content reenacted by the actor). The interplay goes on cumulatively, more learning driving better reasoning and inconsistencies in reasoning driving new learning. Reenacting this on a baby humanoid often makes us remember the alternating "foregrounds" and "backgrounds" as intricately depicted in the several artistic creations of Escher. Simply put, beyond a point a software programmer cannot travel the journey of a cognitive robot like iCub. Instead, like natural cognitive agents, they must also be endowed with mechanisms that enable them to efficiently organize their sensorimotor experiences into their memories, remember, consolidate, forget, and exploit them effectively "when needed" to realize their

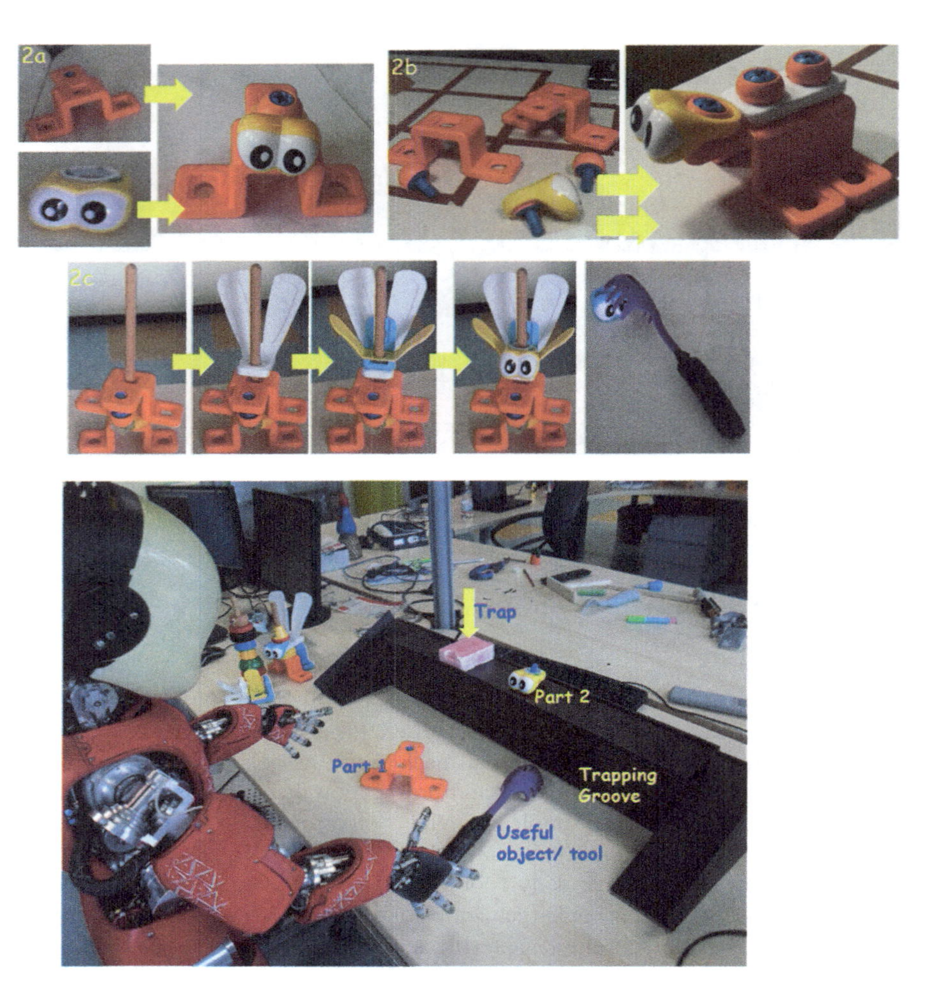

Fig. 7.10 Advanced Darwin scenarios are set up in a range of playful make and break style assembly tasks, also incorporating several elements of goal-directed reasoning, inspired by similar studies in animal and infant cognition

goals and, at the same time, keep learning new things. Open-endedness, cumulatively and growth of a continuously learning system, and gradual emergence of generativity/creativity in their behaviors are natural consequences arising out of such a scheme as different sections in our chapter demonstrate.

In this concluding section, we do not intend to summarize all that has been said so far but instead quickly relate all this to a very fundamental evolutionary function, namely, "navigation," an activity that all living organisms engage in. It is already developed in a sophisticated way in rats, for example, but much more so in humans, with plenty of added/recycled value (green learning!). The computational basis of this added value, at the same time grounded in the biology of the brain and recreated through playful tasks with iCub, was in fact the main subject of this chapter. In the discussion, we attempt to present a perspective that creative "goal-directed generation of behavior itself is navigation" (not in space but in time)!

7.5.1 Traveling in Time vs. Traveling in Space: The Navigating Rat, a Tool-Making Crow, and Darwin Architecture

All living organisms "navigate." There are few exceptions like the sea squirts: after few days of life, the first thing they do is digesting their own brains for nourishment. But as the complexity of the body and the environments in which the species had to survive becomes more complex, their brains also become more and more complex. A rat navigates for food, can remember places where food is found, and finds a path to reach it, sometimes involving novel solutions as demonstrated by several studies on rat navigation. However, with an even more complex body and more complex environment to survive in, higher-order primates need to navigate not only in "space" but also in time. Evolution being always constrained by "energy and space" would have certainly found ways to reorganize the primitive neural substrates engaged in navigating in space already existing in lower-level organisms to be reused to "navigate in time."

Indeed the recent discovery of the default mode network of the brain (both in humans and rats) supports this perspective. There is a wide consensus in the field of neuroscience that the same network is consistently activated while recalling the past (Maguire 2001; Rugg et al 2002) and other activities as diverse as simulating the future (Atance and O'Neill 2001; Addis et al. 2009; Szpunar et al 2007; Schacter et al 2012), spatial navigation (Burgess et al 2002; Suddendorf 2013; Corballis 2013), social cognition (Raichle et al 2001; Frith and Frith 2010), and perspective taking (Mason et al 2007). The essence of these findings is that there is evidence in support of the viewpoint that disparate cognitive functions often treated as distinct might share common underlying processes.

The Darwin architecture being developed looks at the computational basis of how such diverse functions can share resources and enable a cognitive robot to "travel in time" (through its multiple past experiences, the present evolving experience, and the simulated future consequences) to give rise to intelligent goal-directed behavior. In this sense, by mimicking the DMN, we have created a computational framework that enables Darwin robot to travel in time, connect its multiple past experiences to simulate the future, give rise to novel behaviors in unforeseen situations, and learn new things in the process. In this context, what we want to emphasize is that "goal-directed reasoning" is very similar to a path-finding exercise during spatial navigation, but now in "time" not "space."

Let us consider this analogy in detail in the context of this chapter. Goals are distant events in time that have to be reached; past experiences triggered by one's episodic memories give a path in time to reach a future event (which can be remembered based on partial cues). Frequently the paths in time also encounter obstacles, i.e., a contradiction between what the robot expects to ensue in time as a result of its past experience and what is actually happening in the present time. Clearly this is equivalent to getting lost in space, like a rat trapped in a maze. In the present context, the robot gets lost in time instead!

Alternative paths have to be found in time by exploration, in analogy with a rat, engaged in exploring its environment to come up with a new path to its spatial destination. Several cues in the environment are used to guide such exploration. The same applies when obstacles are encountered in time! Just like a train that changes its tracks. Many times there are multiple paths that lead to the same goal, when energy is used as a mechanism to choose the most efficient strategy (PMP mechanism of Sect. 7.2, for instance, which solves the degrees of freedom problem elegantly). The same applies also in the context of the energy of a memory. When we navigate in space, we remember the landmarks. Similarly, events in the episodic memory are landmarks in time. Landmarks in time can be connected by a mechanism of resonance. When landmarks are connected in space, we get a new trajectory to navigate spatially towards the goal. When the dots in time are connected, novel behaviors may emerge (like the examples in Sect. 7.3).

In sum, our memories represent our past, but they can also be used to simulate the future (whether it is while navigating in space or navigating in time). Emergence of creativity and novelty in behavior when encountered with a novel situation is related to the power to "re-invoke" such experiences that otherwise lie dormant in the neural episodic memory based on the present context, connecting the dots between such diverse experiences to find a new path in time. Indeed a navigating rat, a tool-making crow, and iCub share similarities in the way they accomplish their goals. Of course, it may be tough to understand what is going on in the brain of Betty reasoning in time or a rat navigating in space by looking at the neural activations in their brains. But principles can be abstracted from information-rich biology that can help to both "mimic and create" artifacts that show similar competencies.

Embodied developmental robotics helps here provide novel insights, as we computationally attempt to reenact such processes and on the way sometimes manage to abstract "fundamental principles" involved. The discovery of DNA was a result of model building by Watson and Crick, of empirical measurements with X-ray diffraction images by Rosalind Franklin, and the theoretical analysis of chemical bonds by Wolfgang Pauli. The model building direction is what the Darwin goal-directed reasoning framework achieves, using principles that are grounded in the biology of the brain! Of course the discussion does not end here; these were just simple explorations at the tip of the iceberg! Future efforts will be directed to go deeper!

References

Addessi E, Mancini A, Crescimbene L, Padoa-Schioppa C, Visalberghi E (2008) Preference transitivity and symbolic representation in capuchin monkeys (Cebus apella). PLoS One 3 (6):e2414

Addis DR, Schacter DL (2012) The hippocampus and imagining the future: where do we stand? Front Hum Neurosci 5:173. doi:10.3389/fnhum.2011.00173

Addis DR, Pan L, Vu MA, Laiser N, Schacter DL (2009) Constructive episodic simulation of the future and the past: distinct subsystems of a core brain network mediate imagining and remembering. Neuropsychologia 47:2222–2238

Anderson ML (2003) Embodied cognition: a field guide. Artif Intell 149(1):91–130

Asai Y, Tasaka Y, Nomura K, Nomura T, Casadio M, Morasso P (2009) A model of postural control in quiet standing: robust compensation of delay-induced instability using intermittent activation of feedback control. PLoS One 4(7), art. no. e6169

Asatryan DG, Feldman AG (1965) Functional tuning of the nervous system with control of movement or maintenance of a steady posture: I. Mechanographic analysis of the work of the joint or execution of a postural task. Biofizika 10:837–846

Atance CM, O'Neill DK (2001) Episodic future thinking. Trends Cogn Sci 5:533–539

Barabasi AL (2003) Linked: the new science of networks. Perseus Books, Langue. ISBN 0738206679

Barabási A-L (2012) The network takeover. Nat Phys 8:14–16

Barabási A-L, Albert R (1999) Emergence of scaling in random network. Science 286:509–512

Barhen J, Gulati S, Zak M (1989) Neural learning of constrained nonlinear transformations. IEEE Comput 6:67–76

Bernstein N (1935) The problem of the interrelation of coordination and localization. Arch Biol Sci 38:15–59. Reprinted in: Bernstein N (1967) The coordination and regulation of movements. Pergamon Press, Oxford, UK

Bizzi E, Cheung VCK (2013) The neural origin of muscle synergies. Front Comput Neurosci 7(51). doi:10.3389/fncom.2013.00051

Bizzi E, Polit A (1978) Processes controlling arm movements in monkeys. Science 201: 1235–1237

Braitenberg V (1986) Vehicles—experiments in synthetic psychology. MIT Press, Cambridge, MA

Bressler SL, Menon V (2010) Large-scale brain networks in cognition: emerging methods and principles. Trends Cogn Sci 14(6):277–290

Brooks R (1991) Intelligence without representation. Artif Intell J 47:139–159

Buccino G, Binkofski F, Fink GR, Fadiga L, Fogassi L, Gallese V, Seitz RJ, Zilles K, Rizzolatti G, Freund HJ (2001) Action observation activates premotor and parietal areas in a somatotopic manner: an fMRI study. Eur J Neurosci 13(2):400–404

Buckner RL, Carroll DC (2007) Self-projection and the brain. Trends Cogn Sci 2:49–57

Buckner RL, Andrews-Hanna JR, Schacter DL (2008) The brain's default network: anatomy, function, and relevance to disease. Ann N Y Acad Sci 1124:1–38

Burgess N et al (2002) The human hippocampus and spatial and episodic memory. Neuron 35: 625–641

Chiel HJ, Beer RD (1997) The brain has a body: adaptive behavior emerges from interactions of nervous system, body and environment. Trends Neurosci 20:553–557

Churchland MM, Cunningham JP, Kaufman MT, Foster JD, Nuyujukian P, Ryu SI, Shenoy KV (2012) Neural population dynamics during reaching. Nature 487:51–56

Clark A (1997) Being there: putting brain, body and world together again. MIT Press, Cambridge, MA

Coelho CJ, Nusbaum HC, Rosenbaum DA, Fenn KM (2012) Imagined actions aren't just weak actions: task variability promotes skill learning in physical practice but not in mental practice. J Exp Psychol Learn Mem Cogn 38:1759–1764

Cohen MA, Grossberg S (1983) Absolute stability of global pattern-formation and parallel memory storage by competitive neural networks. IEEE Trans Syst Man Cybern 13(5):815–826

Cohen RG, Rosenbaum DA (2011) Prospective and retrospective effects in human motor control: planning grasps for object rotation and translation. Psychol Res 75:341–349
Corballis MC (2013) Mental time travel: a case for evolutionary continuity. Trends Cogn Sci 17:5–6
D'Avella A, Saltiel P, Bizzi E (2003) Combinations of muscle synergies in the construction of a natural motor behavior. Nat Neurosci 6:300–308
Damasio A (2010) Self comes to mind: constructing the conscious brain. Pantheon, New York, NY
Decety J (1996) Do imagined and executed actions share the same neural substrate? Cogn Brain Res 3:87–93
Desmurget M, Sirigu A (2009) A parietal-premotor network for movement intention and motor awareness. Trends Cogn Sci 13:411–419
Diedrichsen J, Classen J (2012) Stimulating news about modular motor control. Neuron 76: 1043–1045
Emery NJ, Clayton NS (2004) The mentality of crows: convergent evolution of intelligence in corvids and apes. Science 306:1903–1907
Frey SH, Gerry VE (2006) Modulation of neural activity during observational learning of actions and their sequential orders. J Neurosci 26:13194–13201
Frith U, Frith C (2010) The social brain: allowing humans to boldly go where no other species has been. Philos Trans R Soc Lond B Biol Sci 365:165–176
Fritzke B (1995) A growing neural gas network learns topologies. In: Tesauro G, Touretzky D, Leen T (eds) Advances in neural information processing systems, vol 7. MIT Press, Cambridge, MA, pp 625–632
Gallese V, Lakoff G (2005) The brain's concepts: the role of the sensory-motor system in reason and language. Cogn Neuropsychol 22:455–479
Gallese V, Sinigaglia C (2011) What is so special with embodied simulation. Trends Cogn Sci 15 (11):512–519
Georgopoulos AP, Schwartz AB, Kettner RE (1986) Neuronal population coding of movement direction. Science 233(4771):1416–1419
Giszter SF, Mussa-Ivaldi FA, Bizzi E (1993) Convergent force fields organized in the frog's spinal cord. J Neurosci 13:467–491
Glenberg AM, Gallese V (2012) Action-based language: a theory of language acquisition, comprehension, and production. Cortex 48:905–922
Grafton ST (2009) Embodied cognition and the simulation of action to understand others. Ann N Y Acad Sci 1156:97–117
Graziano MSA, Botvinick MM (2002) How the brain represents the body: insights from neurophysiology and psychology. In: Prinz W, Hommel B (eds) Common mechanisms in perception and action: attention and performance XIX. Oxford University Press, Oxford, pp 136–157
Graziano MSA, Taylor CSR, Moore T (2002) Complex movements evoked by microstimulation of precentral cortex. Neuron 34:841–851
Grush R (2004) The emulation theory of representation: motor control, imagery, and perception. Behav Brain Sci 27:377–396
Haggard P, Wolpert DM (2005) Disorders of body schema. In: Freund HJ, Jeannerod M, Hallett M, Leiguarda R (eds) Higher-order motor disorders: from neuroanatomy and neurobiology to clinical neurology. Oxford University Press, Oxford, pp 261–271
Hagmann P, Cammoun L, Gigandet X, Meuli R, Honey CJ, Wedeen VJ, Sporns O (2008) Mapping the structural core of human cerebral cortex. PLoS Biol 6:e159
Hassabis D, Maguire EA (2011) The construction system of the brain. In: Bar M (ed) Predictions in the brain: using our past to generate a future. Oxford University Press, New York, NY
Head H, Holmes G (1911) Sensory disturbances in cerebral lesions. Brain 34:102–254
Herbort O, Butz MV (2012) Too good to be true? Ideomotor theory from a computational perspective. Front Psychol 3:494
Hesslow G (2002) Conscious thought as a simulation of behavior and perception. Trends Cogn Sci 6:242–247
Hesslow G, Jirenhed DA (2007) The Inner World of a Simple Robot. J Conscious Stud 14:85–96

Hopfield JJ (1984) Neurons with graded response have collective computational properties like those of 2-state neurons. Proc Natl Acad Sci USA Biol Sci 81(10):3088–3092
Hopfield JJ (2008) Searching for memories, Sudoku, implicit check bits, and the iterative use of not-always-correct rapid neural computation. Neural Comput 20:1119–1164
Iacoboni M (2009) Neurobiology of imitation. Curr Opin Neurobiol 19:661–665
Jeannerod M (2001) Neural simulation of action: a unifying mechanism for motor cognition. Neuroimage 14:103–109
Johnson M (1987) The body in the mind: the bodily basis of meaning, imagination and reason. University of Chicago Press, Chicago, IL
Kandel ER, Tauc L (1965) Heterosynaptic facilitation in neurones of the abdominal ganglion of Aplysia depilans. J Physiol 181:1–27
Kelso JAS, Holt KG (1980) Exploring a vibratory systems analysis of human movement production. J Neurophysiol 43:1183–1196
Kohonen T (1995) Self-organizing maps. Springer, Berlin
Kornysheva K, Sierk A, Diedrichsen J (2013) Interaction of temporal and ordinal representations in movement sequence. J Neurophysiol 109(5):1416–1424
Kuperstein M (1991) Infant neural controller for adaptive sensory-motor coordination. Neural Netw 4(2):131–146
Kutch JJ, Valero-Cuevas FJ (2012) Challenges and new approaches to proving the existence of muscle synergies of neural origin. PLoS Comput Biol 8:e1002434
Lacquaniti F, Terzuolo C, Viviani P (1983) The law relating kinematic and figural aspects of drawing movements. Acta Psychol (Amst) 54:115–130
Lakoff G, Johnson M (1999) Philosophy in the flesh: the embodied mind and its challenge to western thought. Basic Books, New York, NY
Liepmann H (1905) Ueber Störungen des Handelns bei Gehirnkranken. S. Kargen, Berlin
Loram I, Lakie M (2002) Direct measurement of human ankle stiffness during quiet standing: the intrinsic mechanical stiffness is insufficient for stability. J Physiol 545:1041–1053
Lu H, Zou Q, Gu H, Raichle ME, Stein EA, Yang Y (2012) Rat brains also have a default mode network. Proc Natl Acad Sci U S A 109(10):3979–3984
Maguire EA (2001) Neuroimaging studies of autobiographical event memory. Philos Trans R Soc Lond B Biol Sci 356:1441–1451
Maravita A, Iriki A (2004) Tools for the body (schema). Trends Cogn Sci 8:79–86
Marsden CD, Merton PA, Morton HB (1972) Servo action in human voluntary movement. Nature 238:140–143
Martin A (2007) The representation of object concepts in the brain. Annu Rev Psychol 58:25–45
Martin A (2009) Circuits in mind: the neural foundations for object concepts. In: Gazzaniga M (ed) The cognitive neurosciences, 4th edn. MIT Press, Cambridge, MA, pp 1031–1045
Martin VC, Schacter DL, Corballis MC, Addis DR (2011) A role for the hippocampus in encoding future simulations. Proc Natl Acad Sci USA 108:13858–13863
Mason MF et al (2007) Wandering minds: the default network and stimulus-independent thought. Science 315:393–395
McCulloch W, Pitts W (1943) A logical calculus of the ideas immanent in nervous activity. Bull Math Biol 5(4):115–133
Metta G, Natale L, Nori F, Sandini G, Vernon D, Fadiga L, von Hofsten C, Rosander K, Lopes M, Santos-Victor J, Bernardino A, Montesano L (2010) The iCub humanoid robot: an open-systems platform for research in cognitive development. Neural Netw 23:1125–1134
Meyer K, Damasio A (2009) Convergence and divergence in a neural architecture for recognition and memory. Trends Neurosci 32(7):376–382
Mohan V, Morasso P (2011) Passive motion paradigm: an alternative to optimal control. Front Neurorobot 5:4
Mohan V, Morasso P (2012) How past experience, imitation and practice can be combined to swiftly learn to use novel "tools": insights from skill learning experiments with baby

humanoids. In: International conference on biomimetic and biohybrid systems: living machines 2012, Barcelona, 9–12 July 2012
Mohan V, Morasso P, Metta G, Sandini G (2009) A biomimetic, force-field based computational model for motion planning and bimanual coordination in humanoid robots. Auton Robots 27:291–307
Mohan V, Morasso P, Zenzeri J, Metta G, Chakravarthy VS, Sandini G (2011a) Teaching a humanoid robot to draw 'Shapes'. Auton Robots 31(1):21–53
Mohan V, Morasso P, Metta G, Kasderidis S (2011b) The distribution of rewards in growing sensorimotor maps acquired by cognitive robots through exploration. Neurocomputing. doi:10.1016/j.neucom.2011.06.009
Mohan V, Morasso P, Sandini G, Kasderidis S (2013) Inference through embodied simulation in cognitive robots. Cogn Comput 5(1). doi: 10.1007/s12559-013-9205-4
Morasso P (1981) Spatial control of arm movements. Exp Brain Res 42:223–227
Morasso P, Sanguineti V, Frisone F, Perico L (1998) Coordinate-free sensorimotor processing: computing with population codes. Neural Netw 11:1417–1428
Morasso P, Casadio M, Mohan V, Zenzeri J (2010) A neural mechanism of synergy formation for whole body reaching. Biol Cybern 102:45–55
Morasso P, Rea F, Mohan V (2013) A biomimetic framework for coordinating and controlling whole body movements in humanoid robots. In: IEEE EMBC2013, Osaka, 3–7 July, pp 5307–5310
Murata A, Fadiga L, Fogassi L, Gallese V, Raos V, Rizzolatti G (1997) Object representation in the ventral premotor cortex (area f5) of the monkey. J Neurophysiol 78:2226–2230
Mussa Ivaldi FA, Morasso P, Zaccaria R (1988) Kinematic networks. A distributed model for representing and regularizing motor redundancy. Biol Cybern 60:1–16
Mussa-Ivaldi FA (1988) Do neurons in the motor cortex encode movement direction? An alternative hypothesis. Neurosci Lett 91:106–111
Nicoll A, Blakemore C (1993) Patterns of local connectivity in the neocortex. Neural Comput 5:665–680
Overduin SA, D'Avella A, Carmena JM, Bizzi E (2012) Microstimulation activates a handful of muscle synergies. Neuron 76:1071–1077
Patterson K, Nestor PJ, Rogers TT (2007) Where do you know what you know? The representation of semantic knowledge in the human brain. Nat Rev Neurosci 8(12):976–987
Pfeifer R, Scheier C (1998) Representation in natural and artificial agents: an embodied cognitive science perspective. Z Naturforsch C 53(7–8):480–503
Popescu FC, Rymer WZ (2000) End points of planar reaching movements are disrupted by small force pulses: an evaluation of the hypothesis of equifinality. J Neurophysiol 84(5):2670–2679
Pulvermüller F, Fadiga L (2010) Active perception: sensorimotor circuits as a cortical basis for language. Nat Rev Neurosci 11(5):351–360
Raichle ME et al (2001) A default mode of brain function. Proc Natl Acad Sci USA 98:676–682
Reggia JA, D'Autrechy CL, Sutton GG III, Weinrich M (1992) A competitive distribution theory of neocortical dynamics. Neural Comput 4:287–317
Rizzolatti G, Luppino G (2001) The cortical motor system. Neuron 31:889–901
Rizzolatti G, Sinigaglia C (2010) The functional role of the parieto-frontal mirror circuit: interpretations and misinterpretations. Nat Rev Neurosci 11:264–274
Rizzolatti G, Fadiga L, Gallese V, Fogassi L (1996) Premotor cortex and the recognition of motor actions. Cogn Brain Res 3:131–141
Roh J, Cheung VCK, Bizzi E (2011) Modules in the brain stem and spinal cord underlying motor behaviors. J Neurophysiol 106:1363–1378
Rosenbaum DA, Loukopoulos LD, Meulenbroek RGJ, Vaughan J, Engelbrecht SE (1995) Planning reaches by evaluating stored postures. Psychol Rev 102:28–67
Rosenbaum DA, Meulenbroek RG, Vaughan J, Jansen C (2001) Posture-based motion planning: applications to grasping. Psychol Rev 108:709–734

Rugg MD, Otten LJ, Henson RN (2002) The neural basis of episodic memory: evidence from functional neuroimaging. Philos Trans R Soc Lond B Biol Sci 357(1424):1097–1110
Schacter DL, Addis DR, Hassabis D, Martin V, Nathan RS, Szpunar KK (2012) The future of memory: remembering, imagining, and the brain. Neuron 76(4):677–694
Sharma N, Pomeroy VM, Baron J (2006) Motor imagery: a back door to the motor system after stroke? Stroke 37:1941–1952
Sherrington C (1904) The integrative action of the nervous system. Silliman Memorial Lecture
Sporns O (2011) The human connectome: a complex network. Ann N Y Acad Sci 1224:109–125
Sporns O (2013) The human connectome: origins and challenges. Neuroimage 80:53–61
Sporns O, Tononi G, Edelman GM (2002) Theoretical neuroanatomy and the connectivity of the cerebral cortex. Behav Brain Res 20:69–74
Suddendorf T (2013) Mental time travel: continuities and discontinuities. Trends Cogn Sci 17: 151–152
Suddendorf T, Addis DR, Corballis MC (2009) Mental time travel and the shaping of the human mind. Philos Trans R Soc Lond B Biol Sci 364:1317–1324
Suinn RM (1972) Behavior rehearsal training for ski racers. Behav Ther 3:519
Szpunar KK et al (2007) Neural substrates of envisioning the future. Proc Natl Acad Sci USA 104: 642–647
Thompson E (2007) Mind in life: biology, phenomenology and the sciences of mind, no. 1. Harvard University Press, Cambridge, MA, p 568
Tulving E (1972) Episodic and semantic memory. In: Tulving E, Donaldson W (eds) Organisation of memory. Academic, New York, NY, pp 381–403
Tulving E (2002) Episodic memory: from mind to brain. Annu Rev Psychol 53:1–25
van den Heuvel MP, Sporns O (2013) Network hubs in the human brain. Trends Cogn Sci 17 (12):683–696
Varela FJ, Maturana HR, Uribe R (1974) Autopoiesis: the organization of living systems, its characterization and a model. Biosystems 5:187–196
Vernon D, von Hofsten C, Fadiga L (2010) A roadmap for cognitive development in humanoid robots. Springer, Berlin and Heidelberg
Visalberghi E, Tomasello M (1997) Primate causal understanding in the physical and in the social domains. Behav Process 42:189–203
Vygotsky LS (1978) Mind in society: the development of higher psychological processes. Harvard University Press, Cambridge, MA
Watts JD, Strogatz S (1998) Collective dynamics of small world networks. Nature 393(6684): 440–442
Weir AAS, Chappell J, Kacelnik A (2002) Shaping of hooks in New Caledonian crows. Science 297:981–983
Welberg L (2012) Neuroimaging: rats join the 'default mode' club. Nat Rev Neurosci 13(4):223
Whiten A, McGuigan N, Marshall-Pescini S, Hopper LM (2009) Emulation, imitation, overimitation and the scope of culture for child and chimpanzee. Philos Trans R Soc Lond B Biol Sci 364:2417–2428
Wiener N (1948) Cybernetics: or control and communication in the animal and the machine. MIT Press, Cambridge, MA
Woodworth RS (1899) The accuracy of voluntary movement. Psychol Rev Monogr Suppl 3:1–113
Zak M (1988) Terminal attractors for addressable memory in neural networks. Phys Lett 133: 218–222

Chapter 8
Human Machine Interaction and Communication in Cooperative Actions

Gabriel Baud-Bovy, Pietro Morasso, Francesco Nori, Giulio Sandini, and Alessandra Sciutti

8.1 Introduction

Many human activities are performed in groups and require that the individuals in the group coordinate their actions. Joint or cooperative actions can be regarded as any form of social interaction whereby two or more individuals coordinate their activities in space and time to bring about a commonly desired change in the environment (Sebanz et al. 2006). The number and variety of circumstances involving joint actions are countless and might or might not involve physical interaction. For example, carrying bulky objects, dancing, handshaking, and teaching a physical skill are examples of joint actions involving physical interaction. In contrast, workers controlling remotely different parts of a machine, a clinical team performing a surgical operation, musicians playing together in an orchestra, ballet dancers realizing a choreography, and groups of programmers developing software are examples of tasks where all partners need to coordinate their actions to perform the main task in absence of physical interaction. In this Chapter, we will consider joint actions that may or may not involve physical interaction between partners (whether human or robot).

A crucial aspect of joint action is that it requires that the partners share information and communicate to update the information as needed. Without shared information and communication, no form of coordination would be possible. In particular, joint action typically requires knowing or guessing what the other perceives (or does not perceive), and what the other will or should do. It also requires a constant monitoring of one's own action and the state of the interaction, which is far from trivial because the effect of one's action might depend on the action of the two partners. Sebanz et al. (2006) highlight that successful joint actions rest on the abilities to (1) share representations, (2) predict action, and (3) integrate predicted effects of own's and other's action.

G. Baud-Bovy • P. Morasso • F. Nori • G. Sandini (✉) • A. Sciutti
Central Research Laboratory, Istituto Italiano di Tecnologia, Genova, Italy

R. Cingolani (ed.), *Bioinspired Approaches for Human-Centric Technologies*,
DOI 10.1007/978-3-319-04924-3_8,

When analyzing joint action, it is also helpful to consider the distinction between *planned* and *emergent* coordination (Knoblich et al. 2011). In *planned coordination*, the behavior of the partners is driven by representations that specify the desired outcomes of joint action and each partner's own part in achieving these outcomes. For example, some form of explicit planning is involved when two or more individuals play in an orchestra (the plan is the musical score), perform surgery (the plan is the standard sequence of surgical acts), or cooperate in an assembly line according to a blueprint. Planned coordination plays also a central role in new forms of work organization spurred by the development of software to support coordination and cooperation between people working at distance by using a variety of tools, such as bulletin boards, message boards, versioning systems, as well as more sophisticated virtual collaborative environment (Churchill and Snowdon 1998; Bafoutso and Mentzas 2002). Studies on the efficacy of such systems have dealt with topics like the organization of work (planning) and the division of labor (roles) in collaborative work or the importance of face-to-face interaction in these forms of joint actions (Nardi and Whittaker 2002).

In *emergent coordination*, coordinated behavior occurs due to perception–action couplings that make multiple individuals act in similar ways, independently of joint plans. Information might involve the precise timing of an action, the velocity with which a movement is executed, the amount of force that should be employed, etc. Classic examples of emergent coordination include emergent synchronization between the movements of people observing each other (e.g., Schmidt et al. 1990; Oullier et al. 2008). At the neurophysiological level, it is thought that emergent coordination involves some form of resonance between sensory and motor circuits, even in conditions where one of the partners is a simple observer (e.g., Gallese et al. 1996; Fogassi et al. 2005; Jeannerod 2006; Cattaneo et al. 2009).

It is important to note that this information can be communicated and perceived in a more or less explicit manner. For example, during face-to-face collaboration, one might give instructions or explain what she/he is doing or wishes to do, whether verbally or through communicative gestures such as pointing out to an object in the environment with the hand or the eyes. Cleary, explicit communication plays a large role in forms of collaboration that require a large amount of planning. In contrast, emergent coordination is often based on subtle facial or body cues that are picked up almost unconsciously by the partner. Interestingly, these cues can give information about the goal of the action and properties of objects in the environment.

Joint actions that involve physical interaction add a whole new level of communication between partners. As a matter of fact, physical interaction can itself be a communication channel, which can significantly extend the other forms of coordination discussed above. For example, when holding a dance partner, physical interaction is not merely meant to lift the partner or prevent a fall but mainly to guide the partner in a joint performance. A very good example, for our purpose, is *contact improvisation* (CI), which is a partnered modern dance style initially developed by Steve Paxton in the early 1970s, for purposes ranging from social dance, performance art, and therapy. It is an improvised duet that integrates tactile, visual, and vestibular feedback generated by both partners simultaneously and by the forces of motion and gravity. CI directs the dancer's attention to sensation and nonverbal communication rather than execution of specific movement sequences or visible appearance. Remarkably, we know little about how this channel is used to transmit information between partners. To date, only a handful of studies have investigated physical interaction in joint actions (review in Reed 2012).

To a large extent, this chapter focuses on emergent coordination and implicit communication in human–robot joint actions. Because robots differ from humans in several ways, human–robot interactions raise novel questions with respect to human–human interactions:

First, robots in general do not look like humans and, even more often, they do not move like humans. This basic observation raises questions about whether emergent coordination does or can occur in human–robot interaction since this form of coordination is based on subtle cues about the body and the movement of the partners. These questions are addressed in Sect. 8.2, which analyzes whether and under which conditions a robotic device can trigger this form of covert communication with a human partner.

Second, the body of machines and robots differ greatly from the human body, in ways that go well beyond what can be observed visually. As a matter of fact, most robots (e.g., all industrial robots) are rigid and powerful artifacts which are dangerous to interact physically with. Moreover, physical interaction with these robots is limited by the fact that they fully control the movements which must then be passively followed by the partner. This is clearly a strong drawback in robot-assisted rehabilitation where an active participation of the patient is crucial to obtain good results. Section 8.3 is dedicated to physical interaction between humans and machines. Section 8.3.1 proposes a classification scheme of tasks involving physical interaction and a measure of the complexity based on the concept of compliance. In particular, Sect. 8.3.2 reports work done to develop novel compliant actuation technologies that aims at facilitating physical interaction between a robot and a person or its environment. Section 8.3.3 analyzes human control strategies when interacting physically with unpredictable environments simulated by a robot. Section 8.3.4 reports work done to optimize the treatment of people affected by neuromotor diseases like stroke in the context of robot-assisted rehabilitation of the upper limb. The final section emphasizes the importance of human studies for the development of robots that can interact with humans and alludes to the ethical and societal questions that partnerships between humans and robots will have to be addressed as machines play little by little an ever larger role in our daily life.

8.2 Observation-Based Human–Robot Interaction

In the last decades, the use of robotics devices has become more pervasive in society, with robots exiting from confined environments (e.g., segregated compartments in industries) and moving to new applications, as entertainment, telepresence, and rehabilitation at home. A relevant change associated to this evolution is that robots will interact with nonexpert users, who are not interested in how the robot is built and programmed, but want to proficiently collaborate with it, while trusting its safety. This substantial paradigm shift raises the need of changing the interface between humans and robots, with the ideal aim of moving from robot as complex machines to robots as natural interacting partners.

An obvious inspiration to build these interactive machines is represented by humans. Indeed, human beings can be extremely fluid and efficient in their collaboration with each other, so that sometimes even clumsiness can be a human trait with a communicative potential. However, an open question is *what* in the human model triggers the naturalness of the interaction. Such interrogative can in turn be translated into *how* (i.e., *in which aspects*) machines should be biomimetic or, better, humanlike. To date, different researchers have focused on various aspects of humanlikeness Some researchers have built robots with a very humanlike appearance (MacDorman and Ishiguro 2006) or body structure, in terms of biologically plausible muscular structure (e.g., Kozuki et al. 2012). Others have focused on implementing humanlike way of learning new actions (learning by demonstration, Billard et al. 2013) or humanlike language and gestures (Huang and Mutlu 2012; Salem et al. 2012). Although each one of these approaches has produced interesting results, something is still missing to achieve a human–robot interaction as natural as the one with a human partner. In some cases, the choice of humanlikeness has even become an obstacle rather than an advantage in the quest of empathic interaction (see the Uncanny Valley hypothesis, Mori 1970).

We believe that one of the characteristic features specific to human–human interaction still partly missing in robotic implementations is implicit communication, i.e., the mutual understanding that two partners reach with no need of exchanging a word or even a glance. This phenomenon has been extensively studied in the context of gaze. Just by looking around, a person communicates to others which object he is going to use or where his attention is focused. Also with robots, a proper gaze behavior has been shown to modify the way people perceive and interact with the surrounding objects (e.g., Lohan et al. 2012; Boucher et al. 2012; Sciutti et al. 2012), often facilitating the execution of cooperative shared plans.

However, the mechanism of mutual understanding supporting gaze reading encompasses a much wider range of actions. Indeed, often witnessing different partner's actions, as reaching, grasping, or pouring something, is enough to infer what will be his next move and to adapt accordingly the subsequent motion to collaborate. This ability appears very early in our infancy and allows fluid interaction well before language development. During their first year of life, infants already anticipate others' action goals with no need of instructions (e.g., Kanakogi and Itakura 2011, Falck-Ytter et al. 2006), and at around 1 year and a half, they show a natural propensity to instrumentally help others (Warneken et al. 2006), demonstrating that an implicit understanding of others' need is already functional. An important feature of this implicit communication is its integration in the functional motion of the agent. For instance, while one person is just aiming at reaching an object, the way he naturally moves informs the partner about his intention, with no need of an additional dedicated message. This kind of information transfer is particularly efficient, as it is simultaneous with the action and implicitly helps the partner to be motorically prepared to interact.

From a neurophysiological stance, this implicit understanding of the others actions is said to be based on shared motor representations between the human partners and to be directly mediated by dedicated neural mechanisms (Gallese et al. 1996; Cattaneo et al. 2009), as well as accumulated episodic memories (Schacter 2012). Moreover, in the context of the DMN model (Default Mode Network model: Raichle et al. 2001; Buckner et al. 2008), there is wide consensus that a core network of "highly connected" brain areas (referred to as "hubs" in network theory) are consistently activated when subjects perform diverse cognitive functions like recalling past experiences, simulating possible future events (*prospection*), planning goal-directed actions, imagining fictitious scenarios, and interpreting perspectives of other individuals (Buckner and Carroll 2007; Suddendorf et al 2009; Bressler and Menon 2010). We suggest that such effortless understanding is what makes human collaboration so uniquely fluid and efficient. Hence, we propose that if robot behavior could tap into the same mechanisms exploited for humans' action understanding, the fluidity of the interaction would approach that of human collaboration.

Our current research is devoted to analyzing whether and under which conditions a robotic device can trigger this form of covert communication with a human partner, with the dual aim of improving future human–robot interaction and of exploiting a robotic platform, the iCub humanoid robot, as a controllable physical stimulus to investigate the laws of human interactions.

Whether the observation of human and robotic actions elicit similar responses in the observer is a question is under debate in the scientific community (see Chaminade and Cheng 2009; Sciutti et al. 2012 for reviews). Indeed, the evidence is sparse and sometimes conflicting. For instance, the first neuroimaging studies (Perani et al. 2001; Tai et al. 2004) seemed to exclude the activation of neural substrates of this mechanism when the action was performed by a virtual or nonbiological agent. On the contrary, subsequent studies (e.g., Chaminade et al. 2010; Gazzola et al. 2007) have indicated that robotic agents evoke a similar mirror neurons system activity as humans do (or even stronger, Cross et al. 2012). The interrogation is not limited to the neuroimaging domain, though. In fact, motor resonance has behavioral consequences, such as facilitation in performing the same task as observed (e.g., reduced reaction time) and interference in the performance of an incongruent task (e.g., increase in variance). By directly measuring these behavioral phenomena, a few studies found either the absence or a quantitative reduction of the resonance for the observation of robotic agents (e.g. Kilner et al. 2003; Press et al. 2005), while other researchers observed conditions where the motor resonance effect was similar for human and nonhuman agents observation (Liepelt et al. 2010; Press et al. 2007).

In summary, there seems to be the possibility for robotic agents to evoke motor resonance and then induce the action-mediated understanding in a human partner, but the robot shape, the context in which it is immersed, and the way it moves need to be appropriately planned (Fig. 8.1). Moreover, as we are interested in the behavioral consequences of motor resonance, with specific attention to the corresponding facilitation in the interaction, we have to be particularly careful. In fact, if at the neurophysiological level the mirror neuron system activation seems to be present also for very nonbiological stimuli (i.e., when the nonbiological agent moves with a nonbiological kinematics, e.g., Cross et al. 2012; Gazzola et al. 2007), some behavioral effects require a higher degree of human resemblance also in terms of robot motion (Chaminade et al. 2005).

8.2.1 Anticipation of the Robot Action Goal

Having considered the elements in an interaction that might depend on the activation of the resonance mechanism, we focus now on goal anticipation. The ability to understand the actions of others and to attribute intentionality to them is crucial for collaboration, and it has been proposed to depend on motor resonance (Rizzolatti and Sinigaglia 2010; Southgate et al. 2009). Humans' natural tendency to shift their gaze to the action goal before the action is completed is one of the manifestations of such goal attribution. It is important to note that intuitive goal anticipation occurs naturally only in the presence of other people. Previous studies failed to find anticipatory gaze shifts toward the spatial destination of an object moving by itself (Falck-Ytter et al. 2006; Flanagan and Johansson 2003), even if the object movement followed biological rules and the target position was unambiguous. Adult observers exhibited anticipatory gaze behavior in the presence of a nonbiological agent when the latter could be interpreted as a tool they could use (a mechanical claw), while anticipation was not exhibited by young infants (4–10 months old), not as familiar with that tool (Kanakogi and Itakura 2011).

In Sciutti et al. (in press), we addressed the question of whether this kind of intuitive goal understanding can occur not only between humans, but also with humanoid robots. More precisely, we have measured whether human partners instinctively anticipate with their gaze the goal of an action performed by a robot, as they normally would during human observation. Our results, obtained with a humanoid robot following a biologically plausible motion, indicated a similar implicit processing of humans' and robots' actions, yielding the same automatic anticipatory behavior (Sciutti et al. in press). So humans are automatically predicting the partner's action goal, even if he actually is a robot.

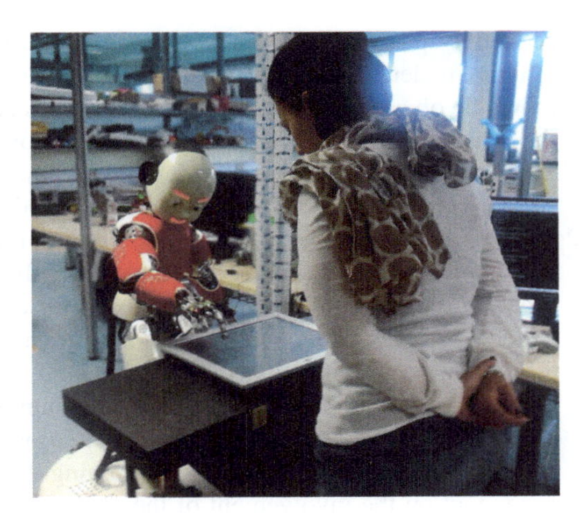

Fig. 8.1 iCub is interacting with a human partner by playing together with a touch screen. The way the robot moves its arm and its gaze has a strong influence on human perception (Sciutti et al. 2013a). Photo by Laura Taverna

8.2.2 Mutual Adaption to Robot Behavior

Another important property of human–human interaction is mutual adaptation. When we walk or work with someone else, we automatically align the speed of our actions to our partners' rhythm. Previous studies have shown that in case of virtual stimuli (e.g., a single dot moving on a screen, ideally representing the finger of an agent), such motor contagion is selectively present only if the motion follows a biologically plausible kinematics (Bisio et al. 2010). We have evaluated whether a similar phenomenon extended also to the interaction with a physical, nonhuman agent, as the robot iCub. In particular, a demonstrator (either human or robot) performed a reaching or a transport action at different speeds. After action observation, subjects were instructed to reach the same target or transport the same object. Motor contagion was assessed by evaluating the influence of the observed speed on the velocity adopted by subjects during their actions. Different parameters of the demonstrator's action were manipulated, including the shape of the trajectory and the kinematics of the motion (biologically plausible or not). Our results suggested that the nature of the agent may have relevance in determining human implicit adaptation, but only as a function of the adopted kinematics (Bisio et al. submitted).

8.2.3 Inferring Object's Properties from Robot Observation

Importantly, through action observation, humans can automatically infer not only others' goals but also the dynamics properties of the objects manipulated by the action partner. For instance, humans are extremely precise at estimating the weight of an object just by observing the lifting action performed by a human partner (Runeson and Frykholm 1981). Moreover, they can also use this information to accurately plan their own next actions on the object (Reichelt et al. 2013). This intuitive understanding is very efficient and allows two collaborators to be prepared to handle objects or tools in common, as they can estimate the weight of the object the other agent is passing to them even before the handover is concluded, also avoiding the potential risk of accepting an object which is too heavy to be held. A similar implicit communication is again mediated by the motor system of the observer (e.g. Senot et al. 2011), being therefore intuitive (or automatic) for the two human action partners. We have recently investigated whether such object property reading could be extended to the observation of a humanoid actor, and at which cost in terms of complexity of robotics action planning. Our results indicated that a simple modification of the humanoid lifting motions trajectories allowed humans to estimate the weight lifted by the humanoid robot with a similar accuracy as the one exhibited during human observation. Furthermore, such ability is intuitive and does not require extensive training. Lastly, weight judgment seems to be dependent on the involvement of the observer's motor system both during human and humanoid observation (Sciutti et al. 2013a). Most importantly, the weight information extracted from action observation facilitates the observer in the planning of his own action on the same object (Sciutti et al. in press). These findings suggest that the neural mechanisms at the basis of human interaction can be extended to human–humanoid interaction, allowing for intuitive and proficient collaboration between humanoid robots and untrained human partners.

8.2.4 Robot Behavior Legibility

It has been suggested that the key to achieve seamless collaboration in human–robot interaction (HRI) stands in the understandability and the intuitiveness of the robotic behavior, defined as transparency or legibility by different authors (e.g., Dragan et al. 2013; Chao et al. 2010). More in general, the need is envisioned for user-friendly or "human-aware" robot design (Sisbot and Alami 2012). For instance, the idea is to make either the goal of the robotic action or the robot's uncertainty about the task at hand easily understandable or its motion compatible with the comfortableness of the human partner.

We suggest that such legibility and comfortableness of the interaction could be expanded to human–robot collaboration when we will be able to activate during HRI the same neural mechanisms that are in place for interacting with humans. This principle applies in particular to the humanoid platforms, as their humanlike structure could induce human observers to expect that the machines would follow the same motor control laws and constraints that apply to human motion. This choice would make interaction with a robot more intuitive and automatic for the nonexpert user, at the cost of taking into account, already at the robot planning level, the need for understanding of the human partner.

We have already proved that this is a viable path, at least in the context of goal anticipation, mutual adaptation, and weight reading. Still many questions are still open for future research. First, it is important to clarify which parameters are relevant in allowing such matching for the wide range of tasks we execute in everyday life and how from single actions this ability could scale to complex activities. Moreover, one needs to investigate how it is possible to generalize this implicit communication, moving from action observation to a continuous interaction, where sometimes complementary—and not purely "resonating"—actions are required and the information exchange is multisensory in nature, travelling not only through vision but across multiple senses.

8.3 Physical Human–Robot Interaction

For machines and in particular robots to make further inroads in natural human environments, contact and physical interaction become necessary and unavoidable. Everyday tasks involve making and breaking contact, with different parts of the body, whether as the result of accidental disturbances or for intentional support for dynamic movement. Critically, robots should be robust enough to cope with unpredictable contact, via safe control mechanisms and compliance. Moreover, robots need the ability to exploit predictable contact to aid in goal achievement, as well as to learn dynamics of contact in order to generalize to novel tasks and domains. This fundamental element of human motor control has not been matched by present-day robots, which are still far from the human capabilities in exploiting predictable events and in coping with uncertainty. Within this context, the gap between humans and robots is particularly apparent in tasks involving unstructured physical interaction with the environment or other agents. Such tasks are among the most important ones for future cognitive robots.

One important difference between humans and robots is that robots have bodies with fundamentally different dynamical properties, beyond those that can be seen visually and that have been analyzed in the previous section. As a matter of fact, most robots have been until quite recently powerful and dangerous machines to interact physically with. Moreover, the way these robots are controlled strongly limit physical interaction to a simple exercise where the partner passively follows the movements of the robot.

A fundamental insight coming from animal and human motor control studies is the importance of compliance for the development of robot–human interaction. Compliance (or the inverse concept of stiffness) is to be understood as the force-displacement characteristic of a contact. Unlike the actuation and control systems of rigid robots, the human motor system is based on agonist–antagonist arrangements of intrinsically compliant muscles and low-level reflex loops. These characteristics of the motor apparatus provide animals and humans with a built-in capacity to deal with contacts and possible external perturbations that greatly simplifies the control. While the important role of compliance was first recognized in the context of human motor control studies (e.g., Feldman 1966; Polit and Bizzi 1979), compliance is nowadays a very active research area in robotics (Hogan 1984), as widely discussed in Chaps. 5 and 6 for the Coman and ICub platforms. In particular, the importance of adjustable compliance to deal with unpredictable tasks has been the focus of several recent behavioral and robotic studies. Already in early experiments, it has been shown (Shadmehr and Mussa-Ivaldi 1994) that humans learn and adapt internal dynamical models of their own arm in interaction with the environment. Such internal models appear to be crucial in predicting how muscle activations produce hand movements and therefore may play an essential predictive role in movement planning. However, Burdet and co-workers (2001) have shown that when prediction is not a viable strategy, humans rely on arm compliance regulation (by means of muscle co-activation) to cope with the unpredictability that naturally arises from feedback delays when performing arm-reaching movements in unstable environments. Basic research and robotics technology appear ready to extend such insights from single limb movements to whole-body interaction and the validation of these models appears feasible.

As mentioned in the introduction of this chapter, joint action requires shared representations and the transmission of information. This also holds true in the case of joint action involving physical interaction. While scenarios involving physical interaction do not exclude explicit planning and the uses of verbal instruction and miscellaneous visual cues for coordination, physical interaction provides an additional communication channel between the partners. Unfortunately, little is known about how contact and interaction forces are used to transmit information about the goal of the action or the intention and state of each partner (review in Reed 2012).

Most of the research on physical interaction has focused on haptic dyads, i.e., scenarios where two persons interact physically to achieve some goal. Haptic dyads are very common in human activities, like physical collaboration in handling bulky objects (Reed and Peshkin 2008; Van der Wel et al. 2011) or in performing arts, like dancing (Gentry and Murray-Smith 2003). Interestingly, it has been found that dyads produce much more overlapping forces than individuals, especially for tasks with higher coordination requirements, thus suggesting that dyads use larger forces in the joint action to generate a haptic information channel.

A limited number of studies have analyzed human-robot haptic dyads in cooperative tasks. For example, Corteville et al. (2007) investigated a human-inspired robot assistant for fast point-to-point movements: the robot scaled the offered level of assistance in order to give the operator the opportunity to gradually learn how to interact with the system. The results of the study showed a bidirectional, synergic influence: while the robot was programmed to adapt to the human motion, the operator also adapted to the offered assistance, inducing a highly natural type of interaction. In a shared virtual object manipulation task, performance-related energy exchange in haptic dyadic interaction has been analyzed, and the results indicate that the interacting partners benefit from role distribution which can be associated with different energy flows (Feth et al. 2009). On the other hand, in physical collaborative tasks, it has been found that it may be beneficial to switch continuously between two distinct extreme behaviors (leader and follower), thus creating an implicit bilateral coupling within the dyad (Evrard and Kheddar 2009). In a similar vein, it has been found (Oguz et al. 2010) that in order to facilitate the arousal of a natural sense of collaboration in a robot guidance mechanism, it is appropriate to supplement the haptic guidance with a role exchange mechanism, which allows the computer to adjust the forces it applies to the user in response to his/her actions. In general, a recent review on bilateral haptic interaction systems (Passenberg et al 2010) shows that the incorporation of environment, operator, or task-specific information in the controller structure can improve robustness and performance, but such benefits are application dependent to a large extent.

In the rest of this section, we propose first a taxonomy for haptic interaction which could potentially be used both for human-human and human-robot haptic dyads. Then, we discuss in more detail the implications that the differences between a musculo-skelettal system for humans and traditional actuators for robots bring have from a motor control point of view, and the consequences for physical interaction. A novel actuator, inspired by the structure of the musculo-skelettal system is described. Finally, we consider one application domain - robot-assisted physical therapy - where decoding the information in the physical interaction about the state and interaction of the partner is of utmost importance to identify the right level of assistance to the patient.

8.3.1 A Metrics to Measure Physical Interaction Complexity

To classify the various situations involving physical interaction and measure the complexity of the challenge from a control point of view, we propose a metric based on the well-known concept of compliance. More specifically, we propose to classify physical-interaction scenarios according to two essential components of contacts: external and internal compliance (see Fig. 8.2). The adjective internal as opposed to external here refers to the interactive agent, in other words “the self” as opposed to “the other.” For convenience, we will use the term self-compliance when referring to internal compliance and the term external compliance when referring to “the other” compliance. Self- and external compliance are the two sides of the interaction. It is therefore crucial to understand how these two concepts become intertwined once contacts are established. From here on, we will introduce the concept of contact compliance, which corresponds to the overall compliance obtained once the external and the self-compliance become coupled with the contact establishment. At a coarse representational level, establishing a contact can be seen as the serial connection of two compliances, one representing the external compliance, the other representing the self-compliance. We propose to classify physical interaction according to the degree of compliance involved on both sides of the interaction and to measure the complexity of the interaction with contact compliance. Remarkably, the compliance of a serial interconnection is simply the linear sum of the individual compliances.[1] Therefore, roughly speaking,

[1] If we consider the simple example of two springs serially interconnected, it is well known that the stiffness of the serial interconnection $k_{\text{series}}$is associated to the stiffness of the individual springs

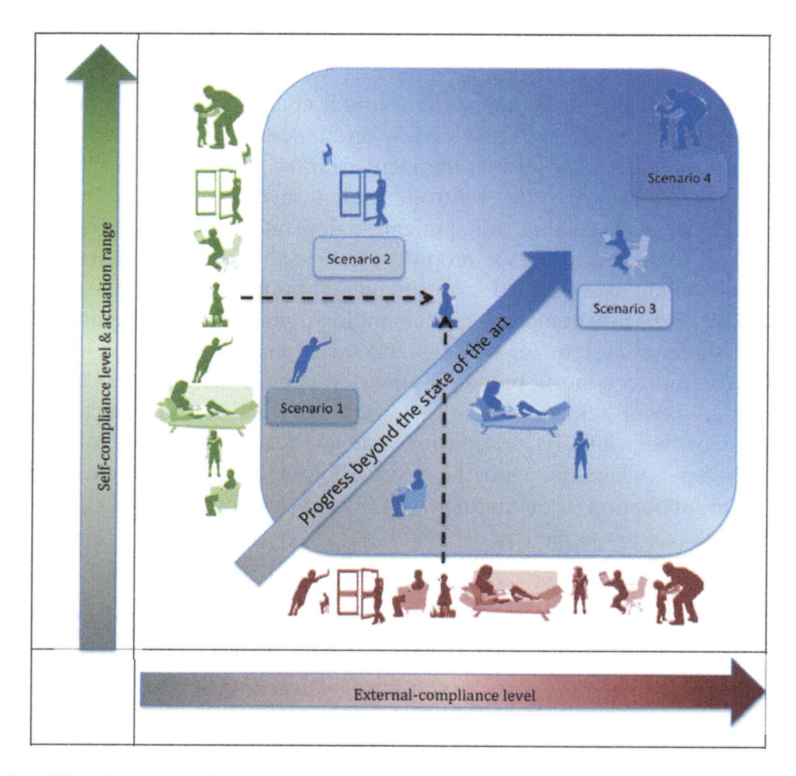

Fig. 8.2 Visualization of the metric space to be used in order to classify physical interaction complexity. Interaction is always the intertwined combination of two components, external and self-compliance, both contributing to the concept of contact compliance

the contact compliance does not significantly change when the external and self-compliance are changed simultaneously by an equal and opposite quantity. Each agent has control only on its own side of the interaction, what we call the "self" (internal) compliance. Therefore, each agent has only partial control the contact compliance. Yet it possible to adapt self-compliance to the environment compliance and the ability to actively regulate the internal compliance has been only recently implemented on multi-degrees-of-freedom robots.

The horizontal axis sorts possible scenarios according to a progressively increasing external compliance level. The bottom level of this subdivision (left-hand side in Fig. 8.2) clusters scenarios that involve noncompliant (rigid) external contacts. The intermediate level corresponds to scenarios with compliant external contacts. This second category is extremely wide in consideration of the multitude of possible compliant behaviors that can be experienced: from the linear force-displacement

k_1, k_2 by the following equation: $1/k_{\text{series}} = 1/k_1 + 1/k_2$. If instead of stiffness we consider compliance g, defined as the inverse of the stiffness $g = 1/k$, we have: $g_{\text{series}} = g_1 + g_2$.

characteristic of a linear spring to the complex nonlinear characteristic of a pillow. Scenarios within this category practically overlap with the first category, but rigid contacts are replaced by nonrigid contacts. In these two categories, the agent (or "the self", represented with a human silhouette) is always interacting with inanimate objects (the external contacts: a chair, a sofa, the floor, etc.). In the last category, "the self" and "the other" are both humans (left-hand side in Fig. 8.2).

The vertical axis instead orders the same scenarios by means of increasing self-compliance levels and actuation ranges[2]: tasks involving minimal self-compliance regulation or low levels of compliance are shown at the bottom[3]; tasks involving wide self-compliance regulation ranges including high compliance levels are at the top. The self-compliance regulation represents the proactive and cognitive component of the interaction and therefore gives the robot an enhanced degree of autonomy to be exploited in handling situations not anticipated at design time. In this sense, the self-compliance level and actuation range can be used to classify physical interaction scenarios. At the very first level of this classification, we will consider scenarios that do not require significant self-compliance regulation as they typically involve dynamically stable situations. Such situations involve, for example, dynamically stable tasks, which substantially require direct control of stable postures. The second level of the classification includes tasks that require a certain level of active compliance either to stabilize unstable systems (e.g., balancing) or to compensate for unpredictable interaction characteristics (e.g., standing hand in hand with another agent). Finally at the highest level of this classification, we consider highly complex tasks characterized by strong requirements in terms of "self"-compliance planning and regulation.

8.3.2 *Interaction and Novel Actuations Technologies*

Recently, robotic research has shown a growing interest in studying human motor control to understand how humans are capable of performing motor skills well beyond current robot motor capabilities. In particular, recent findings in human motor control have suggested that co-contraction, or the human ability to change the intrinsic musculoskeletal compliance, might play a crucial role when dealing

[2] In evaluating the self-compliant component, we explicitly refer not only to the self-compliance level but also to the regulation range. This is a necessary clarification, which is motivated by the fact that "the self" is always an agent (human or robot) capable of regulating its own compliance. Therefore ranges of regulation are much more fundamental than in the case of external compliance which, in most of the cases, is not assumed to be regulated unless we consider "the other" to be human.

[3] An extreme example, not shown in Fig. 8.2, is represented by a human (the other) moving a completely passive robot (the self). In this case, the robot compliance level is high but the compliance regulation is absent. Therefore, such a scenario would be at the very bottom of the vertical axis in Fig. 8.2.

with uncertainties and unpredictability. It is therefore reasonable to understand if and consequently why we need to replicate this capability in the robots of the next generation since the ability of changing the system mechanical impedance is nowadays not available in most of the robots.

The present section focuses on systems capable of varying their intrinsic compliance. As previously discussed, the human musculoskeletal system possesses this property via muscular co-contraction. Recently, a number of robotic actuators capable of actively regulating the overall system compliance have been proposed (see also Chaps. 5 and 6). Different motivations have been behind the design of these actuators: safety (Alami et al. 2006), energy storing (Au et al. 2009), and force regulation (Pratt and Williamson 1995) to cite a few. We propose here a rather different point of view suggested by recent results from human motor control which have proposed that variable compliance can be interpreted as a tunable, high-bandwidth reaction strategy. In this paper, we suggest that a relevant advantage of variable compliance becomes apparent when considering the intrinsic latencies typical of a distributed control system. Within this context, it is worth observing that both humans and robots share qualitatively similar (but quantitatively different) control issues. Generally speaking, signal transmissions are never instantaneous, neither in robots nor in humans. Latencies typically augment with distances, and therefore, as a rule of thumb, (a) local (distributed) controls are typically affected by relatively small latencies, and (b) global (centralized) controllers are necessarily affected by significant delays in signal propagation (Fig. 8.3).

The idea investigated by several authors is that co-contraction in humans can be interpreted as a distributed and local control strategy not affected by delays. Our goal will be to show that the ability of actively varying the system compliance can prevent the disadvantages of delayed feedback if coupled with a global and centralized feedforward motor plan which exploits muscle co-contraction to achieve (feedback free) disturbance rejection. Similar characteristics will be simulated in robots equipped with passive variable impedance actuators (VIA) where the ability of actively regulating the stiffness can be seen as an analogous of muscle co-contraction.

Previous works within the field of motor control have demonstrated that humans have at least two different control strategies to compensate for external disturbances: disturbance compensation via motor plan adaptation (Shadmehr and Mussa-Ivaldi 1994) and disturbance rejection via muscle co-contraction (Burdet et al. 2001).

When the disturbance is deterministic and predictable, it can be compensated by a proper adjustment of the feedforward motor plan. In particular, Mussa-Ivaldi and collaborators (Shadmehr and Mussa-Ivaldi 1994) have shown that humans are able to compensate for the disturbance due to a velocity dependent force field. Evidence suggests that disturbs are compensated by a motor plan adaptation (i.e., feedforward control adjustment) since a sudden removal of the pertubation produces an incorrect movement execution, the so-called aftereffect. If the disturbance compensation were the result of an increased musculoskeletal compliance (i.e., an increased muscle co-contraction), then the aftereffect should not be noticeable; its presence therefore has been classically interpreted as an evidence for the adaptation of the motor plan to the applied disturbance.

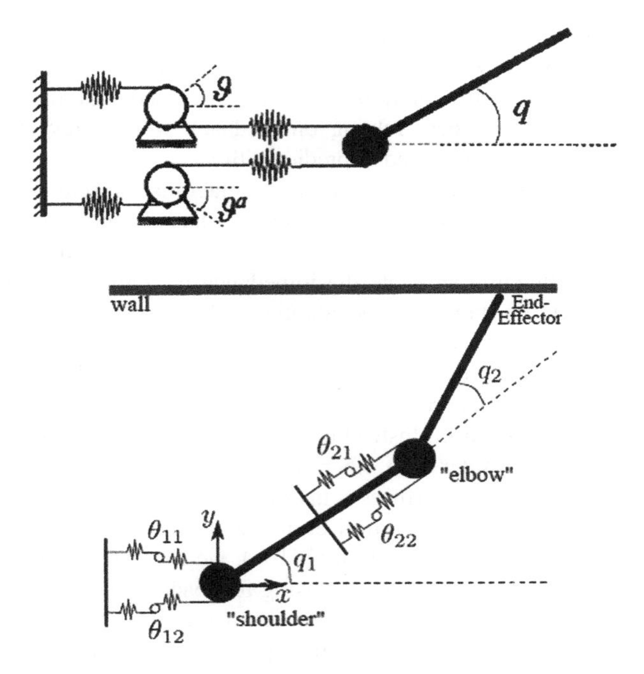

Fig. 8.3 The *top image* sketches the basic structure of the variable stiffness actuator (VSA) recently proposed in Berret et al. (2012) as a mean to obtain passive noise rejection (see text). The *bottom part* shows a two-degrees-of-freedom manipulator equipped with these actuators. Preliminary simulation results (Berret et al. 2013) show that the proposed solution outperforms conventional solutions in handling interaction tasks in presence of uncertainties

When the disturbance is stochastic and unpredictable, augmenting the musculoskeletal stiffness via muscle co-contraction can compensate it. Burdet and collaborators (2001) have shown that when executing a reaching movement in a divergent force field, the initial task failures gradually disappear as a consequence of an increased stiffness, which compensates for the instability caused by the force field. Differently from the disturbance proposed by Mussa-Ivaldi, it is likely to expect that a divergent force field is unpredictable as a consequence of the fact that little (i.e., nonmeasurable) positioning errors either produce a perturbing force in one direction or in the opposite direction. Changing the motor plan would be inefficient in this context, because it is practically impossible to decide a priori on which side of the divergent field the movement will fall. Even motor plan adaptation strategies relying on a (delayed) feedback will not be useful, because the divergent field intensity was tuned so that typical reaction delays in the central nervous system were not sufficiently fast to react on time before the arm was driven away from the target trajectory. The observed behavior, an increase of the muscle co-contraction to modify the intrinsic musculoskeletal compliance, was therefore reasonable to expect given the task specifications.

Remarkably, classical neurophysiological experiments have already shown that disturbance rejection does not necessarily pass through proprioceptive feedback. Polit and Bizzi (1979) have demonstrated that both intact and deafferented monkeys correctly perform goal-directed reaching movements even in the presence of unexpected displacement of the arm (prior to movement initialization). These results have been classically interpreted as an evidence for the so-called “equilibrium point hypothesis” suggesting that the central nervous system controls both the body equilibrium and the stiffness via proper agonist/antagonist muscles co-contraction. It is worth stressing here that even if deafferentation (i.e., total removal of feedback) is just an extreme situation, we just discussed that there might be tasks (Burdet et al. 2001) where relying on feedback would prevent the task achievement in presence of delays and unpredictability.

The importance of the agonist/antagonist muscle arrangement in dealing with the minimization of uncertainties has been recently studied in Mitrovic et al. (2010a). In particular, it was shown that the tool of stochastic optimal control can efficiently simulate the impedance regulation principles observed in humans performing stationary and adaptive tasks. Similar to the work presented in Mitrovic et al. (2010a), we will make extensive use of a state-of-the-art optimization tool (ILQG, Todorov and Li 2005) to solve the problem of planning movements in presence of uncertainties but extending results to two-degrees-of-freedom models of the human arm. Instead of focusing only on realistic models of human muscles, we will consider also other actuators whose dynamical model covers a number passive variable stiffness actuators recently designed for robotic applications (Wolf and Hirzinger 2008; Jafari et al. 2010). Moreover, differently from the approach proposed in Mitrovic et al. (2010b), we focus on purely feedforward control thus neglecting the possibility of using feedback to correct online the motor plan.

Driven by the considerations above, roboticists in the last decade have started studying mechanical solutions capable of controlling the system structural stiffness by proposing a number of solutions, which fall under the broad category of passive variable stiffness actuators (pVSA). All these systems use different principles (cam mechanisms, nonlinear springs, etc.) to change the rigidity between actuator and joint in order to mimic human ability to change the body compliance by regulating the muscle co-activation. Although the proposed designs possess interesting features, it has been recently pointed out that available solutions strongly rely on feedback control strategies and differ (as to this concern) from human muscles (Berret et al. 2011). Specifically, simulations conducted by Berret et al. (2011) indicate that muscle models outperform available pVSA solutions in dealing with unpredictable (i.e., stochastic) perturbations. These results motivated the design of a different type of pVSA (Berret et al. 2012; Nori et al. 2012, Fig. 8.4) possessing a novel property that we named passive noise rejection variable stiffness actuators (pnrVSA). The design was inspired by recent motor control experiments showing that humans adopt muscle co-activation as a strategy to deal with highly unstable force fields in the presence of significant proprioceptive delays. Preliminary results (Berret et al. 2013) show that the proposed solution outperforms conventional solutions in handling interaction tasks in presence of uncertainties.

8.3.3 *Stiffness vs. Feedback Strategy in Unstable Interactions*

Although modulation of the musculoskeletal stiffness via muscle co-contraction can compensate stochastic and unpredictable disturbances, as shown in the already

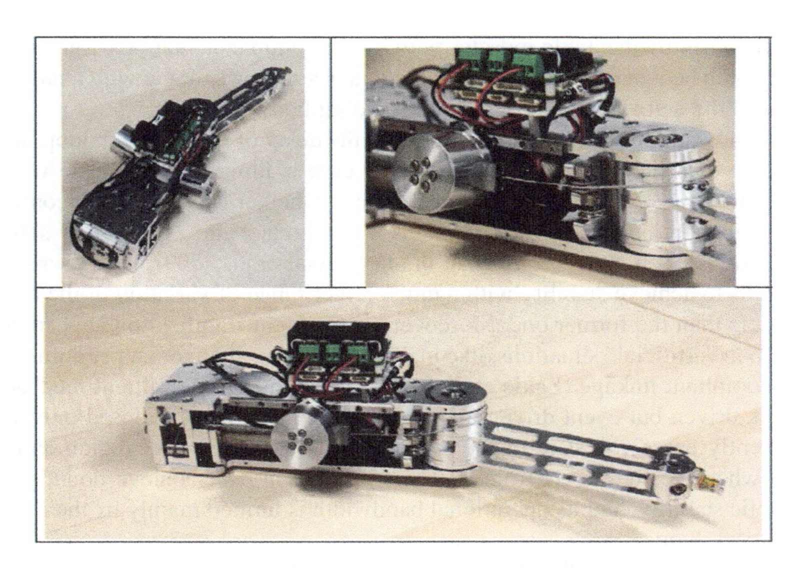

Fig. 8.4 Pictures of the pnrVSA (passive noise rejection variable stiffness actuator) prototype realized at the Istituto Italiano di Tecnologia. The device is capable of rejecting noise without explicitly relying on feedback

quoted experiments by Burdet et al. (2001) on reaching movements of the arm in a divergent force field, this is not a universal strategy. As a matter of fact, two requirements are necessary for making co-contraction an effective strategy for modulating joint impedance: (1) the length–tension curve of skeletal muscles must be nonlinear, typically quadratic in the physiological range in such a way to have a linear increase of stiffness with muscle stretch, and (2) the stiffness of tendons, which have an approximately linear length–tension curve, must be much greater than the range of stiffness achievable by the corresponding muscles. If both requirements are satisfied, the overall muscle–tendon stiffness is dominated by muscle properties, and co-contraction of antagonist muscles will increase the corresponding joint stiffness, because muscles and the attached tendons are mechanically linked in series. However, this is not always the case: in particular, it may happen that tendon stiffness is significantly smaller than muscle stiffness, as in the Achilles tendon (Loram et al. 2007), with the consequence that co-contraction of the ankle muscles has little effect on the overall ankle stiffness. As a matter of fact, co-contraction of ankle muscles is never observed in quiet standing humans but what really matters, from the behavioral point of view, is that ankle stiffness is significantly smaller than the rate of growth of the gravity-driven toppling torque (Casadio et al. 2005), which is analogous to the force generated by the divergent force field of the experiment by Burdet et al. (2001). In other words, the feedforward stiffness strategy is not functional for the stabilization of the standing posture, and thus, human subjects are forced to use a feedback strategy that supplements the insufficient stabilization torque provided for free and instantaneously by the ankle muscles with motor commands that take into account the mismatch between the goal state, namely, a desired sway angle with a null sway speed, and the actual state of the human standing body.

The weak point of the feedback strategy is the delay of the feedback loop, which is a source of instability by itself and in any case is limiting in a drastic way the bandwidth of the control. The point of debate is whether such feedback controller operates in continuous or discontinuous/intermittent time. The latter solution appears to be much more robust than the first (Asai et al. 2009), in the sense that it succeeds to achieve stability with a much larger range of variation of the control parameters than the former one. Moreover, intermittent stabilization appears to be used also in "artificial" situations, like manual balancing an inverted pendulum with a very compliant linkage (Lakie et al. 2003). This kind of intermittent feedback is not clock driven but event driven, namely, the feedback loop is closed only when the currently perceived state of the system enters a "dangerous" region and it is opened when the state exits from it. The strategy can only achieve bounded, not asymptotic stability, and its operational bandwidth is limited mainly by the delay in the feedback loop.

One may wonder why the feedforward stiffness strategy is not the natural choice in all situations, given its clear superiority in terms of dynamic performance in the compensation of unpredictable disturbances. For example, in the case of upright standing, why did phylogenetic development favor a soft compliant Achilles tendon instead of a strong rigid one, thus complicating the stabilization of the standing posture? A biomechanical explanation is suggested by the fact that when a powerful disturbance is resisted by a pair of elastic elements connected in series, the amount of energy absorbed by each of them is inversely proportional to their stiffness. This means that when jumping or running, at each impact with the ground, the Achilles tendon is absorbing much more energy than the dorsal flexors of the ankle and thus operates as a kind of mechanical fuse, protecting the delicate muscle tissue from overload.

In general, when dealing with unpredictable interactions, different elements must be played one against the other in order to make the "optimal" choice as regards the compensation of disturbances. If the primary requirement is movement precision, then operating with a high stiffness level is apparently the optimal choice. If the danger of overloading muscles is the main concern, then it is better to operate with a low stiffness level. If the task is extended in time, one must take into account the effect of fatigue and the fact that muscle noise grows with muscle contraction; thus, even in precision tasks, the level of stiffness must not be kept at its maximum all the time but must be modulated, thus alternating phases characterized by a high stiffness strategy with phases dominated by a low stiffness, feedback strategy. Modulation of stiffness and alternation of stiffness vs. feedback strategies is far from trivial and requires a complex process of motor learning and, more generally, motor cognition.

The human ability of switching strategy in a complex interactive environment was investigated by Saha and Morasso (2012) by using a bimanual underactuated compliant tool in an unstable environment. The tool, which is simulated by a pair of force-controlled manipulanda, consists of a mass (the "tool-tip") and two handheld nonlinear springs. The tool-tip operates in an unstable environment, characterized by a saddlelike force field, with mediolaterally oriented unstable manifold and anteroposterior oriented stable manifold. The nonlinearity of the two springs allows the users to affect size and orientation of the tool stiffness ellipse, by using different patterns of bimanual coordination of the two spring terminals: minimal stiffness occurs when the two spring terminals are aligned and the stiffness size grows by stretching apart the two terminals. The tool parameters are set such that minimal stiffness is insufficient to provide stable equilibrium of the tool-tip, but asymptotic stability can be achieved with sufficient stretching, although at the expense of a larger effort. As a consequence, tool users have two possible strategies for stabilizing the tool-tip in different regions of the workspace: (1) high stiffness strategy aiming at asymptotic stability and (2) low stiffness positional strategy aiming at bounded stability, similar to the manual stabilization of an inverted pendulum. The behavior of naïve users is spontaneously clustered into two groups of approximately equal size: a stiffness strategy group and a feedback strategy group (Saha and Morasso 2012). In a following study (Zenzeri et al. 2013) subjects were trained to become expert users of both strategies in a discrete reaching task. Then the generalization capabilities were tested by means of a continuous stabilization task which consists of tracking a target in the unstable workspace: the results show that human subjects can learn to master complex interaction tasks alternating different interaction strategies.

8.3.4 Human–Robot Interaction in Neuromotor Rehabilitation

Robot therapy is slowly emerging as an acceptable technique for the routine treatment of people affected by neuromotor diseases like stroke (Mehrholz et al. 2012; Krebs and Hogan 2012). However, there is still little agreement on the theoretical background that is necessary for overcoming the current empirical approach and for attempting to optimize and personalize the treatment provided by the robot. This is indeed the topic which is currently the focus of the research carried out in the MLRR-lab.

After the studies on animal models of stroke by Nudo (2006, 2007), it has become clear that beyond time-dependent spontaneous neurological recovery, the principal process responsible for functional recovery is the *use-dependent reorganization* of neural mechanisms made possible by *neural plasticity*. So neural plasticity is important, but is it the effect of intensive and repetitive robot therapy or the other way around? We are in favor of the latter option, because in our opinion such fundamental property of neural tissue is the prerequisite for assuming that robot therapy may have a chance of success, inducing a reorganization of the damaged brain of the patient via appropriate physical interaction patterns.

The second issue coming out from the animal studies quoted above, namely, the requirement of use-dependent reorganization, means that promotion of active movements should be preferred to passive mobilization for inducing relearning and functional recovery. This is not to say that passive mobilization should be always avoided: it is known indeed that it can help contrasting the deterioration of the thixotropic properties of the collagen matrix of the muscle tissue that is a secondary consequence of the functional immobilization of the paretic limbs of the stroke patient. Thus, although some degree of passive mobilization is acceptable in a treatment routine, considered as a technique of dynamic splinting, the core of treatment should be based on smooth and minimal patterns of assistance, capable to recruit neural plasticity by inducing active participation of the subjects.

The rationale of emphasizing the patient's active participation to the treatment process comes also from the discovery that during motor adaptation human subjects behave as greedy optimizers (Emken et al. 2007), in the sense that they tend to decrease the active participation as a function of the degree of assistance, what is described as slacking behavior (Wolbrecht et al. 2008). As a matter of fact, one of the main cybernetic effects of brain damage after stroke is to break the intrinsic coherence of purposive actions, namely, the causal relation or volitional loop between intended actions, actual movements, and the corresponding feedback reafference: the motor program that drives the muscles in agreement with a given task can successfully unfold its control patterns only if the sensory consequences of them (the sensory reafferences) match the expected motion patterns. In severely impaired subjects, who are unable to carry out simple reaching movements or have a strongly reduced ROM (range of motion), these movements must be supported by carefully regulated assistance. The purpose of such assistance is not to carry out the movements in place of the subject. On the contrary, robot assistance must help recreating the volitional loop mentioned above. This means that the assisting force generated by the robot must match the subject's intention to move and must be modulated in such a way to complement the voluntary neuromuscular commands in order to produce physiologically consistent reafferent signals. In other words, the relation between the stroke patient and the robot/human therapist can be viewed as a haptic dyad, characterized by bidirectional interaction.

According to Gibson (1966), the human haptic system is the sensibility of the individual to the world adjacent to his body by use *of his body*. This implies a close link between haptic perception and body movement, suggesting that haptic perception is not a *passive* sensory modality but, different from other modalities, is intrinsically active, integrating sensory and motor aspects at the same time. Force and touch are indeed constituent elements of haptic perception, and it is well known that both afferent and efferent signals contribute to force perception (Jones 1986).

The main difference between human–robot interaction systems used in therapy and cooperative handling is that we may assume that in the latter case the human part of the dyad has intact sensorimotor capabilities, thus simplifying the learning/adaptation process between the human and robot. In this case, for example, there is no danger of slacking because with insufficient participation by the human partner cooperative tasks could not be carried out successfully. In contrast, in the clinical

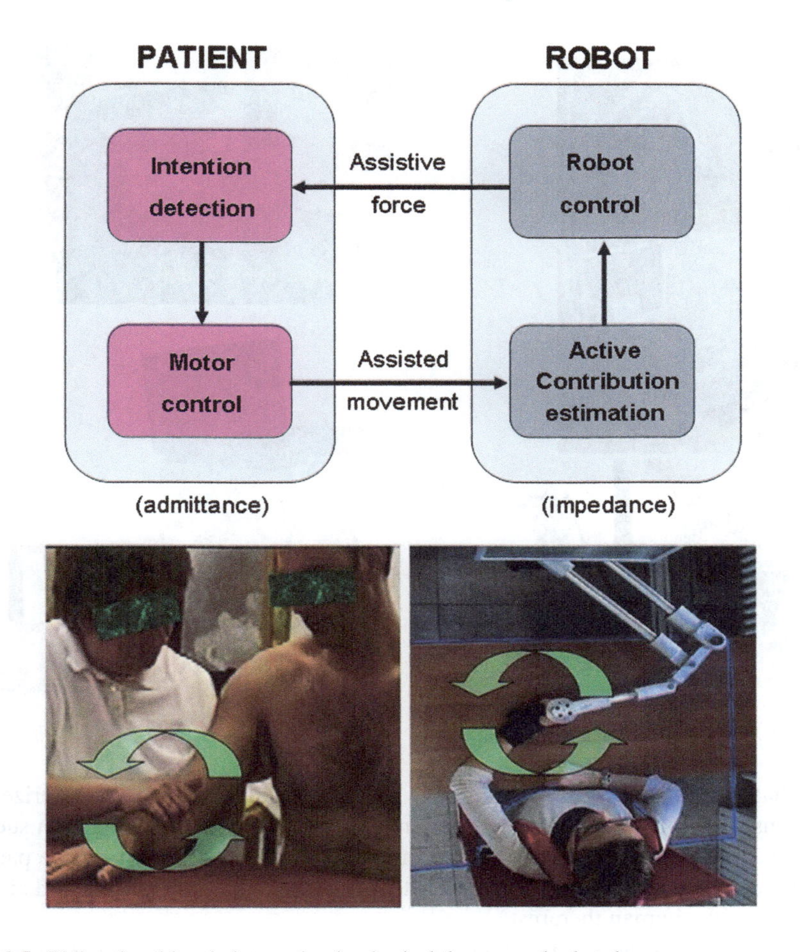

Fig. 8.5 Bidirectional haptic interaction in physical therapy and robot therapy

case, the human is the weak part of the dyad, unable to carry out the task being alone; in this situation the robot must do most of the job but in a clever way, i.e., by avoiding slacking and promoting the emergence of active participation. Moreover, as a further important side-effect, balanced bidirectional interaction provides a reinforcement of proprioceptive awareness which is the other side of neuromotor impairment in stroke patients.

Such general concepts are summarized in Fig. 8.5. In the dyadic interaction the robot plays the role of an impedance and the patient the role of an admittance. The robot provides assistive force patterns related to the assisted movement. The forces activate tactile and proprioceptive channels of the patient, who is required to estimate from them the intention of the robot therapist. The assisted movements measured by the robot are analyzed in order to estimate an index of active contribution and from this the assistive force generation module can be modulated for reinforcing active and precise control of the patient.

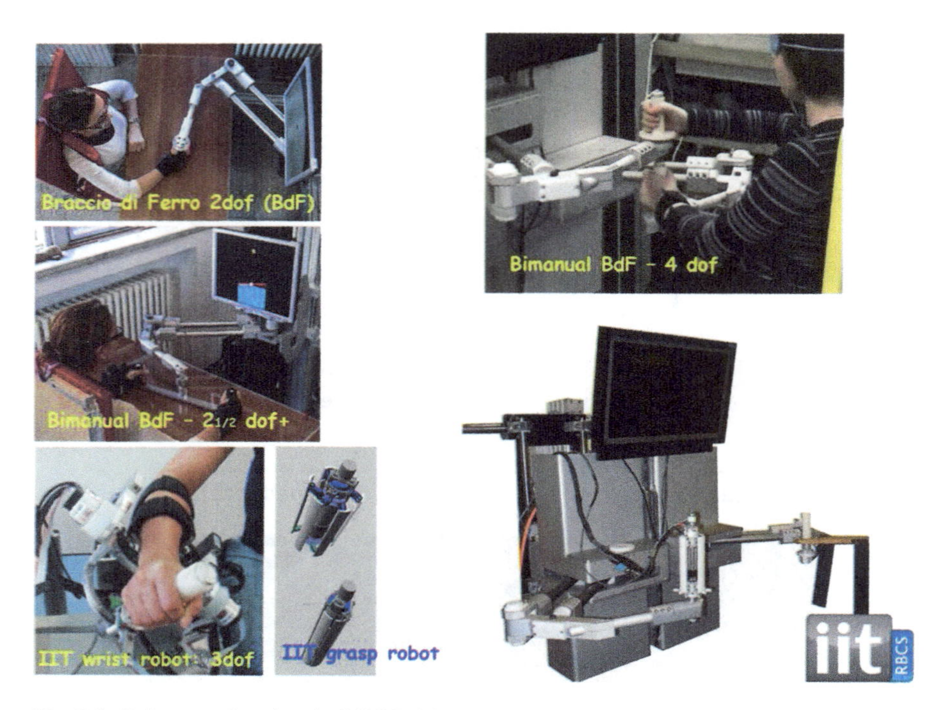

Fig. 8.6 Robots employed at the MLRR-lab

What is important is that bidirectional haptic interaction should characterize the relationship between the stroke patient and the human or robot therapist, in such a way to avoid passive mobilization and thus enhancing the degree of active participation of the patient. In a sense, the controller of the robot therapist should aim at mimicking the human therapist.

Figure 8.6 illustrates some of the haptic devices which have been developed and employed in a number of pilot clinical studies, involving adult patients (Casadio et al. 2007, 2009a, b; Masia et al. 2009, 2011; Vergaro et al. 2010; Piovesan et al. 2012; Squeri et al. 2014). In the near future, this approach will be extended to the pediatric area, adapting the developed methodologies to the special needs of children and designing new devices for robotized haptic assistance aimed at children.

8.4 Concluding Remarks

At some point in the future, technological progress will allow robots to understand speech, recognize actions, move in the house or at the work place, and act dexterously on the environment. However, to be able to serve as technical assistants or domestic helpers, to participate to the many human activities that require some form of cooperation, and, more generally, to fulfill their potential as partners (or servants), robots will have to cooperate closely with humans.

This chapter shows that cooperative actions is based not only on explicit planning but also on more subtle forms of coordination that involve the way we look, move, and interact physically. These forms of communications play an important role in cooperative actions as they allow partners to understand each other, guess what one is (or is not) perceiving and wants to do, receive and provide guidance, synchronize the action, etc.

The challenge that we face to endow robots with these capacities has many facets. As a matter of fact, the robot must not only be able to identify and understand these cues as they are exhibited by the human partner but also display them so that the human partner understands what the robot is actually doing. To achieve such a result, considerable work is still needed to understand this form of communication between humans.

In Sect. 8.2, we mentioned that humans are able to pick up very subtle cues and can perceive the slightest change in the kinematics of other people's movements. Moreover, it has been demonstrated that even the simple observation of an action evokes widespread activities at the cortical level that include primary sensory and motor areas. The research illustrated in this section constitutes a step forward figuring out the extent to which the appearance and behavior of the robot must match the human one.

Robots will also need to be able to exploit physical interaction to communicate with their human partners. To that end, the body of the robots will have to satisfy constraints that go beyond what can be perceived visually. Recent research has shown that mechanical properties like compliance and the ability to regulate it play a central role in human motor control together with the ability of humans to exploit the dynamics of their body and of the environment. However, the technology that might allow robots to interact safely with humans, a prerequisite to be able to exploit physical interaction to communicate, is still under development. Moreover, additional research is needed to understand how humans switch strategies when interacting with different partners not only to control their own movement but also to communicate with them. This need is particularly well illustrated by the current development of robots for the sensorimotor rehabilitation of people affected by neuromotor diseases like stroke, where the robot—like the therapist—must understand the level of assistance that is needed by the patient and adjust its behavior in consequence.

To conclude, the research on human–robot interaction presented in this chapter is closely inspired by our current understanding of the human sensory, motor, and cognitive systems. As a matter of fact, a deep understanding of humans' body and mind appears to be crucial to develop machines and robots, whether they have a humanoid appearance or not, that can interact closely and cooperate with humans. While this was not the main focus of this chapter, it is also important to note that our understanding of the sensory and, in particular, motor systems benefits greatly from the tools and theoretical concepts that are developed in engineering to address the challenges that one faces when trying to build such a machines. Moreover, a future of closely interacting robots and humans opens social and ethical questions beyond these addressed in this chapter (Lin et al. 2012). At the societal level, the impact of these synergies on the image of one self and humankind, the possibility of emotional bounds between robots and humans, questions like who is legally responsible for possible robot malfunctions, the degree of autonomy and the rights that might be granted to robots, the role that they might play in war, and whether they should have moral standards are not anymore only the realm of science fiction but start to be discussed in various public forums by researchers and philosophers. In this framework, we believe that biomimetism is a crucial feature in human–robot interaction to be explored and implemented at multiple levels, from the bodily "superficial" appearance to the "hidden" cognitive architecture that allows the accumulation of memory, knowledge, and, ultimately, mutual understanding.

References

Alami R, Albu-Schaeffer A, Bicchi A, Bischoff R, Chatila R, Luca AD, Santis AD, Giralt G, Guiochet J, Hirzinger G, Ingrand F, Lippiello V, Mattone R, Powell D, Sen S, Siciliano B, Tonietti G, Villani L (2006) Safe and dependable physical human-robot interaction in anthropic domains: state of the art and challenges. In: Bicchi A, Luca AD (eds) Proceedings of the IROS'06 workshop on pHRI—physical human-robot interaction in anthropic domains. IEEE

Asai Y, Tasaka Y, Nomura K, Nomura T, Casadio M et al (2009) A model of postural control in quiet standing: robust compensation of delay-induced instability using intermittent activation of feedback control. PLoS One 4:e6169Au

Au SK, Weber J, Herr H (2009) Powered ankle-foot prosthesis improves walking metabolic economy. Trans Robot 25:51–66

Bafoutso G, Mentzas G (2002) Review and functional classification of collaborative systems. Int J Inf Manage 22(4):281–305

Berret B, Ivaldi S, Nori F, Sandini G (2011) Stochastic optimal control with variable impedance manipulators in presence of uncertainties and delayed feedback. In: IEEE/RSJ international conference on intelligent robots and systems (IROS), pp 4354–4359

Berret B, Sandini G, Nori G (2012) Design principles for muscle-like variable impedance actuators with noise rejection property via co-contraction. In: IEEE-RAS international conference on humanoid robots (HUMANOIDS2012)

Berret B, Yung I, Nori F (2013) Open-loop stochastic optimal control of a passive noise-rejection variable stiffness actuator: application to unstable tasks. In: 2013 IEEE/RSJ international conference on intelligent robots and systems (IROS). Tokyo, Japan, 3–7 Nov 2013, pp 3029–3034

Billard A, Calinon S, Dillmann R (2013) Learning from human demonstration. Handbook of robotics. MIT Press, Cambridge, MA

Bisio A, Sciutti A, Nori F, Metta G, Fadiga L, Sandini G, Pozzo T (submitted) Motor contagion during human-human and human-robot interaction

Bisio A, Stucchi N, Jacono M, Fadiga L, Pozzo T (2010) Automatic versus voluntary motor imitation: effect of visual context and stimulus velocity. PLoS One 5(10):e13506

Boucher JD, Pattacini U, Lelong A, Bailly G, Elisei F, Fagel S, Dominey PF, Ventre-Dominey J (2012) I reach faster when I see you look: gaze effects in human–human and human–robot face-to-face cooperation. Front Neurorobot 6:1–11

Bressler SL, Menon V (2010) Large-scale brain networks in cognition: emerging methods and principles. Trends Cogn Sci 14(6):277–290

Buckner RL, Carroll DC (2007) Self-projection and the brain. Trends Cogn Sci 2:49–57
Buckner RL, Andrews-Hanna JR, Schacter DL (2008) The brain's default network: anatomy, function, and relevance to disease. Ann N Y Acad Sci 1124:1–38
Burdet E, Osu R, Franklin DW, Milner TE, Kawato M (2001) The central nervous system stabilizes unstable dynamics by learning optimal impedance. Nature 414(6862):446–449
Casadio M, Morasso P, Sanguineti V (2005) Direct measurement of ankle stiffness during quiet standing: implications for control modelling and clinical application. Gait Posture 21:410–424
Casadio M, Sanguineti V, Solaro C, Morasso P (2007) A haptic robot reveals the adaptation capability of individuals with multiple sclerosis. Int J Robot Res 26:1225–1234
Casadio M, Giannoni P, Morasso P, Sanguineti V (2009a) A proof of concept study for the integration of robot therapy with physiotherapy in the treatment of stroke patient. Clin Rehabil 23:217–228
Casadio M, Morasso P, Sanguineti V, Giannoni P (2009b) Minimally assistive robot training for proprioception enhancement. Exp Brain Res 194:219–231
Cattaneo L, Caruana F, Jezzini A, Rizzolatti G (2009) Representation of goal and movements without overt motor behavior in the human motor cortex: a transcranial magnetic stimulation study. J Neurosci 29(36):11134–11138
Chaminade T, Cheng G (2009) Social cognitive neuroscience and humanoid robotics. J Physiol 103(3–5):286–295
Chaminade T, Franklin D, Oztop E, Cheng G (2005) Motor interference between humans and humanoid robots: effect of biological and artificial motion. In: Proceedings of the 4th international conference on development and learning, pp 96–101
Chaminade T, Zecca M, Blakemore S-J, Takanishi A, Frith CD, Micera S, Dario P, Rizzolatti G, Gallese V, Umiltà MA (2010) Brain response to a humanoid robot in areas implicated in the perception of human emotional gestures. PLoS One 5(7):e11577
Chao C, Cakmak M, Thomaz AL (2010) Transparent active learning for robots. In: Proceedings of the international conference on human-robot interaction (HRI), pp 317–324
Churchill EF, Snowdon D (1998) Collaborative virtual environments: An introductory review of issues and systems. Virtual Real 3(1):3–15
Corteville B, Aertbelien E, Bruyninckx H, De Schutter J (2007) Human-inspired robot assistant for fast point-to-point movements. In: Proceedings of the IEEE conference on robotics and automation (ICRA'07), pp 33639–33644
Cross ES, Liepelt R, Hamilton AF, Parkinson J, Ramsey R, Stadler W, Prinz W (2012) Robotic movement preferentially engages the action observation network. Hum Brain Mapp 33 (9):2238–2254
Dragan AD, Lee KC, Srinivasa SS (2013) Legibility and predictability of robot motion. In: Proceedings of the 8th ACM/IEEE international conference on human-robot interaction, pp 301–308
Emken JL, Benitez R, Sideris S, Bobrow JE, Reinkensmeyer DJ (2007) Motor adaptation as a greedy optimization of error and effort. J Neurophysiol 97(6):3997–4006
Evrard P, Kheddar A (2009) Homotopy switching model for dyad haptic interaction in physical collaborative tasks. In: Proceedings of the world haptics conference, 2009, pp 45–50
Falck-Ytter T, Gredebäck G, von Hofsten C (2006) Infants predict other people's action goals. Nat Neurosci 9(7):878–879
Feldman AG (1966) Functional tuning of the nervous system with control of movement or maintenance of a steady posture. Biophysics 11:565–578
Feth D, Groten R, Peer A, Hirche S, Buss M (2009) Performance related energy exchange in haptic human-human interaction in a shared virtual object manipulation task. In: Proceedings of the world haptics conference, 2009, pp 338–343
Flanagan JR, Johansson RS (2003) Action plans used in action observation. Nature 424 (6950):769–771
Fogassi L, Ferrari PF, Gesierich B, Rozzi S, Chersi F, Rizzolatti G (2005) Parietal lobe: from action organization to intention understanding. Science 308(5722):662–667

Gallese V, Fadiga L, Fogassi L, Rizzolatti G (1996) Action recognition in the premotor cortex. Brain 119(Pt 2):593–609

Gazzola V, Rizzolatti G, Wicker B, Keysers C (2007) The anthropomorphic brain: the mirror neuron system responds to human and robotic actions. Neuroimage 35(4):1674–1684

Gentry S, Murray-Smith R (2003) Haptic dancing: human performance at haptic decoding with a vocabulary. In: Proceedings of the IEEE systems, man, cybernetics conference, vol 4, pp 3432–3437

Gibson JJ (1966) The senses considered as perceptual systems. Houghton Mifflin, Boston, MA

Hogan N (1984) Adaptive control of mechanical impedance by coactivation of antagonist muscles. IEEE Trans Auto Control 29:681–690

Huang CM, Mutlu B (2012) Robot behavior toolkit: generating effective social behaviors for robots. In: Proceedings of the seventh annual ACM/IEEE international conference on human-robot interaction, pp 25–32

Jafari A, Tsagarakis NJ, Vanderborght B, Caldwell D (2010) A novel actuator with adjustable stiffness (AwAS). In: IEEE/RSJ international conference on intelligent robots and systems (IROS 2010), Taipei, pp 4201–4206

Jeannerod M (2006) Motor cognition: what actions tell to the self. Oxford University Press, Oxford

Jones L (1986) Perception of force and weight: theory and research. Psychol Bull 100:29–42

Kanakogi Y, Itakura S (2011) Developmental correspondence between action prediction and motor ability in early infancy. Nat Commun 2:341

Kilner JM, Paulignan Y, Blakemore SJ (2003) An interference effect of observed biological movement on action. Curr Biol 13(6):522–525

Knoblich G, Butterfill S, Sebanz N (2011) Psychological research on joint action: theory and data. In: Ross B (ed) The psychology of learning and motivation, vol 54. Academic, Burlington, VT, pp 59–101

Kozuki T, Mizoguchi H, Asano Y, Osada M, Shirai T, Urata J, Nakanishi Y, Okada K, Inaba M (2012) Design methodology for thorax and shoulder of human mimetic musculoskeletal humanoid kenshiro—a thorax with rib like surface. In: Proceedings of the 2012 IEEE/RSJ international conference on intelligent robots and systems, pp 4367–4372

Krebs HI, Hogan N (2012) Robotic therapy: the tipping point. Am J Phys Med Rehabil 91(11 suppl 3):S290–S297

Lakie M, Caplan N, Loram ID (2003) Human balancing of an inverted pendulum with a compliant linkage: neural control by anticipatory intermittent bias. J Physiol 551:357–370

Liepelt R, Prinz W, Brass M (2010) When do we simulate non-human agents? Dissociating communicative and noncommunicative actions. Cognition 115(3):426–434

Lin P, Abney K, Bekey GE (2012) Preface. In: Lin P, Abney K, Bekey GA (eds) Robot ethics the ethical and social implications of robotics. MIT Press, Cambridge, MA

Lohan K, Rohlfing KJ, Pitsch K, Saunders J, Lehmann H, Nehaniv CL, Fischer K, Wrede B (2012) Katrin Lohan tutor spotter: proposing a feature set and evaluating it in a robotic system. Int J Soc Robot 4:131–146

Loram ID, Maganaris CN, Lakie M (2007) The passive, human calf muscles in relation to standing: the non-linear decrease from short range to long range stiffness. J Physiol 584:661–675

MacDorman K, Ishiguro H (2006) The uncanny advantage of using androids in cognitive and social science research. Interact Stud 7(3):297–337

Masia L, Casadio M, Giannoni P, Sandini G, Morasso P (2009) Performance adaptive training control strategy for recovering wrist movements in stroke patients: a preliminary, feasibility study. J Neuroeng Rehabil 6(44):1–11

Masia L, Frascarelli F, Morasso P, Di Rosa G, Castelli E, Cappa P (2011) Reduced short term adaptation to robot generated dynamic environment in children affected by congenital hemiparesis. J Neuroeng Rehabil 8:28

Mehrholz J, Hädrich A, Platz T, Kugler J, Pohl M (2012) Electromechanical and robot-assisted arm training for improving generic activities of daily living, arm function, and arm muscle

strength after stroke. Cochrane Database Syst Rev 6, CD006876. doi:10.1002/14651858.CD006876.pub3
Mitrovic D, Klanke S, Osu R, Kawato M, Vijayakumar S (2010a) A computational model of limb impedance control based on principles of internal model uncertainty. PLoS One 5(10):e13601
Mitrovic D, Nagashima S, Klanke S, Matsubara T, Vijayakumar S (2010b) Optimal feedback control for anthropomorphic manipulators. In: ICRA 2010, pp 4143–4150
Mori M (1970) Bukimi no tani—the uncanny valley (MacDorman KF, Minato T, Trans.). Energy 7 (4):33–35
Nardi BA, Whittaker S (2002) The place of face-to-face communication in distributed work. In: Hinds PJ, Kiesler S (eds) Distributed work. MIT Press, Cambridge, MA, pp 83–113
Nori F, Berret B, Fiorio L, Parmiggiani A, Sandini G (2012) Control of a single degree of freedom noise-rejecting variable impedance. In: Proceedings of the 10th international IFAC symposium on robot control (SYROCO), pp 473–478
Nudo RJ (2006) Mechanisms for recovery of motor function following cortical damage. Curr Opin Neurobiol 16:638–644
Nudo RJ (2007) Postinfarct cortical plasticity and behavioral recovery. Stroke 38:840–845
Oguz SO, Kucukyilmaz A, Sezgin TM, Basdogan C (2010) Haptic negotiation and role exchange for collaboration in virtual environments. In: Proceedings of the IEEE haptics symposium, 2010, pp 371–378
Oullier O, de Guzman GC, Jantzencb KJ, Lagarded J, Kelso JAS (2008) Social coordination dynamics: measuring human bonding. Soc Neurosci 3(2):178–192
Passenberg C, Peer A, Buss M (2010) A survey of environment-, operator-, and task-adapted controllers for teleoperation systems. J Mechatron 20:787–801
Perani D, Fazio F, Borghese NA, Tettamanti M, Ferrari S, Decety J, Gilardi MC (2001) Different brain correlates for watching real and virtual hand actions. Neuroimage 14(3):749–758
Piovesan D, Morasso P, Giannoni P, Casadio M (2012) Arm stiffness during assisted movement after stroke. IEEE Trans Neural Syst Rehabil 21(3):454–465
Polit A, Bizzi E (1979) Characteristics of motor programs underlying arm movements in monkeys. J Neurophysiol 42(1):183–194
Pratt G, Williamson M (1995) Series elastic actuators. In: 1995 IEEE/RSJ international conference on intelligent robots and systems. Human robot interaction and cooperative robots, vol 1. IEEE Computer Society Press, Los Alamitos, CA, pp 399–406
Press C, Bird G, Flach R, Heyes C (2005) Robotic movement elicits automatic imitation. Cogn Brain Res 25(3):632–640
Press C, Gillmeister H, Heyes C (2007) Sensorimotor experience enhances automatic imitation of robotic action. Proc Biol Sci 274(1625):2509–2514
Raichle ME, MacLeod AM, Snyder AZ, Powers WJ, Gusnard DA, Shulman GL (2001) A default mode of brain function. Proc Natl Acad Sci USA 98:676–682
Reed KB (2012) Cooperative physical human-human and human-robot interaction. In: Peer A, Giachritsis CD (eds) Immersive multimodal interactive presence, Springer series on touch and haptic systems. Springer, London, pp 105–127
Reed KB, Peshkin MA (2008) Physical collaboration of human-human and human-robot teams. IEEE Trans Haptics 1:1–13
Reichelt AF, Ash AM, Baugh LA, Johansson RS, Flanagan JR (2013) Adaptation of lift forces in object manipulation through action observation. Exp Brain Res 228(2):221–234
Rizzolatti G, Sinigaglia C (2010) The functional role of the parieto-frontal mirror circuit: interpretations and misinterpretations. Nat Rev Neurosci 11(4):264–274
Runeson S, Frykholm G (1981) Visual perception of lifted weight. J Exp Psychol Hum Percept Perform 7:733–740
Saha D, Morasso P (2012) Stabilization strategies for unstable dynamics. PLoS One 7(1):e30301
Salem M, Kopp S, Wachsmuth I, Rohlfing KJ, Joublin F (2012) Generation and evaluation of communicative robot gesture. Int J Social Robot 4(2):201–217
Schacter DL (2012) Constructive memory: past and future. Dialogues Clin Neurosci 14:7–18

Schmidt RC, Carello C, Turvey MT (1990) Phase transitions and critical fluctuations in the visual coordination of rhythmic movements between people. J Exp Psychol Hum Percept Perform 16:227–247

Sciutti A, Patanè L, Nori F, Sandini G Understanding object weight from human and humanoid lifting actions. In: IEEE transactions on autonomous mental development (in press)

Sciutti A, Bisio A, Nori F, Metta G, Fadiga L, Pozzo T, Sandini G (2012) Measuring human-robot interaction through motor resonance. Int J Soc Robot 4(3):223–234

Sciutti A, Del Prete A, Natale L, Burr D C, Sandini G, Gori M (2013a) Perception during interaction is not based on statistical context. In: Proceedings of the 8th ACM/IEEE international conference on human-robot interaction, pp 225–226

Sciutti A, Patanè L, Nori F, Sandini G (2013b) Do humans need learning to read humanoid lifting actions? In: Proceedings of the third joint IEEE international conference of development and learning and on epigenetic robotics

Sciutti A, Bisio A, Nori F, Metta G, Fadiga L, Sandini G (in press) Robots can be perceived as goal-oriented agents. Interact Stud

Sebanz N, Bekkering H, Knoblich G (2006) Joint action: bodies and minds moving together. Trends Cogn Sci 10(2):70–76

Senot P, D'Ausilio A, Franca M, Caselli L, Craighero L, Fadiga L (2011) Effect of weight-related labels on corticospinal excitability during observation of grasping: a TMS study. Exp Brain Res 211(1):161–167

Shadmehr R, Mussa-Ivaldi FA (1994) Adaptive representation of dynamics during learning of a motor task. J Neurosci 14(5 Pt 2):3208–3224

Sisbot EA, Alami R (2012) A human-aware manipulation planner. IEEE Trans Robot 28(5):1045–1057

Southgate V, Johnson MH, Osborne T, Csibra G (2009) Predictive motor activation during action observation in human infants. Biol Lett 5(6):769–772

Squeri V et al (2014) Wrist rehabilitation in chronic stroke patients by means of adaptive, progressive robot aided therapy. IEEE Trans Neural Syst Rehab Eng 22(2):1–14

Suddendorf T, Addis DR, Corballis MC (2009) Mental time travel and the shaping of the human mind. Philos Trans R Soc Lond B Biol Sci 364:1317–1324

Tai YF, Scherfler C, Brooks DJ, Sawamoto N, Castiello U (2004) The human premotor cortex is 'mirror' only for biological actions. Curr Biol 14(2):117–120

Todorov E, Li W (2005) A generalized iterative lqg method for locally-optimal feedback control of constrained nonlinear stochastic systems. In: Proceedings of American control conference, June, vol 1, pp 300–306

Van der Wel RP, Knoblich G, Sebanz N (2011) Let the force be with us: dyads exploit haptic coupling for coordination. J Exp Psychol Hum Percept Perform 37:1420–1431

Vergaro E, Casadio M, Squeri V, Giannoni P, Morasso P, Sanguineti V (2010) Self-adaptive robot-training of stroke patients for continuous tracking movements. J Neuroeng Rehabil 7:13

Warneken F, Chen F, Tomasello M (2006) Cooperative activities in young children and chimpanzees. Child Dev 77:640–663

Wolbrecht ET, Chan V, Reinkensmeyer DJ, Bobrow JE (2008) Optimizing compliant, model-based robotic assistance to promote neurorehabilitation. IEEE Trans Neural Syst Rehabil Eng 16(3):286–297

Wolf S, Hirzinger G (2008) A new variable stiffness design: matching requirements of the next robot generation. In: ICRA 2008, pp 1741–1746

Zenzeri J, De Santis D, Morasso P (2013) Strategy switching in the stabilization of unstable dynamics. PLoS One (submitted)

Chapter 9
Complexity and Computation at the Synapse: Multilayer Architecture and Role of Diffusion in Shaping Synaptic Activity and Computation

Andrea Barberis and Fabio Benfenati

The nervous system confers living organisms the ability to perceive and appropriately respond to external signals. At any given moment, a multitude of different stimuli are received, processed, and integrated by the brain. The correct handling of this huge amount of information requires the coordination of extraordinary number of diverse events at both cellular and network levels. The basis of this extremely complex regulation lays on synapses, the specific contact sites between neurons. At the presynaptic level, electrical stimuli are translated into chemical signals, i.e., the release of neurotransmitters, which are recognized and translated into an appropriate biological response (either electric or metabolic, or both) at the postsynaptic level. The combined action of synapses acting in distinct brain areas is ultimately responsible for the generation and shaping of higher brain functions such as learning and memory. The molecular mechanisms modulating synaptic function have been the subject of intense investigation since the earliest days of modern neuroscience. Initially, synapses were thought to be "static" structures where presynaptic stimuli are linearly converted into neurotransmitter release and action potentials. This idea has now been replaced by a more modern view, whereby synapses represent extremely dynamic sites whose activity can be modified by a vast array of signals coming from the presynaptic, postsynaptic, and extracellular compartments as well as by the previous history of the neuron. This new view of synaptic functioning has been obtained by the application of novel advanced techniques that allow interrogating the synapses in live neurons under various environmental conditions. Among these are patch-clamp electrophysiology, dynamic electron microscopy, and innovative imaging and optogenetic techniques coupled with high-resolution and super-resolution live imaging approaches.

A. Barberis (✉) • F. Benfenati
Central Research Laboratory, Istituto Italiano di Tecnologia, Genova, Italy
e-mail: andrea.barberis@iit.it

R. Cingolani (ed.), *Bioinspired Approaches for Human-Centric Technologies*,
DOI 10.1007/978-3-319-04924-3_9, © Springer International Publishing Switzerland 2014

9.1 Diffusion as a Computational Operator

Diffusion is a fundamental process in nature and a key mechanism in biology. At the body level, diffusion governs the exchange of gases and nutrients in our tissues, but if we zoom into the cell or at the subcellular level, we can observe that diffusion is fully involved in regulating cell physiology by driving the motion of organelles and molecules within the cytoplasm as well as that of macromolecules in the membrane bilayer. When the organelles or the molecules experiencing diffusion have an informational role, then diffusion becomes a key process shaping information content and transfer. At the synapse, this is the case for (1) synaptic vesicles (SVs), small organelles storing and releasing neurotransmitter in a quantal fashion by regulated exocytosis; (2) neurotransmitter molecules released into the synaptic cleft that, based on the dynamics of release, will bind to postsynaptic receptors, but also diffuse out in the extracellular space, carrying their message through the tissue volume; and (3) neurotransmitter receptors that undergo both trafficking between a membrane-exposed pool and an intracellular "inactive" pool, as well as diffusion in the plane of the membrane between synaptic and extrasynaptic domains (Fig. 9.1). From the ensemble of these parallel processes that are layered across the serial sequence of synaptic events, a new multilayer architecture of synaptic transmission and plasticity emerges with higher complexity and computational abilities.

9.2 Synaptic Vesicle Pools and Superpool: Synaptic Vesicle Diffusion, Trafficking, and Sharing

Presynaptic terminals contain many SVs, small organelles (40–50 nm diameter) of surprisingly homogeneous size that store and release a discrete amount of small neurotransmitter molecules (e.g., acetylcholine, glutamate, GABA; about 5,000–10,000 molecules/vesicle). SVs are clustered within the terminal and contact the presynaptic membrane at the active zone, a specialized area where exocytosis preferentially occurs. Such SV clusters, together with SV recycling mechanisms, allow nerve terminals to faithfully convert action potentials into neurotransmitter secretion over a large firing range.

On a morphological basis, ultrastructure of central synapses shows that a limited number of SVs are physically docked to the active zone, while the majority of SVs is distributed in clusters that fill the terminal at various distances from the active zone. However, on a functional basis, SVs can be divided into "functional pools" that do not have a close morphological correspondence. On the basis of patch-clamp electrophysiology and fluorescent reporters of SV cycling (see below), there is a large consensus on the existence of three SV pools that are characterized by distinct functions and, possibly, molecular features of SVs. Synaptic vesicles docked to the active zone and characterized by an already assembled fusion complex (composed of SNARE proteins, complexins, and Ca^{2+} sensor) are primed

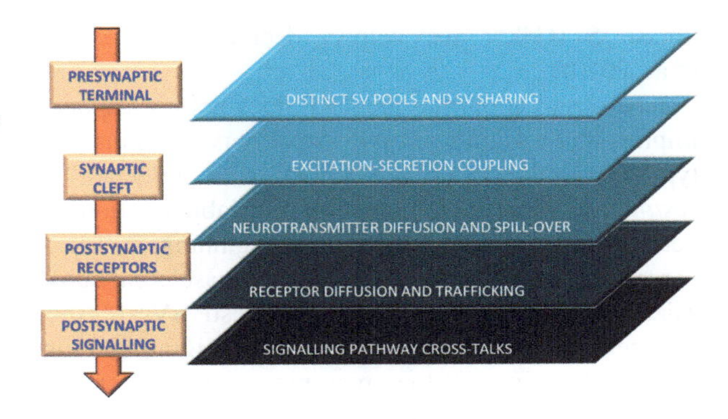

Fig. 9.1 Schematic representation of the multilayer architecture of synaptic transmission and of the parallel processes occurring at the various levels through diffusion. For further details, see text

for fusion and constitute the *readily releasable pool* (RRP) (Jahn and Fasshauer 2012). Based on their release probability, these SVs can be immediately released in response to the action potential and in general are completely discharged after 1–2 s at 20–40 Hz or by a hypertonic stimulus (sucrose; Fatt and Katz 1952) that destabilizes the bilayer in a Ca^{2+}-independent fashion. Depleted RRP is refilled by a second pool of SVs, the *recycling pool* (RP) that represents a large reserve of SV that are not immediately releasable. This pool is maintained by endocytosis of released SVs and is responsible for the continued release occurring after complete RRP depletion. RRP and RP represent all SVs capable of undergoing release and constitute the so-called total recycling pool (TRP) (Alabi and Tsien 2012) that serves evoked neurotransmitter release. In hippocampal synapses, 5–9 SVs form the RRP, while the TRP can represent at most 60–70 % of the total SV population and the RP is about 3–5-fold the RRP size (Murthy and Stevens 1999). The transition of SVs from the RP to the RRP is a rate-limiting reaction during sustained activity, and its kinetics impacts synaptic transmission. The time constant of RRP replenishment under basal conditions is in the order of seconds, and its speed and extent can be significantly modulated by activity (von Gersdorff and Matthews 1997).

The interplay of SVs between functional pools represents a mechanism of paramount importance to adapt the response of the nerve terminal to the action potential on the basis of the previous history of the neuron and the parallel activity of signal transduction pathways. Transitions of SVs in and out of the various pools are fueled by second messengers and phosphorylation/dephosphorylation of specific SV substrates that favor association/dissociation of the SVs with the cytoskeleton and the active zone scaffold components, as well as their mobility within the terminal. Phosphorylation of synapsin I by Ca^{2+}/calmodulin-dependent kinases I and II, as well as by protein kinase A and neurotrophin-dependent extracellular-regulated kinase (MAPK/Erk), increases the availability of SVs for refilling the RRP and therefore contributes to the expression of short-term plasticity phenomena by enhancing post-tetanic potentiation and limiting depression through a positive effect on the quantal content (Cesca et al. 2010; Valente et al. 2012), while phosphorylation of synapsin I by the tyrosine kinase Src or by cyclin-dependent kinase 5 (Cdk5; see below) decreases SV availability for release (Messa et al. 2010).

The observation that the TRP does not correspond to the total number of SVs implies that a significant portion of nerve terminal SVs are not releasable by any type of stimulation and are defined to be "reluctant" for fusion. This pool, named *resting pool* (RestP), accounts for a variable fraction of the total SV content ranging between 30 % and 85 %. In the beginning, it was surprising that such a large percentage of SVs was "useless for release", but subsequent studies have hypothesized several possible functions for RestP SVs: (1) they can dynamically exchange between terminals as members of a migrating "superpool" of SVs shared by adjacent boutons; (2) they may represent a buffer for trapping/supplying proteins during SV recycling; (3) they can sustain spontaneous release, while evoked release is administered by the TRP; and (4) although not immediately usable on a stimulus-to-stimulus basis, they may represent a "savings" of SVs that can undergo homeostatic transitions to the RP on the basis of the sustained activity status of the neuron, thus regulating the release capability of the terminal in the long term.

It has been clarified that the transition between releasable and reluctant SVs reflects the equilibrium between the kinase Cdk5 and the phosphatase calcineurin dephosphorylating Cdk5 substrates, with Cdk5 favoring the recruitment of SVs from the TRP to the RestP and calcineurin catalyzing the release of SVs from the RestP to increase the TRP size. Cdk5 is present at nerve terminal and phosphorylates a large array of substrates involved in the exo-endocytotic cycle of SVs (such as the dephosphins dynamin-1, amphiphysin-1, intersectin, and phosphatidylinositol kinase-Iγ, as well as the other presynaptic substrates CASK, Munc-18, Pictaire-1, Sept5, N-type Ca^{2+} channels, and synapsin I; Barnett and Bibb 2011). However, the Cdk5 substrates mediating the transition of SVs have not been identified yet, although a strong indication exists for a key role of N-type Ca^{2+} channels and synapsin I. Cdk5/calcineurin represents a very efficient push–pull mechanism for the long-term regulation of the size of the TRP, which adapt the exocytosis power of nerve terminal to the environmental conditions. It has been shown that prolonged neuronal silencing with the Na^+ channel blocker tetrodotoxin markedly decreases Cdk5 activity and expression at nerve terminals, thus decreasing the RestP size and increasing SV availability for release (Kim and Ryan 2010, 2013). On the contrary, sustained hyperactivity with the GABA receptor blocker bicuculline increases Cdk5 activity, thus sequestering SVs into the RestP and decreasing the pool of releasable SVs (Verstagen et al. under review).

The description of the intraterminal functional pools of SVs is likely to be an oversimplification, as SVs do not spend all their life in a single bouton, but are capable to navigate and reach adjacent terminals as far as tens of μm away (Westphal et al. 2008; Staras et al. 2010). Indeed, dynamic imaging has revealed that this *superpool* of SVs, deriving from both the RP and the RestP, collectively accounts for about 4 % of total SV trafficking (Staras and Branco 2010). Since this inter-terminal trafficking occurs at a relatively high rate, it implies that SVs are significantly turned over at individual synapses. Many of these SVs have been found to be functional and to contribute to exocytosis of their new presynaptic host.

Axons of primary hippocampal neurons typically form en passant synaptic terminals at relatively short pitches (2–10 μm), indicating that (1) SV migration by stochastic or regulated lateral diffusion could represent an important informational cross talk among adjacent terminals and (2) SV traffic may not be limited to immediately adjacent synapses, but rather SVs can be shared across multiple nerve terminals. The existence of functional SV sharing among different synapses provides novel perspectives for synaptic physiology: migrating SVs could supply a reservoir for synaptic release to depressed synapses or contribute to the regulation of synaptic strength through remodeling of SV pools at host synapses. Moreover, since heterogeneity among SV populations exists, the SV sharing mechanism could involve SV populations that are specific for distinct release modalities, thus propagating SV heterogeneity among distinct synapses. It is tempting to speculate that lateral diffusion of SVs carries activity signals and modifies host synapses based on the previous history of their neighbors. At present, the regulatory mechanisms that might control the release/capture of SVs at individual terminals are unknown. One such candidate could be BDNF that was reported to induce a TrkB-linked SV declustering (Bamji et al. 2006; Staras et al. 2010). In the opposite direction, synapsin I and synapsin II, in addition to their involvement in the structural organization of synapses, represent an inhibitory clamp to SV diffusion by reversibly tethering SVs to the synaptic region in a phosphorylation-dependent fashion. Accordingly, genetically altered mice in which either or both synapsin genes have been deleted exhibit a decreased density of SVs at individual boutons and an increased size of the superpool of SVs migrating along the axonal shafts (Fig. 9.2; Fornasiero et al. 2012; Orenbuch et al. 2012).

Advanced imaging techniques allow to investigate in detail not only the quantal parameters of release, but also the dynamic trafficking of SVs within the terminal. The latter techniques include: (1) super-resolution optical imaging techniques, such as STED confocal microscopy that allow to resolve, under optimal conditions and with suitable fluorophores, the size of single SVs or of very small SV clusters (Galiani et al. 2012); (2) dynamic electron microscopy in which nerve terminals are "frozen" under specific stimulation paradigms and in the presence of extracellular tracers (e.g., horseradish peroxidase) that are taken up by SVs during exo-endocytotic cycling (Fig. 9.3; Lignani et al. 2013); and (3) genetically encoded reporters of SV cycling represented by superecliptic pH-sensitive GFP (pHluorin) targeted to the intravesicular space of SVs by fusion with the intravesicular domains of either VAMP2, synaptophysin, or VGLUT1. The pHluorin fluorescence ($pK_a = 7.1$) is quenched at the acidic pH of the SV interior and strongly increases when exposed to the neutral extracellular medium during exocytosis (Miesenböck et al. 1998; Sankaranarayanan et al. 2000; Burrone et al. 2006). The latter tool allows an extremely detailed kinetic analysis of exocytosis from the RRP, depletion of the RP, endocytosis, and respective size of the three pools of SVs. Acute addition of the proton pump inhibitor bafilomycin blocks reacidification of SVs after endocytosis and thus allows the study of the net exocytotic traffic, while intracellular basification with ammonia/ammonium chloride unquenches both recycling and

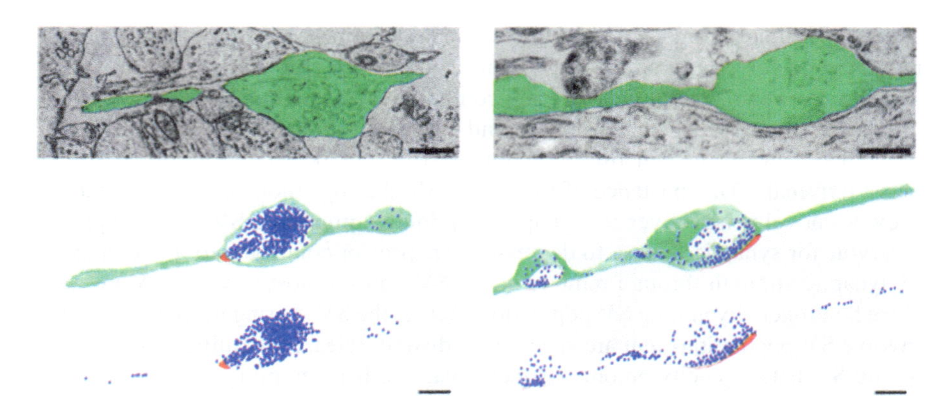

Fig. 9.2 Analysis of SV dispersion along the preterminal axon by electron microscopy. Three-dimensional reconstruction of synapses from serial sections of primary hippocampal neurons and morphometric analysis of synaptic and extrasynaptic SVs. *Upper panel:* Representative images of the serial sections used for the reconstruction (with the analyzed neuron in *green*). *Lower panels:* Three-dimensional reconstruction of SV distribution in the synapse and the surrounding axon (*green*, plasma membrane; *blue*, SVs; *red*, active zone). To appreciate SV dispersion and sharing among adjacent terminals, only SVs and AZs are shown in the *bottom images* (from Fornasiero et al. 2012)

non-recycling pHluorin-labeled SVs, thus allowing to determine the total SVs complement of the nerve terminal.

9.3 Neurotransmitter Release Dynamics

Synaptic transmission is initiated when an action potential reaching the nerve terminal triggers exocytosis of one or more SVs. The action potential induces the opening of Ca^{2+} channels, resulting in a transient Ca^{2+} influx triggering exocytosis. After exocytosis, SVs are endocytosed and locally recycled to undergo further rounds of exocytosis. The action potential-driven neurotransmitter release has been extensively studied and represents the basis of our current understanding of signaling and information processing in the nervous system. However, central synapses can operate neurotransmission in several modalities: (1) spontaneous neurotransmitter release in which single SVs are released in the absence of an action potential, (2) synchronous/fast neurotransmitter release that is tightly coupled to the action potential, and (3) asynchronous neurotransmitter release that is slower, delayed with respect to the stimulus, and long lasting (tens to hundreds milliseconds after repolarization) (Pang and Südhof 2010; Walter et al. 2011; Kavalali et al. 2011).

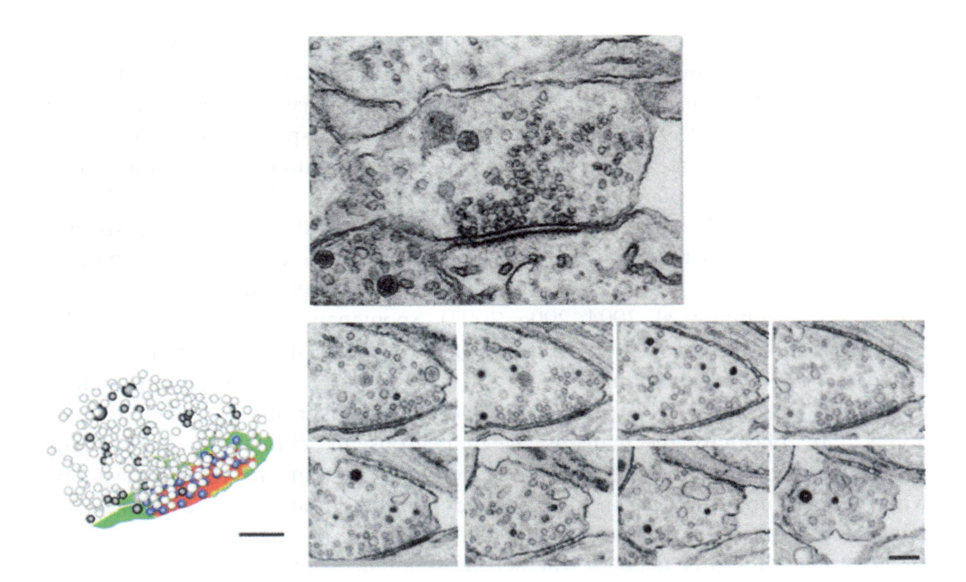

Fig. 9.3 Electron microscopy analysis of the SV uptake of an extracellular tracer (horseradish peroxidase) in serial sections after stimulation at 1 Hz for 30 s. Representative 60-nm-thick serial sections and their respective three-dimensional reconstructions. Recycled SVs are easily recognizable in the images due to their electron-dense lumen. In the three-dimensional reconstructions, total SVs, HRP-positive SVs, and physically docked SVs are depicted as *transparent*, *black*, and *blue spheres*, respectively. Scale bar, 200 nm (from Lignani et al. 2013)

9.3.1 Spontaneous Release

Spontaneous transmission is defined as neurotransmission occurring at very low rate independently of action potentials. Spontaneous transmission has been fundamental to the discovery of the quantal nature of neurotransmitter release. Studying the postsynaptic response to the spontaneous exocytosis of a single SV, the so-called miniature postsynaptic current (mPSC), has allowed to formulate the quantal theory of synaptic transmission and to dissect changes occurring in its distinct determinants, namely *quantal size* (the response to the release of a single quantum), *quantal content* (number of active release sites), and *probability of release* (the probability for a single SV to undergo fusion after the action potential). Besides its historical value, spontaneous transmission has recently attracted significant attention. Traditionally, both evoked and spontaneous forms of release are believed to occur at the active zone and to activate the same set of postsynaptic receptors. Moreover, unitary release events share similar features with their evoked counterparts recorded under low-probability conditions (e.g., low extracellular Ca^{2+}). This indicates that also spontaneous release events are largely Ca^{2+} dependent, although very low cytoplasmic Ca^{2+} concentrations are sufficient to trigger them.

Recent experimental evidence indicates that spontaneous transmission serves important roles in neuronal communication. Spontaneous GABA release provides continuous background inhibition and sets the inhibitory tone of postsynaptic neurons (Otis et al. 1991; Lu and Trussell 2000), and spontaneous release has been hypothesized to regulate receptor clustering and neuronal excitability particularly at high levels of input resistance (Saitoe et al. 2001; Carter and Regehr 2002; Sharma and Vijayaraghavan 2003). Convincing evidence exists that spontaneous release affects the local dendritic signal transduction systems and protein translation machinery (Sutton et al. 2007), thereby modulating postsynaptic responsivity (Sutton et al. 2004, 2006, 2007). Spontaneous release represents the only cross talk between the presynaptic and the postsynaptic neuron in silent synapses, with a central trophic role for the postsynaptic neuron, triggering signaling, maturation, and stability of neural networks. Moreover, it is the main target of homeostatic plasticity mechanisms: when neurons are chronically deprived of activity or subjected to prolonged hyperactivity, spontaneous release responds with compensatory changes in the frequency and amplitude of the events, trying to rescue the initial set point of synaptic activity.

Several studies have debated whether the spontaneous release activity depends on a specific pool of SVs endowed with distinct molecular markers present in all synapses (e.g., Vti1a or VAMP7 positive) or reflects a specialization of certain populations of synapses that exhibit a very low probability for evoked release (Ramirez and Kavalali 2011). Interestingly, spontaneous neurotransmission seems to use specific postsynaptic pathways for information transfer. Indeed, a subset of ionotropic NMDA-type glutamate receptors appears to be selectively activated by this particular modality of release. Treatment with MK-801, a high-affinity use-dependent open channel blocker of NMDA receptors, strongly reduces miniature NMDA-mediated currents, leaving NMDA receptor activation in response to subsequent evoked release unaffected. Multichannel parallel signaling is a common feature of ICT networks. These parallel communication channels cooperate with the main, time-locked information transfer channel (i.e., the synchronous release) and ensure error correction, maintenance, and connectivity. Thus, it is likely that spontaneous transmission, far from simply being the expression of the stochastic overcoming of the fusion energy barrier for exocytosis (basal *fusion willingness* of SVs) or *synaptic noise*, plays a key function in maintaining a tight synaptic homeostasis and connectivity within a large dynamic range for reliable information transfer and storage.

9.3.2 Synchronous and Asynchronous Release

Fast neurotransmitter release is tightly time-locked (less than 0.5–1 ms delay) to the action potential (Sabatini and Regehr 1996). Such a process is fundamental for the timing and high fidelity of neuronal communication. However, neurotransmitter quanta are also released with some delay in response to Ca^{2+} entry in a sustained,

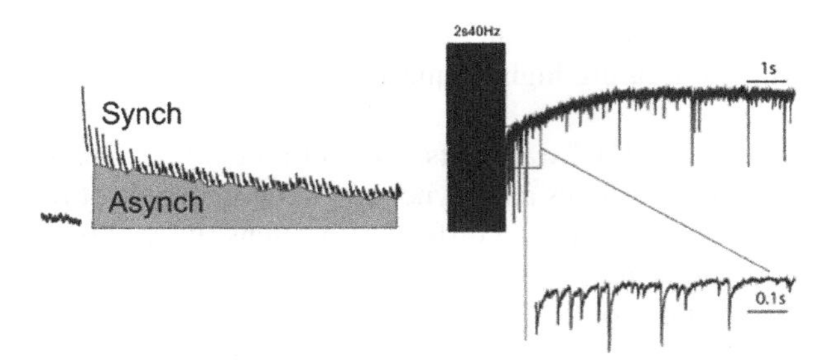

Fig. 9.4 *Left panel:* Model of charge analysis to differentiate asynchronous and synchronous charge transferred during a high-frequency train (from Lignani et al. 2013). *Right panel:* Representative traces of the inhibitory delayed asynchronous response in dentate gyrus granule cells after high-frequency stimulation (2 s at 40 Hz) of the medial perforant path. *Inset* represents the recording during the first second after the end of the stimulation (from Medrihan et al. 2013)

loosely coupled fashion. Although asynchronous release is mostly evident during high-frequency activity and for a while after the cessation of the train stimulation, it also occurs after a single action potential (Fig. 9.4; Iremonger and Bains 2007; Medrihan et al. 2013). Asynchronous neurotransmitter release has been proposed to be important for information discrimination, and its increase in synaptotagmin-1 knockdown mice was found to be associated with alterations in the frequency of hippocampal theta oscillations (Buzsáki 2012). Moreover, when the asynchronous/synchronous balance was deranged in the prefrontal cortex, fear memory retrieval was significantly impaired (Xu et al. 2012). These data indicate that the two modes of release participate in the dynamics of network activities and that asynchronous release may serve as a low-pass filter in some brain areas, while in others it may regulate distinct patterns of information coding (Buzsáki 2012).

9.3.3 Ca^{2+} Dependence of the Release Dynamics and Role of Heterogeneities in the Machinery of Release

Phasic transmitter release in response to single action potentials in the nerve terminal is triggered and driven by intense Ca^{2+} transients that occur at nanometric distances from the cytoplasmic "mouth" of the voltage-gated Ca^{2+} channels concentrated at the active zone, as long as they stay open before membrane repolarization. Ca^{2+} concentrations decay very steeply away from the Ca^{2+} channels, and the local Ca^{2+} signal breaks down quickly after the closure of the channels. Thus, both the steep spatial gradient and the fast temporal decay of the Ca^{2+} concentration are responsible for the high temporal and spatial precision of synchronous release. In addition to spatial redistribution of Ca^{2+} and equilibration with fast cytoplasmic buffers, a much lower and spatially averaged concentration Ca^{2+} is left at the active zone (about 0.5 μM; residual Ca^{2+}) and decays with a slower kinetics (10–100 ms) by binding to slow buffers such as parvalbumin and secondary active extrusion from the cell. Due to its long half-life, residual Ca^{2+} can easily build up by temporal and spatial summation during high-frequency repetitive activity to reach levels in the low μM range.

Due to the kinetics of Ca^{2+} transients, two not mutually exclusive mechanisms can account for the synchronous and asynchronous components of release, namely: (1) an "allosteric model" based on a different Ca^{2+} sensitivity of the two processes, but with a homogeneous machinery and (2) the "two-Ca^{2+} sensor model," based on selective genetic deletions of Ca^{2+} sensors, holding that different sensors present in distinct SV pools or coexisting in the same SVs mediate the two forms of release: a low-affinity sensor with fast on/off rates that sustains fast synchronous release and a high-affinity sensor with slow off rate that is involved in sustaining asynchronous release (Kochubey et al. 2011; Walter et al. 2011). According to this view, a *countinuum* of Ca^{2+} concentration levels would direct the spectrum of the release modes. While synchronous release requires high concentrations (10–50 μM) at the channel nanodomains with very fast dynamics and strong cooperativity, spatially averaged/slow decaying residual Ca^{2+} buildup following high-frequency activity and/or release from intracellular stores triggers asynchronous release, characterized by linear dependence on the Ca^{2+} concentration. Even lower basal Ca^{2+} concentrations facilitate spontaneous release. Notably, the same mechanisms triggering asynchronous release also promote the expression of short-term plasticity.

Synchronous release has been so far intensely connected with members of the synaptotagmin (Syt) family of SV Ca^{2+} sensors. Out of 16 isoforms of synaptotagmin that were identified, only Syt 1–9 bind Ca^{2+} through specific Ca^{2+}/ phospholipid binding domains (C2 domains; Pang and Südhof 2010). Among the latter group, Syt-1, Syt-2, and Syt-9 are considered fast sensors mediating synchronous release. Deletions of Syt-1, Syt-2, or of the SNARE complex-associated protein complexin lead to a complete loss of synchronous release at both excitatory and inhibitory synapses, while asynchronous release is preserved and even enhanced at high stimulation frequencies. The knockdown of Syt-7 at the zebrafish neuromuscular junction reduces asynchronous release; however, it has no effect on synchronous/asynchronous release in central synapses.

The mechanisms behind asynchronous release are still far from being understood, but recent work has proposed several hypotheses. One potential mechanism involves a distinct slow presynaptic Ca^{2+} sensor, Doc2, that binds Ca^{2+} with slower kinetics, and its knockdown in hippocampal cultures results in reduced asynchronous release (Yao et al. 2011). Another recent report proposes that the SNARE protein VAMP2 drives synchronous release, while its isoform VAMP4 boosts asynchronous release. Moreover, it was also recently shown that both voltage-gated presynaptic Cav-2.1 and Cav-2.2 channels that conduct P/Q-type and N-type Ca^{2+} currents, respectively, are characterized by a prolonged Ca^{2+} current that promotes asynchronous release (Few et al. 2012). In this respect, we have recently shown that the SV phosphoprotein synapsin II constitutively enhances asynchronous GABA release by specifically interacting with the P/Q-type channel, while its isoform synapsin I has the opposite effect and boosts synchronous GABA release (Medrihan et al. 2013). Although most studies agree that the synchronous and asynchronous components of release compete for the same pool of SVs, the presence of presynaptic protein isoforms favoring one type or the other of release indicates that heterogeneity exists between distinct subpopulations of SVs within the same nerve terminals or among synapses exhibiting a distinct complements of Ca^{2+} channel subtypes and/or SV protein isoforms.

Asynchronous release in inhibitory synapses may play an important role in the volume control of excitability. Changes in GABA asynchronous release between specific neurons from human epileptic and non-epileptic tissue have been recently reported. Interestingly, long-lasting inhibitory PSCs generated by asynchronous GABA release, occurring with significant delays after trains of action potentials or in some cases just one action potential, can increase the effectiveness of inhibition. GABA spillover and GABA concentrations in the interstitial fluid mainly result from asynchronous release, whose charge as a function of time can provide a more continuous supply of neurotransmitter to the extracellular space. In this respect, synapsin knockout mice strongly defective in asynchronous release also lack tonic inhibition (Farisello et al. 2013). Interestingly, in central synapses, asynchronous GABA release apparently allows an inhibitory compensatory tuning proportional to the extent of presynaptic activity and is markedly increased when synapses are stimulated with behaviorally relevant high-frequency patterns.

The availability of genetically encoded fluorescent Ca^{2+} indicators that specifically target synaptic boutons allows relating the dynamics of Ca^{2+} transients with the dynamics of release. The sensor GCaMP2, for example, has been efficiently fused to the cytoplasmic end of the SV proteins synaptotagmin or synaptophysin, thus reporting nerve terminal Ca^{2+} transients with high spatial and temporal precision and a linear response over a wide range of action potential frequencies (Dreosti et al. 2009). Moreover, we are currently engineering an array of microbial opsins (such as the excitatory opsins ChETA and CATCH derivatives of channelrhodopsin or the inhibitory opsin halorhodopsin; Mattis et al. 2011; Prakash et al. 2012) to target their expression to presynaptic terminals by fusion with the SNARE protein SNAP-25. A similar targeting strategy has also been applied to the photoswitchable kainate receptor LiGluK2 (see below) that can be commanded to open and close (binding and unbinding of the cross-linked azido-glutamate) by illumination with distinct wavelengths (Szobota et al. 2007; Gorostiza and Isacoff 2008). While in the case of the fast cationic channel ChETA or the Cl^- pump halorhodopsin, the respective inward and outward currents can affect the temporal profile of depolarization and the activation kinetics of voltage-gated Ca^{2+} channels, CATCH and LiGliK2 are directly permeable to Ca^{2+} and therefore can directly affect the intraterminal Ca^{2+} concentrations. The use of these targeted tools, together with genetically encoded targeted Ca^{2+} indicators, will soon allow switching from one mode of release to another one by light to further dissect the mechanisms and functional roles of spontaneous, synchronous, and asynchronous release.

9.4 Neurotransmitter Diffusion

While the mechanisms of transmitter release and the functioning of synaptic receptors have been extensively investigated, the dynamics of neurotransmitter diffusion in the synaptic cleft has received less attention. Indeed, it was assumed that, after the synaptic release, the neurotransmitter in the cleft would reach a supersaturating concentration, thus representing an all-or-none mechanism. In contrast, an increasing body of evidence has revealed that the fine modulation of the spatiotemporal profile of neurotransmitter concentration significantly impacts on the amplitude and duration of the unitary postsynaptic signals, being an important determinant for synaptic transmission. In addition, it has also been shown that neurotransmitter released at a given synapse can diffuse and activate neighboring synapses representing an efficient mechanism for synaptic cross talk. In this section, we will review the role of neurotransmitter diffusion in modulating and coordinating the synaptic function.

9.4.1 Estimating the Dynamics of Neurotransmitter Diffusion in the Synaptic Cleft

To date, the direct measurement of the neurotransmitter concentration profile in the synaptic cleft remains a major challenge. Typically, at central synapses, the width of synaptic cleft is ~20 nm, thus precluding the placement of a measuring device within the synapse to monitor the agonist time course. Due to this limitation, the current knowledge of the neurotransmitter dynamics is mainly derived from indirect measurements that infer the synaptic neurotransmitter waveform by analyzing the susceptibility of the postsynaptic response to pharmacological agents (Barberis et al. 2011). This approach is based on the concept that the degree of postsynaptic receptor block by competitive blockers closely depends on the concentration profile of neurotransmitter in the cleft: indeed, strong synaptic neurotransmitter exposures will overcome the current block by displacing the competitive blockers (generating mild current block), while weak synaptic exposures will determine a more pronounced current block. Thus, by estimating the degree of synaptic current reduction induced by competitive blockers, it is possible to infer the neurotransmitter waveform in the synaptic cleft that elicits synaptic current. This approach, referred as "deconvolution," consistently revealed that, after the vesicle release, the neurotransmitter concentration peaks in the cleft at 1–3 mM and decays exponentially with main time constant of ~0.1 ms (Clements et al. 1992; Clements 1996; Diamond and Jahr 1997; Mozrzymas et al. 1999; Overstreet et al. 2003; Barberis et al. 2004, 2005; Beato 2008).

Another strategy to study the spatiotemporal profile of neurotransmitter synaptic concentration exploits computer model simulations that simulate the neurotransmitter diffusion by using Fick's equation solved for boundary conditions reflecting the spatial structure of the synapse and the diffusion constrains in its surroundings. The estimations of neurotransmitter concentration and clearance provided by this in silico approach confirmed the substantial match of those obtained with "deconvolution" experiments (Holmes 1995; Clements 1996; Kleinle et al. 1996; Wahl et al. 1996; Glavinovíc 1999; Franks et al. 2002; Ventriglia and Maio 2003; Petrini et al. 2011). In addition, these studies highlighted a critical dependence of these values on several factors including the following (1) number of released molecules, (2) synaptic geometry, (3) number of binding sites (neurotransmitter receptors and transporters), (4) neurotransmitter reuptake, and (5) neurotransmitter diffusion coefficient.

The neurotransmitter concentration time course also depends on the modality of presynaptic release. The aforementioned model simulations assume the "full-collapse fusion," the main release mode described at central synapses that involve the complete fusion of the vesicle membrane into the presynaptic plasma membrane. However, it has been proposed that synaptic vesicles may fuse transiently and incompletely with the plasma membrane by forming a reversible "fusion pore" connecting the vesicle lumen with the synaptic cleft, a releasing mechanism referred to as "kiss-and-run" or "continuous-release" (Heuser and Reese 1973; Ceccarelli and Hurlbut 1980; Harata et al. 2006). The impact of this latter mechanism of release has been addressed by Kleinle et al. (1996) by adding to the Fick's equation a "release function" that describes the neurotransmitter escape from the vesicle through a fusion pore formed by the synaptic vesicle and the presynaptic membrane. The authors found that in conditions of simulated "continuous release," the neurotransmitter concentration only peaked at 0.37 mM and decayed in ~2 ms, more than one order of magnitude slower than in the conventional "full collapse" mode. Overall, the experimental and modeling studies indicate that, following typical synaptic release, the neurotransmitter peaks at very high concentration (mM range) and, due to diffusion, lasts in the synaptic cleft for only few hundreds of microseconds, similar to an "explosion" at the nanometric scale. It has to be born in mind, however, that the profile of concentration in the synaptic cleft can be highly diverse in specific synaptic subtypes, neuronal developmental stages, and physiological conditions (Barberis et al 2005; Karayannis et al. 2010).

9.4.2 *Functional Implications of Fast Neurotransmitter Diffusion*

Synaptic neurotransmitter exposure in the range of ~100 ms represents a time considerably briefer than that needed for the full activation of most fast ligand-gated postsynaptic receptors (AMPA, $GABA_A$, and glycine receptors ~300–400 ms). As a consequence, unitary synaptic currents evoked by the release of a single vesicle quantum are elicited under conditions of substantial *nonequilibrium*. The most important conceptual consequence of "nonequilibrium activation" concerns the definition of "effective neurotransmitter concentration." According to classical "equilibrium" pharmacology, the relative current amplitude is univocally determined by the agonist concentration: conversely, in nonequilibrium conditions, the degree of receptor activation depends on both the *concentration* and the *duration* of the agonist exposure. For instance, 1–3 mM GABA is supersaturating in equilibrium conditions, but is no longer saturating if applied for only 100 μs. Another consequence of "nonequilibrium conditions" is that the amplitude of synaptic current is extremely susceptible to the duration of the neurotransmitter exposure. The experimental evidence of this latter point has been obtained by using polymers such as dextran that, by increasing the viscosity of the extracellular medium, slows down neurotransmitter diffusion thereby prolonging the presence of neurotransmitter in the synaptic cleft. In these conditions of reduced neurotransmitter clearance, indeed, the peak amplitude of synaptic current both at glutamatergic and GABAergic synapses significantly increased, confirming the general idea that the brief synaptic exposure represents a limiting factor for the activation of postsynaptic receptors (Min et al. 1998; Perrais and Ropert 2000; Barberis et al. 2004).

Nonequilibrium conditions have also been demonstrated to influence the kinetics of synaptic current decay. $GABA_A$ receptors ($GABA_ARs$) require the binding of two agonist molecules to fully activate. However, it has been proposed that $GABA_ARs$ can open in the monoliganded state mediating currents decaying almost one order of magnitude faster than that elicited in the double bound state (Macdonald et al. 1989; Jones et al. 1995; Petrini et al. 2011). By using model simulations, we examined the impact of these two $GABA_AR$ activation modes at the synapse and found that "synaptic-like" GABA exposures favored the $GABA_AR$ activation in the singly bound state, especially at the periphery of the postsynaptic disk where the GABA concentration is almost one order of magnitude lower than that observed in front of the releasing site (Petrini et al. 2011). In these conditions, the duration of the neurotransmitter exposure can efficiently tune the decay kinetics of synaptic current by modulating the ratio of singly bound vs. doubly bound activation of $GABA_AR$.

Another "receptor gating feature" that can be unmasked in nonequilibrium conditions concerns the specific role of $GABA_AR$ desensitization. It is well established that the decay time of GABAergic currents is heavily shaped by desensitization (Jones et al. 1995; Jones and Westbrook 1998). Indeed, after the agonist removal, the current deactivation is prolonged by the time needed to exit from desensitized state(s). Thus, the length of agonist exposure modulates the degree of receptor desensitization accumulation, hence controlling the duration of synaptic currents (Jones et al. 1995; Petrini et al. 2011). The kinetics of currents mediated by glutamatergic kainate receptors has also shown clear dependence upon the transmitter exposure time. Indeed, although currents mediated GluK2/GluK5 heteromeric receptors show fast decay kinetics when elicited by "long" (100 ms) pulses of saturating glutamate, they display a singnificantly slower deactivation time course upon "brief" (~1 ms) glutamate exposures (Barberis et al. 2008). The molecular mechanism of this relation between glutamate exposure and current decay kinetics has been explained by the fact that GluK2/K5 receptors possess two different types of binding sites showing distinct affinity and desensitization properties. In particular, glutamate binding to the high-affinity sites induces poor desensitization, while activation of low-affinity binding sites determines fast and profound GluK2/K5 desensitization (Mott et al. 2010). During fast synaptic activation, therefore, the high-affinity/poorly desensitizing binding site is preferentially activated, mediating hence slow decaying responses.

Another interesting dependence of GABAergic current kinetics upon the time course of presynaptic GABA is provided by the slow inhibitory postsynaptic currents (slow IPSCs) first observed in the CA1 regions of the hippocampus (Pearce 1993; Banks et al. 1998). These particular forms of GABAergic synaptic current, characterized by slow onset and decay kinetics, have been shown to be mediated by the neurogliaform cells (NGFCs), specific interneuron subtype located in the *stratum lacunosum moleculare*. Ultrastructural and electrophysiological investigations clarified that the presynaptic boutons of NGFCs are distant from the postsynaptic element, thus determining GABA "volume release" (Szabadics et al. 2007; Oláh et al. 2009). Karayannis et al. (2010), using a quantitative approach, demonstrated that slow IPSCs are, by a slow and low-concentration GABA transient (1–60 μM, 20–200 ms), compatible with the "volume release" from NGFC boutons to pyramidal cells.

9.4.3 Neurotransmitter Diffusion Outside the Synaptic Cleft

In conventional synaptic transmission, the information transfer mediated by neurotransmitter release is believed to be restricted to the pre- and postsynaptic elements of the same synapse. It has been argued that these conditions of "synapse independence" would maximize the information storage capacity of the brain (Barbour 2001). However, several lines of evidence indicate that, after synaptic release, neurotransmitter can diffuse out the synaptic cleft thus activating both postsynaptic receptors belonging to neighbor synapses and receptors expressed at the presynaptic level (Trussell et al. 1993; Rusakov and Kullmann 1998; Isaacson 1999; Digregorio et al. 2002; Arnth-Jensen et al. 2002; Chalifoux and Carter 2011; Scanziani et al. 1997; Mitchell and Silver 2000a, b). This phenomenon, referred to as "neurotransmitter spillover," has been shown to play a central role in the modulation of the synaptic activity.

At the presynaptic level, the activation of high-affinity neurotransmitter receptors (mGluR, GABAB) reduces the glutamate release (Mitchell and Silver 2000a, b) and increases the threshold for LTP (Vogt and Nicoll 1999). At the postsynaptic level, neurotransmitter spillover has been extensively demonstrated to activate the high-affinity NMDA glutamate receptors at Asztely et al. (1997), Arnth-Jensen et al. (2002), and Chalifoux and Carter (2011). Rusakov and Kullmann (1998) by using model simulations estimated that a single quantum of glutamate can escape the synaptic cleft and reach (although to a considerably lower concentration) neighboring glutamatergic synapses (spaced by ~500 nm) and suggested that, due to its high-affinity and perisynaptic location, NMDA receptor is an optimal candidate to mediate synaptic responses induced by glutamate spillover. In line with this, at excitatory synapses in CA1 pyramidal neurons, Asztely et al. (1997) demonstrated that spillover can activate NMDA but not AMPA receptors, while at dendrodendritic synapses in the olfactory bulb, spillover activation of NMDA receptors contributes in synchronizing the activity of olfactory principal cells (Isaacson 1999). Scimemi et al. (2004), in the hippocampus, isolated specific molecular players for NMDA receptor-mediated synaptic cross talk by demonstrating that 30–35 % of NMDA receptors are activated by glutamate spillover and that only NR2B receptors were activated by spillover, while NR2A receptors mediated conventional synaptic transmission. More recently, it has been also shown in the layer 5 of the mouse prefrontal cortex that glutamate spillover mediates the initiation of NMDA dendritic spikes with important implications for the dendritic signal processing and computation (Chalifoux and Carter 2011).

Besides the synaptic cross talk mediated by high-affinity receptors, glutamate released from neighboring synapses has been shown to contribute to the activation of low-affinity AMPAR during a single excitatory postsynaptic current (EPSC). This phenomenon has been mainly described in the cerebellum at synapses formed by mossy fibers and granule cells. These synapses, in which an individual mossy fiber terminal innervates several granule cells, are encapsulated in a glomerular structure that limits the neurotransmitter diffusion, thus favoring synaptic cross talk. DiGregorio et al. (2002), indeed, demonstrated that excitatory postsynaptic currents (EPSCs) recorded at granule cells are evoked both by conventional point-to-point AMPA receptor activation and by glutamate spillover to AMPA receptor belonging to neighboring synapses. In the same study, it has been shown that glutamate spillover evokes both "pure spillover EPSCs" (characterized by slow rise and decay kinetics) and contributes to slow down the decaying phase of conventional EPSCs, accounting for the ~70 % of the total charge transfer at granule cells. These results were corroborated by modeling studies that simulated the glutamate diffusion within the cerebellar glomerulus (Nielsen et al. 2004). Such synaptic cross talk has been shown to reduce the trial-to-trial fluctuations and to increase the efficacy of synaptic transmission. In addition, a more recent study focusing on NMDA receptors at the glomerulus indicates that glutamate spillover activates the high-affinity NMDA receptors equally to direct glutamate release, corroborating the idea of increased synaptic reliability by synaptic cross talk (Mitchell and Lee 2011). Besides the glomerular glutamate diffusion, following tetanic stimulation of cerebellar parallel fibers, glutamate spillover activates AMPA receptors at glutamatergic synapses of stellate interneurons in the cerebellar molecular layer, exerting an efficient frequency-dependent modulation of cerebellar microcircuits (Carter and Regehr 2000). Overall, the non-conventional activation of synaptic receptors by neurotransmitter spillover contributes to refine synaptic transmission by increasing its versatility, thus expanding the computational properties of neuronal circuits.

9.5 Receptor Lateral Diffusion

In the classical view of the synapse, postsynaptic receptors are fixed and clustered in front of releasing terminals due to action of scaffold proteins that structurally link the receptors with the neuronal cytoskeleton. Over the last decade, conversely, the analysis of the synaptic plasticity mechanisms revealed that the number of receptors expressed at postsynaptic sites may vary in response to external stimuli, clearly challenging the static view of postsynaptic receptor organization. In particular, several studies showed that the number of receptors expressed at synapses after plasticity induction was associated to changes in the receptor exocytosis and/or endocytosis suggesting a dynamic exchange between synaptic receptors and a pool of intracellular receptors, thus emphasizing the concept of receptor "trafficking". The evidence that both receptor endocytosis and exocytosis occurred in specialized zones outside the synapse indicated that, in order to be inserted or removed from synapses, neurotransmitter receptors must laterally diffuse in the plane of the membrane. It is now clear that receptor lateral diffusion not only represents a step of receptor recycling but is crucial in the fast redistribution of neurotransmitter receptors at the different sub-compartments at the neuronal surface (Tovar and Westbrook 2002; Shi et al. 1999). The technological advancement that allowed the direct visualization of the trajectories of individual receptors diffusing both in the synaptic and extrasynaptic space clarified that lateral mobility is a major determinant for both short- and long-term modulation of synaptic strength.

9.5.1 Single-Particle Tracking Technique

Having established that neurotransmitter receptors are mobile, a considerable effort has been made to characterize and quantify the diffusion properties of receptors on the neuronal surface. By using a pharmacological approach, Tovar and Westbrook (2002) found that synaptic current mediated by NMDA receptors could recover after irreversible block of the open channel blocker MK-801 indicating replacement of synaptic "blocked NMDA receptors" with naïve extrasynaptic receptors indicating exchange between synaptic and extrasynaptic receptors by lateral diffusion. Using a similar approach at GABAergic synapses, the activity-dependent block of GABAA receptors by MTSES revealed the exchange rate of GABAA receptors at synapses of hippocampal pyramidal neurons. Other approaches for the measurement of receptor "population mobility" exploited live imaging of receptors tagged with fluorescent reporters. For instance, Shi et al. (1999) using two-photon imaging found that, following high-frequency stimulation of neurons in organotypic cultures, synapses were enriched with GFP-tagged AMPA receptors indicating receptor redistribution to glutamatergic spines. In the fluorescence recovery after photobleaching technique (FRAP), following photobleaching of a small spot on the neuron induced by sustained laser illumination, the time needed for fluorescent-tagged receptors to fill the fluorescence gap is related to the rate of receptor lateral diffusion (although other sources of fluorescence recovery including direct exocytosis of receptors in the bleached area cannot be neglected) (Jacob et al. 2005; Holcman and Triller 2006; Petrini et al. 2009). Another bulk measurement of the molecule diffusion exploits the fluorescence correlation spectroscopy (FCS) that infers the mobility of the molecule of interest by its time of residence in small detection volumes (Schwille et al. 1999).

A major breakthrough in the study of receptor lateral mobility is represented by the advent of the single-particle tracking techniques (SPTs) that allow the direct visualization of receptor diffusion at the single-molecule level. This was first achieved through the tracking of latex beads of 500 nm diameter coupled to the receptors of interest by means of primary antibodies to reveal the trajectories of individual receptors diffusing on the neuronal surface (Meier et al. 2001; Borgdorff and Choquet 2002). This approach, first used at both glycine and AMPA receptors, described the basic properties of receptor diffusion that are characterized by high- and low-mobility periods correlating with the receptor diffusion in the extrasynaptic and synaptic compartments, respectively. These pioneering studies also revealed that receptor Brownian diffusion (induced by thermal agitation) is strongly influenced by transient interactions with scaffold proteins. Under the hypothesis that, due to its large size, the latex bead may preclude the study of receptor dynamics at synapses, small organic fluorescent dyes (~1 nm) have been used as a reporter of the receptor mobility. However, this nanoprobes undergo rapid photobleaching (<10 s), thus limiting the visualization of the receptor diffusion to short receptor displacements.

The use of semiconductor quantum dots (QDs), fluorescent nanoprobes of 15–25 nm, represents the best trade-off between size and photostability. QDs, indeed, are much smaller than latex beads and, differently to organic dyes, they show very low photobleaching, allowing the tracking of receptors for long periods of time, an essential requirement for the study of receptor diffusion in processes such as long-term synaptic plasticity (Triller and Choquet 2005, 2008) (Fig. 9.5). Technological advances allowed to further decrease the QD size to 10–12 nm (Howarth et al. 2008) to ensure better access to the highly packed synaptic structure. Gold particles of ~5 nm have also been used to track AMPA receptor in live neurons (Lasne et al. 2006). These probes are extremely small and do not undergo photobleaching, but, differently from latex beads of fluorescent reporters, they can only be detected by photothermal imaging, a technique that requires complex experimental setup (Berciaud et al. 2004). Interestingly, these QDs derive from the same colloidal technology described in Chap. 1 for the nanoparticle drug delivery and in Chaps. 2 and 3 for the various nanocomposite materials and Ag nanoparticle-based wound-healing materials, once again witnessing the impressive cross fertilization between nanotechnology, materials science, and life science. The combination of single-particle techniques with super-resolution microscopy, like the "single-particle tracking photoactivated localization microscopy" (sptPALM), permits to simultaneously perform single-particle trajectories and population measurement (Manley et al. 2008), obtaining a real-time dynamic representation of the

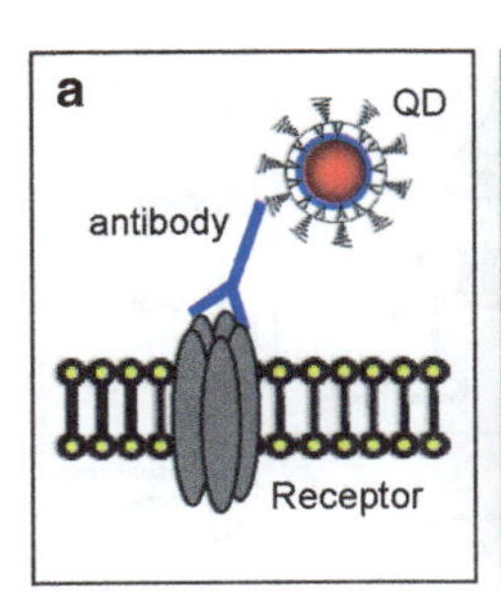

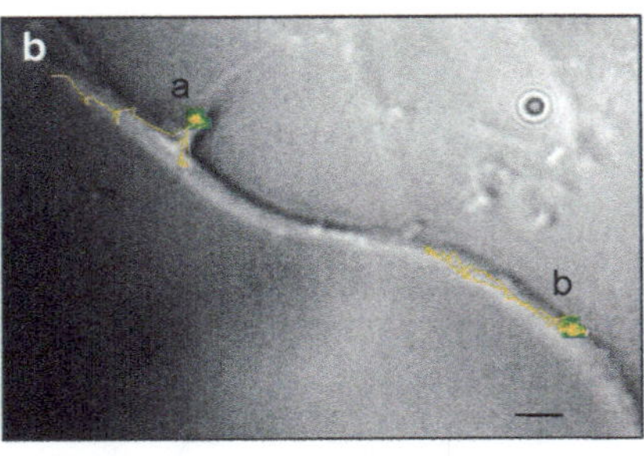

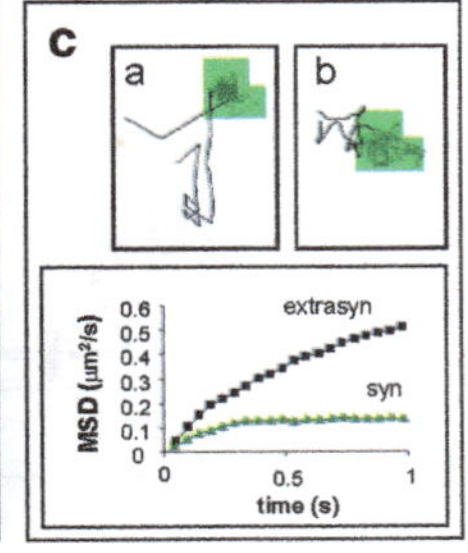

Fig. 9.5 Experimental approach of single-particle tracking. (**A**) Diagram of surface receptor labeling with a quantum dot (QD) through a specific antibody directed against an extracellular epitope of the receptor of interest. (**B**) Visualization of surface receptor diffusion (*yellow trajectories*) in the dendrite of a cultured hippocampal neuron. *Green spots* represent glutamatergic synapses visualized by transfection with fluorescent PSD-95. The "differential interference contrast" image is superimposed to QD trajectories and the GFP fluorescence. Scale bar 5 μm. (**C**) *Upper panels:* Magnification of QD-receptor complex diffusing at synapses "a" and "b" shown in panel **B**. *Lower panel:* Mean square displacement curve (MSD) of receptors at synaptic (*green*) and extrasynaptic (*black*) areas. The steady state reached by the *green curve* indicates that receptors are confined in synaptic areas, while the linear MSD curve describing the receptor mobility in the extrasynaptic space indicates free Brownian diffusion outside synapses. Scale bar = 1 μm

diffusion of several individual molecules resolved at sub-diffraction-limited pointing accuracy (Nair et al. 2013; Giannone et al. 2013).

9.5.2 *Implications of Receptor Diffusion in Short-Term Plasticity*

At conventional central synapses, during repetitive synaptic activation, the postsynaptic response typically decreases in a frequency-dependent manner. At the presynaptic level, indeed, the fatigue of the machinery release depresses the neurotransmitter release, while at the postsynaptic side the accumulation of receptor desensitization may limit receptor activation (Zucker and Regehr 2002). After neurotransmitter release, indeed, postsynaptic receptors are readily open, producing a postsynaptic response, but following their activation, they enter nonconductive (desensitized) state(s) that can persist for hundreds of milliseconds. In this situation, a second event of neurotransmitter release (in tens of millisecond time range) will generate a lower response due to the fact that some receptors are nonresponsive. By assuming fast receptor exchange between extrasynaptic and synaptic receptor, after the first release event, desensitized receptors at the synapses are replaced by extrasynaptic naïve receptors with consequent reduction of the synaptic response depression (Fig. 9.6a). This mechanism represents a form of short-term synaptic plasticity that may significantly modulate the availability of activatable receptors at

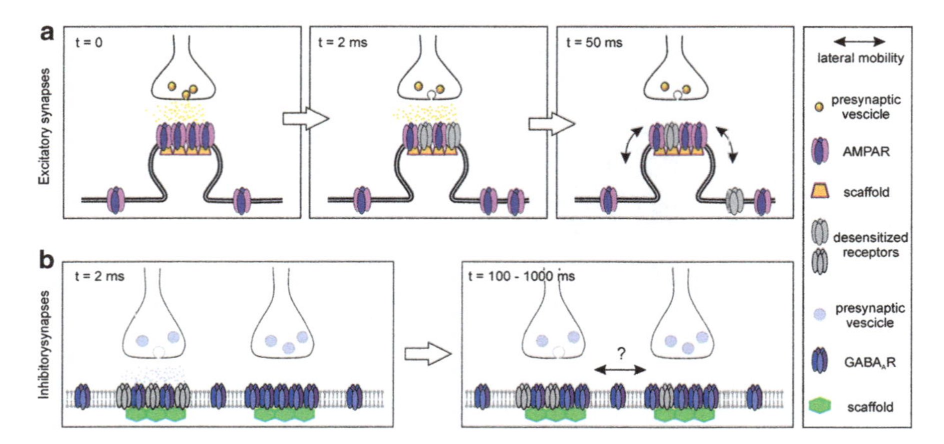

Fig. 9.6 Functional role of lateral diffusion in the fast modulation of synaptic response. (**a**) Diagram of fast AMPA receptor exchange at synapses during synaptic transmission: following glutamate release (*left panel*), some AMPA receptors undergo desensitization (*middle panel*). After 50 ms, due to lateral mobility, desensitized receptors are partially replaced by naïve extrasynaptic receptors, thus limiting the depression of synaptic current due to accumulation of desensitization (*right panel*). (**b**) Hypothetical redistribution of desensitized receptors at inhibitory synapses after GABA release. GABAA receptors possess long-living desensitized states that can persist up to 1 s. In these conditions, GABAA receptors in the desensitized state may diffuse to neighboring GABAergic synapses determining "functional cross talk"

synapses. This finding emphasizes the crucial importance of receptor diffusion in synaptic transmission and adds a further level of complexity in the modulation of postsynaptic signal at sub-millisecond time scale. Indeed, in particular during sustained synaptic activity, the level of the steady-state current will be influenced not only by the equilibrium between desensitized and non-desensitized state (dictated by presynaptic release and receptor gating) but also from the rate of exchange between postsynaptic and extrasynaptic receptors. Receptor diffusion, thus, is a key player in modulating the fidelity of synaptic transmission with crucial implications in the neuronal signal processing.

9.5.3 Implications of Receptor Diffusion in Long-Term Plasticity

Besides its role in the fast tuning of receptor availability at synapses, at longer time scale, lateral diffusion has been extensively implicated in setting the number of postsynaptic receptors expressed at postsynaptic sites in response to external stimuli, thus representing an important determinant for postsynaptic long-term plasticity. As demonstrated in the first studies describing the diffusion of receptors at single-molecule level (Meier et al. 2001; Borgdorff and Choquet 2002), the lateral mobility of receptors at synapses is strongly influenced by interactions with scaffold proteins that limit the receptor diffusion by acting as "diffusion traps". At glutamatergic synapses, several studies have highlighted that long-term potentiation (LTP) is largely dictated by lateral diffusion-mediated dendritic redistribution of AMPA receptors that are likely stabilized at synapses due to increased interaction with scaffold proteins at the glutamatergic postsynaptic density (PSD) (Makino and Malinow 2009; Petrini et al. 2009; Opazo et al. 2010, 2012). However, it has not been established yet whether after plasticity induction the increased AMPA receptor anchoring occurs through either increased receptor affinity or higher availability of "anchoring slots." Bats et al. (2007) demonstrated that the binding between stargazin (transmembrane AMPA receptor regulatory protein (TARP)) and PSD95, the main component of glutamatergic density, is crucial for the immobilization of AMPA receptors at synapses. More recently, it has been shown that the stargazin-PSD95 interaction, if favored by the stargazin phosphorylation by the CaMKII kinase (Opazo et al. 2010), suggesting that, during LTP, CaMKII activity promotes the stabilization of AMPAR-stargazin onto preexisting "PSD95 slots" (Opazo et al. 2012).

Besides interaction with scaffold proteins, other "diffusive mechanisms" have been described to play an important role of AMPA receptor stabilization at synapses. Petrini et al. (2009) demonstrated that a local the presence of endocytic zones (EZs) adjacent to glutamatergic synapses establishes a "local receptor recycling" that maintains a pool of mobile receptors at synapses crucial for the accumulation of receptors at synapses during synaptic plasticity. Furthermore, EZs, by reversibly trapping AMPA receptors, act as diffusional barriers limiting the dispersion of receptors from glutamatergic synapses.

At GABAergic synapses, the role of diffusion on the changes of synaptic strength has been mainly analyzed during long-term depression (LTD). Sustained neuronal activity, indeed, has been demonstrated to decrease inhibitory synaptic currents due to reduced GABAA receptor and gephyrin clustering (Bannai et al. 2009). In the same study, this observation was associated with increased mobility and decreased confinement of GABAA receptor at synapses. Similar results are shown in Muir et al. (2010) where activation of glutamatergic synapses (with consequent calcium entry through NMDA receptors) led to mobilization and dispersal of GABAA receptors at GABAergic synapses. Interestingly, these two studies highlight the role of the phosphatase calcineurin in this form of synaptic depotentiation. In particular, Muir et al. (2010) found that the lower interaction of GABA receptors at GABAergic PSD and its consequent higher synaptic lateral diffusion is due to the dephosphorylation of the residue Serine 327 on the $\gamma 2$ subunit of GABAA receptors, a residue already reported to interfere with GABAA receptor stability at synapses (Wang et al. 2003). It is interesting to point out that neuronal activity with consequent increase of intracellular [Ca^{++}] immobilizes AMPA receptors (Borgdorff and Choquet 2002) while increasing the diffusion of GABAA receptors. This opposite effect may play an important functional role in the coordination of the activity of excitatory and inhibitory systems. Indeed, as LTP and LTD are associated to immobilization and mobilization of synaptic receptors, respectively, it may be argued that local calcium increase may concomitantly induce LTP at glutamatergic synapses and LTD at GABAergic synapses leading to a strong unbalance tipped toward excitation.

9.5.4 Future Perspectives

It has been shown that, as postulated by the Bienestock–Cooper–Munro (BCM) rule, at glutamatergic synapses, high calcium increase would lead to LTP, while moderate calcium entry would trigger LTD (Lisman 2001). At GABAergic synapses, conversely, sustained calcium entry leads to synaptic depression (Lu et al. 2000; Bannai et al. 2009) while moderate calcium may lead to LTP (Marsden et al. 2010; Petrini personal communication). This opposite "calcium rule" at glutamatergic and GABAergic synapses may determine a complex scenario in which calcium spread from glutamatergic synapses may induce different plasticity at neighboring GABAergic synapses according to the concentration reached by calcium. In this context, due to intracellular calcium diffusion, the relative distance of GABAergic synapses from glutamatergic synapses may play an important role in setting the calcium concentration that induced LTD or LTP, linking the distribution of glutamatergic and GABAergic synapses on the neuronal dendrites to the activity-dependent tuning of synaptic strength and excitatory to inhibitory (E/I) balance. As mentioned above, it has been shown that the amplitude of synaptic current can be modulated by fast exchange between synaptic and extrasynaptic receptors.

Very likely this concept can be further extended, assuming that by diffusing between two or more synapses (transsynaptic diffusion), a receptor can bring to the next synapse the "history" of its experience in the previous synapse, creating a cross talk between synapses. For example, if a given synapse undergoes sustained activity, the consequent accumulation of desensitized receptors could reduce the short-term efficacy of adjacent synapses through lateral transsynaptic diffusion of desensitized receptors. A requirement for such diffusion-mediated "information exchange" between synapses is that specific receptor states (e.g., open or desensitized) persist long enough to allow receptor diffusion between two or more synapses. This condition is fulfilled by desensitized states of $GABA_ARs$ that can persist up to 1–10 s. According to measurements of diffusion coefficients of $GABA_AR$ and glutamate in extrasynaptic compartments (0.2–1 $\mu m^2/s$), we estimate that, during the desensitized state, those receptors can cover distances in the range of 0.9–6.3 μm, on par with the typical distance between adjacent synapses, e.g., 1.5–2 μm in hippocampal dendrites (Fig. 9.6b). To explore our hypothesis, we are currently exploiting light-gated glutamate receptors (LiGluK2), an optogenetic tool developed in the Isacoff Lab, that can be effectively switched to either the open/desensitized or closed state by illuminating with 380 nm or >460 nm light, respectively. By activating LiGluK2 receptors at individual synapses, indeed, it is possible to explore the receptor diffusion in "controlled conformational states" and to test the functional effect of their insertion onto neighboring synapses. Optogenetic experiments aimed at studying receptors at the level of the synapse typically exploit (single or two-photon) diffraction-limited UV laser spots of ~250 nm diameter. However, since the synapse size is in the range of 100 nm, this spatial resolution is not adequate to perform single-synapse stimulation.

To overcome this technical limitation, new illumination devices capable to focus light in sub-diffraction-limited spots need to be developed. The methodology for constructing a highly focused beam of light is based on the increment of the localized electric field occurring when a laser beam interacts with a metallic surface with a sharp nanostructure. This phenomenon is at the basis of plasmon polariton technology (Raether 1988). The methodological innovation consists in the combination and utilization of nanofabrication techniques to develop structures with spatial control at the nanoscale and nanopositioning such as piezo-manipulator or AFM scanning probe. The spatial confinement of light in the near field is comparable to the radius of curvature of tapered nanowires, generating the highly localized beam of light in the order of 20–30 nm (Fig. 9.7) (De Angelis et al. 2011; Giugni et al. 2013). By directing the tapered nanoprobe to synapses expressing fluorescent light-gated receptors, it will be possible to restrict the illumination to individual synapses. In particular by using electrophysiological and single-particle techniques, one can study the dynamics and the redistribution of "pure synaptic receptors" onto to adjacent synapses. The understanding of the transsynaptic receptor dynamics is crucial to assess the "independence of the synapse," a long debated issue in neuroscience. A quantitative assessment of the impact of transsynaptic receptor exchange at glutamatergic and GABAergic synapses can significantly contribute to identify the rules of signal integration and computation in neuronal dendrites.

9.6 Conclusions

The astonishing development of the understanding of synaptic physiology that occurred in the last few years would not have been possible without the application of new techniques allowing to approach the tiny synaptic region in live, behaving neuronal networks both in vitro and in vivo. The coupling of patch-clamp electrophysiology with fluorescent reporters of neuronal activity (Ca^{2+} sensors, voltage-sensitive molecules, pHluorin reporters of SV cycling) and light-dependent actuators (microbial opsins and light-switchable ion channels) now allows to stimulate and record synaptic responses with an unprecedented spatial and temporal resolution. The possibility to synaptically target sensors and actuators, track single molecules in their activity-dependent navigation, bring resolution of confocal microscopy to the nanodomain with the STED technique, and physically go below the diffraction limit of light microscopy using the plasmon polariton

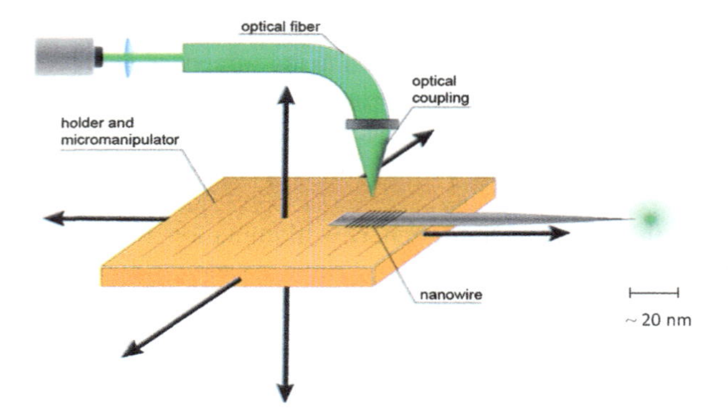

Fig. 9.7 The spatial confinement of light in the near field. This illumination device is composed of a single nanowire excited from one end by a highly focused laser beam that, through a "backfire coupling," generates a highly localized optical field at the other end of the nanowire. This focused light acts as optical exciting source of light-sensitive receptors expressed at synapses

technology is providing invaluable weapons to extend our knowledge of synaptic functions and dysfunctions in the healthy and diseased brain.

References

Alabi AA, Tsien RW (2012) Synaptic vesicle pools and dynamics. Cold Spring Harb Perspect Biol 4(8):a013680

Arnth-Jensen N, Jabaudon D, Scanziani M (2002) Cooperation between independent hippocampal synapses is controlled by glutamate uptake. Nat Neurosci 5(4):325–331

Asztely F, Erdemli G, Kullmann DM (1997) Extrasynaptic glutamate spillover in the hippocampus: dependence on temperature and the role of active glutamate uptake. Neuron 18(2):281–293

Bamji SX, Rico B, Kimes N, Reichardt LF (2006) BDNF mobilizes synaptic vesicles and enhances synapse formation by disrupting cadherin-beta-catenin interactions. J Cell Biol 174(2):289–299

Banks MI, Li TB, Pearce RA (1998) The synaptic basis of GABAA, slow. J Neurosci 18(4):1305–1317

Bannai H, Lévi S, Schweizer C, Inoue T, Launey T, Racine V, Sibarita JB, Mikoshiba K, Triller A (2009) Activity-dependent tuning of inhibitory neurotransmission based on GABAAR diffusion dynamics. Neuron 62(5):670–682

Barberis A, Petrini EM, Cherubini E (2004) Presynaptic source of quantal size variability at GABAergic synapses in rat hippocampal neurons in culture. Eur J Neurosci 20(7):1803–1810

Barberis A, Lu C, Vicini S, Mozrzymas JW (2005) Developmental changes of GABA synaptic transient in cerebellar granule cells. Mol Pharmacol 67(4):1221–1228

Barberis A, Sachidhanandam S, Mulle C (2008) GluR6/KA2 kainate receptors mediate slow-deactivating currents. J Neurosci 28(25):6402–6406

Barberis A, Petrini EM, Mozrzymas JW (2011) Impact of synaptic neurotransmitter concentration time course on the kinetics and pharmacological modulation of inhibitory synaptic currents. Front Cell Neurosci 5:6

Barbour B (2001) An evaluation of synapse independence. J Neurosci 21(20):7969–7984

Barnett DG, Bibb JA (2011) The role of Cdk5 in cognition and neuropsychiatric and neurological pathology. Brain Res Bull 85(1–2):9–13

Bats C, Groc L, Choquet D (2007) The interaction between Stargazin and PSD-95 regulates AMPA receptor surface trafficking. Neuron 53(5):719–734
Beato M (2008) The time course of transmitter at glycinergic synapses onto motoneurons. J Neurosci 28(29):7412–7425
Berciaud S, Cognet L, Blab GA, Lounis B (2004) Photothermal heterodyne imaging of individual nonfluorescent nanoclusters and nanocrystals. Phys Rev Lett 93(25):257402
Borgdorff AJ, Choquet D (2002) Regulation of AMPA receptor lateral movements. Nature 417 (6889):649–653
Burrone J, Li Z, Murthy VN (2006) Studying vesicle cycling in presynaptic terminals using the genetically encoded probe synaptopHluorin. Nat Protoc 1:2970–2978
Buzsáki G (2012) How do neurons sense a spike burst? Neuron 73(5):857–859
Carter AG, Regehr WG (2000) Prolonged synaptic currents and glutamate spillover at the parallel fiber to stellate cell synapse. J Neurosci 20(12):4423–4434
Carter AG, Regehr WG (2002) Quantal events shape cerebellar interneuron firing. Nat Neurosci 5 (12):1309–1318
Ceccarelli B, Hurlbut WP (1980) Vesicle hypothesis of the release of quanta of acetylcholine. Physiol Rev 60(2):396–441
Cesca F, Baldelli P, Valtorta F, Benfenati F (2010) The synapsins: key actors of synapse function and plasticity. Prog Neurobiol 91(4):313–348
Chalifoux JR, Carter AG (2011) Glutamate spillover promotes the generation of NMDA spikes. J Neurosci 31(45):16435–16446
Clements JD (1996) Transmitter time course in the synaptic cleft: its role in central synaptic function. Trends Neurosci 19:163–171
Clements JD, Lester RA, Tong G, Jahr CE, Westbrook GL (1992) The time course of glutamate in the synaptic cleft. Science 258:1498–1501
De Angelis F, Liberale C, Coluccio ML, Cojoc G, Di Fabrizio E (2011) Emerging fabrication techniques for 3D nano-structuring in plasmonics and single molecule studies. Nanoscale 3(7): 2689–2696
Diamond JS, Jahr CE (1997) Transporters buffer synaptically released glutamate on a submillisecond time scale. J Neurosci 17(12):4672–4687
DiGregorio DA, Nusser Z, Silver RA (2002) Spillover of glutamate onto synaptic AMPA receptors enhances fast transmission at a cerebellar synapse. Neuron 35(3):521–533
Dreosti E, Odermatt B, Dorostkar MM, Lagnado L (2009) A genetically encoded reporter of synaptic activity in vivo. Nat Methods 6(12):883–889. doi:10.1038/nmeth.1399
Farisello P, Boido D, Nieus T, Medrihan L, Cesca F, Valtorta F, Baldelli P, Benfenati F (2013) Synaptic and extrasynaptic origin of the excitation/inhibition imbalance in the hippocampus of synapsin I/II/III knockout mice. Cereb Cortex 23(3):581–593
Fatt P, Katz B (1952) Spontaneous subthreshold activity at motor nerve endings. J Physiol 117 (1):109–128
Few AP, Nanou E, Watari H, Sullivan JM, Scheuer T, Catterall WA (2012) Asynchronous Ca^{2+} current conducted by voltage-gated Ca^{2+} (CaV)-2.1 and CaV2.2 channels and its implications for asynchronous neurotransmitter release. Proc Natl Acad Sci USA 109(7):E452–E460
Fornasiero EF, Raimondi A, Guarnieri FC, Orlando M, Fesce R, Benfenati F, Valtorta F (2012) Synapsins contribute to the dynamic spatial organization of synaptic vesicles in an activity-dependent manner. J Neurosci 32(35):12214–12227
Franks KM, Bartol TM Jr, Sejnowski TJ (2002) A Monte Carlo model reveals independent signaling at central glutamatergic synapses. Biophys J 83(5):2333–2348
Galiani S, Harke B, Vicidomini G, Lignani G, Benfenati F, Diaspro A, Bianchini P (2012) Strategies to maximize the performance of a STED microscope. Opt Express 20(7):7362–7374
Giannone G, Hosy E, Sibarita JB, Choquet D, Cognet L (2013) High-content super-resolution imaging of live cell by uPAINT. Methods Mol Biol 950:95–110

Giugni A, Torre B, Toma A, Francardi M, Malerba M, Alabastri A, Proietti Zaccaria R, Stockman MI, Di Fabrizio E (2013) Hot-electron nanoscopy using adiabatic compression of surface plasmons. Nat Nanotechnol 8:845–852
Glavinovíc MI (1999) Monte Carlo simulation of vesicular release, spatiotemporal distribution of glutamate in synaptic cleft and generation of postsynaptic currents. Pflugers Arch 437(3): 462–470
Gorostiza P, Isacoff EY (2008) Optical switches for remote and noninvasive control of cell signaling. Science 322(5900):395–399
Harata NC, Aravanis AM, Tsien RW (2006) Kiss-and-run and full-collapse fusion as modes of exo-endocytosis in neurosecretion. J Neurochem 97(6):1546–1570
Heuser JE, Reese TS (1973) Evidence for recycling of synaptic vesicle membrane during transmitter release at the frog neuromuscular junction. J Cell Biol 57(2):315–344
Holcman D, Triller A (2006) Modeling synaptic dynamics driven by receptor lateral diffusion. Biophys J 91(7):2405–2415
Holmes WR (1995) Modeling the effect of glutamate diffusion and uptake on NMDA and non-NMDA receptor saturation. Biophys J 69:1734–1747
Howarth M, Liu W, Puthenveetil S, Zheng Y, Marshall LF, Schmidt MM, Wittrup KD, Bawendi MG, Ting AY (2008) Monovalent, reduced-size quantum dots for imaging receptors on living cells. Nat Methods 5(5):397–399
Iremonger KJ, Bains JS (2007) Integration of asynchronously released quanta prolongs the postsynaptic spike window. J Neurosci 27(25):6684–6691
Isaacson JS (1999) Glutamate spillover mediates excitatory transmission in the rat olfactory bulb. Neuron 23(2):377–384
Jacob TC, Bogdanov YD, Magnus C, Saliba RS, Kittler JT, Haydon PG, Moss SJ (2005) Gephyrin regulates the cell surface dynamics of synaptic GABAA receptors. J Neurosci 25(45): 10469–10478
Jahn R, Fasshauer D (2012) Molecular machines governing exocytosis of synaptic vesicles. Nature 490(7419):201–207
Jones MV, Westbrook GL (1998) Defining affinity with the GABAA receptor. J Neurosci 18(21): 8590–8604
Jones MV, Sahara Y, Dzubay JA, Westbrook GL (1995) Desensitized states prolong GABAA channel responses to brief agonist pulses. Neuron 15(1):181–191
Karayannis T, Elfant D, Huerta-Ocampo I, Teki S, Scott RS, Rusakov DA, Jones MV, Capogna M (2010) Slow GABA transient and receptor desensitization shape synaptic responses evoked by hippocampal neurogliaform cells. J Neurosci 30(29):9898–9909
Kavalali ET, Chung C, Khvotchev M, Leitz J, Nosyreva E, Raingo J, Ramirez DM (2011) Spontaneous neurotransmission: an independent pathway for neuronal signaling? Physiology 26(1):45–53
Kim SH, Ryan TA (2010) CDK5 serves as a major control point in neurotransmitter release. Neuron 67(5):797–809
Kim SH, Ryan TA (2013) Balance of calcineurin Aα and CDK5 activities sets release probability at nerve terminals. J Neurosci 33(21):8937–8950
Kleinle J, Vogt K, Lüscher HR, Müller L, Senn W, Wyler K, Streit J (1996) Transmitter concentration profiles in the synaptic cleft: an analytical model of release and diffusion. Biophys J 71(5):2413–2426
Kochubey O, Lou X, Schneggenburger R (2011) Regulation of transmitter release by Ca(2+) and synaptotagmin: insights from a large CNS synapse. Trends Neurosci 34(5):237–246
Lasne D, Blab GA, Berciaud S, Heine M, Groc L, Choquet D, Cognet L, Lounis B (2006) Single nanoparticle photothermal tracking (SNaPT) of 5-nm gold beads in live cells. Biophys J 91 (12):4598–4604
Lignani G, Raimondi A, Ferrea E, Rocchi A, Paonessa F, Cesca F, Orlando M, Tkatch T, Valtorta F, Cossette P, Baldelli P, Benfenati F (2013) Epileptogenic Q555X SYN1 mutant

triggers imbalances in release dynamics and short-term plasticity. Hum Mol Genet 22(11): 2186–2199

Lisman JE (2001) Three Ca2+ levels affect plasticity differently: the LTP zone, the LTD zone and no man's land. J Physiol 532:285

Lu T, Trussell LO (2000) Inhibitory transmission mediated by asynchronous transmitter release. Neuron 26(3):683–694

Lu YM, Mansuy IM, Kandel ER, Roder J (2000) Calcineurin-mediated LTD of GABAergic inhibition underlies the increased excitability of CA1 neurons associated with LTP. Neuron 26 (1):197–205

Macdonald RL, Rogers CJ, Twyman RE (1989) Kinetic properties of the GABAA receptor main conductance state of mouse spinal cord neurones in culture. J Physiol 410:479–499

Makino H, Malinow R (2009) AMPA receptor incorporation into synapses during LTP: the role of lateral movement and exocytosis. Neuron 64(3):381–390

Manley S, Gillette JM, Patterson GH, Shroff H, Hess HF, Betzig E, Lippincott-Schwartz J (2008) High-density mapping of single-molecule trajectories with photoactivated localization microscopy. J Nat Methods 5(2):155–157

Marsden KC, Shemesh A, Bayer KU, Carroll RC (2010) Selective translocation of Ca^{2+}/calmodulin protein kinase II alpha (CaMKIIalpha) to inhibitory synapses. Proc Natl Acad Sci USA 107 (47):20559–20564

Mattis J, Tye KM, Ferenczi EA, Ramakrishnan C, O'Shea DJ, Prakash R, Gunaydin LA, Hyun M, Fenno LE, Gradinaru V, Yizhar O, Deisseroth K (2011) Principles for applying optogenetic tools derived from direct comparative analysis of microbial opsins. Nat Methods 9(2):159–172

Medrihan L, Cesca F, Raimondi A, Lignani G, Baldelli P, Benfenati F (2013) Synapsin II desynchronizes neurotransmitter release at inhibitory synapses by interacting with presynaptic calcium channels. Nat Commun 4:1512

Meier J, Vannier C, Sergé A, Triller A, Choquet D (2001) Fast and reversible trapping of surface glycine receptors by gephyrin. Nat Neurosci 4(3):253–260

Messa M, Congia S, Defranchi E, Valtorta F, Fassio A, Onofri F, Benfenati F (2010) Tyrosine phosphorylation of synapsin I by Src regulates synaptic-vesicle trafficking. J Cell Sci 123 (Pt 13):2256–2265

Miesenböck G, De Angelis DA, Rothman JE (1998) Visualizing secretion and synaptic transmission with pH-sensitive green fluorescent proteins. Nature 394:192–195

Min MY, Rusakov DA, Kullmann DM (1998) Activation of AMPA, kainate, and metabotropic receptors at hippocampal mossy fiber synapses: role of glutamate diffusion. Neuron 21: 561–570

Mitchell CS, Lee RH (2011) Synaptic glutamate spillover increases NMDA receptor reliability at the cerebellar glomerulus. J Theor Biol 289:217–224

Mitchell SJ, Silver RA (2000a) GABA spillover from single inhibitory axons suppresses low-frequency excitatory transmission at the cerebellar glomerulus. J Neurosci 20(23): 8651–8658

Mitchell SJ, Silver RA (2000b) Glutamate spillover suppresses inhibition by activating presynaptic mGluRs. Nature 404(6777):498–502

Mott DD, Rojas A, Fisher JL, Dingledine RJ, Benveniste M (2010) Subunit-specific desensitization of heteromeric kainate receptors. J Physiol 588(Pt 4):683–700

Mozrzymas JW, Barberis A, Michalak K, Cherubini E (1999) Chlorpromazine inhibits miniature GABAergic currents by reducing the binding and by increasing the unbinding rate of GABAA receptors. J Neurosci 19:2474–2488

Muir J, Arancibia-Carcamo IL, MacAskill AF, Smith KR, Griffin LD, Kittler JT (2010) NMDA receptors regulate GABAA receptor lateral mobility and clustering at inhibitory synapses through serine 327 on the γ2 subunit. Proc Natl Acad Sci USA 107(38):16679–16684

Murthy VN, Stevens CF (1999) Reversal of synaptic vesicle docking at central synapses. Nat Neurosci 2(6):503–507

Nair D, Hosy E, Petersen JD, Constals A, Giannone G, Choquet D, Sibarita JB (2013) Super-resolution imaging reveals that AMPA receptors inside synapses are dynamically organized in nanodomains regulated by PSD95. J Neurosci 33(32):13204–13224
Nielsen TA, DiGregorio DA, Silver RA (2004) Modulation of glutamate mobility reveals the mechanism underlying slow-rising AMPAR EPSCs and the diffusion coefficient in the synaptic cleft. Neuron 42(5):757–771
Oláh S, Füle M, Komlósi G, Varga C, Báldi R, Barzó P, Tamás G (2009) Regulation of cortical microcircuits by unitary GABA-mediated volume transmission. Nature 461(7268):1278–1281
Opazo P, Labrecque S, Tigaret CM, Frouin A, Wiseman PW, De Koninck P, Choquet D (2010) CaMKII triggers the diffusional trapping of surface AMPARs through phosphorylation of stargazin. Neuron 67(2):239–252
Opazo P, Sainlos M, Choquet D (2012) Regulation of AMPA receptor surface diffusion by PSD-95 slots. Curr Opin Neurobiol 22(3):453–460
Orenbuch A, Shalev L, Marra V, Sinai I, Lavy Y, Kahn J, Burden JJ, Staras K, Gitler D (2012) Synapsin selectively controls the mobility of resting pool vesicles at hippocampal terminals. J Neurosci 32(12):3969–3980
Otis TS, Staley KJ, Mody I (1991) Perpetual inhibitory activity in mammalian brain slices generated by spontaneous GABA release. Brain Res 545(1–2):142–150
Overstreet LS, Westbrook GL, Jones MV (2003) Measuring and modeling the spatiotemporal profile of GABA at the synapse. In: Quick MW (ed) Transmembrane transporters. Wiley, New York, pp 259–275
Pang ZP, Südhof TC (2010) Cell biology of Ca^{2+}-triggered exocytosis. Curr Opin Cell Biol 22 (4):496–505
Pearce RA (1993) Physiological evidence for two distinct GABAA responses in rat hippocampus. Neuron 10(2):189–200
Perrais D, Ropert N (2000) Altering the concentration of GABA in the synaptic cleft potentiates miniature IPSCs in rat occipital cortex. Eur J Neurosci 12(1):400–404
Petrini EM, Lu J, Cognet L, Lounis B, Ehlers MD, Choquet D (2009) Endocytic trafficking and recycling maintain a pool of mobile surface AMPA receptors required for synaptic potentiation. Neuron 63(1):92–105
Petrini EM, Nieus T, Ravasenga T, Succol F, Guazzi S, Benfenati F, Barberis A (2011) Influence of GABAAR monoliganded states on GABAergic responses. J Neurosci 31(5):1752–1761
Prakash R, Yizhar O, Grewe B, Ramakrishnan C, Wang N, Goshen I, Packer AM, Peterka DS, Yuste R, Schnitzer MJ, Deisseroth K (2012) Two-photon optogenetic toolbox for fast inhibition, excitation and bistable modulation. Nat Methods 9(12):1171–1179
Raether H (1988) Surface plasmons. Springer, New York
Ramirez DM, Kavalali ET (2011) Differential regulation of spontaneous and evoked neurotransmitter release at central synapses. Curr Opin Neurobiol 21(2):275–282
Rusakov DA, Kullmann DM (1998) Extrasynaptic glutamate diffusion in the hippocampus: ultrastructural constraints, uptake, and receptor activation. J Neurosci 18(9):3158–3170
Sabatini BL, Regehr WG (1996) Timing of neurotransmission at fast synapses in the mammalian brain. Nature 384(6605):170–172
Saitoe M, Schwarz TL, Umbach JA, Gundersen CB, Kidokoro Y (2001) Absence of junctional glutamate receptor clusters in Drosophila mutants lacking spontaneous transmitter release. Science 293(5529):514–517
Sankaranarayanan S, De Angelis D, Rothman JE, Ryan TA (2000) The use of pHluorins for optical measurements of presynaptic activity. Biophys J 79:2199–2208
Scanziani M, Salin PA, Vogt KE, Malenka RC, Nicoll RA (1997) Use-dependent increases in glutamate concentration activate presynaptic metabotropic glutamate receptors. Nature 385 (6617):630–634
Schwille P, Haupts U, Maiti S, Webb WW (1999) Molecular dynamics in living cells observed by fluorescence correlation spectroscopy with one- and two-photon excitation. Biophys J 77(4): 2251–2265

Scimemi A, Fine A, Kullmann DM, Rusakov DA (2004) NR2B-containing receptors mediate cross talk among hippocampal synapses. J Neurosci 24(20):4767–4777

Sharma G, Vijayaraghavan S (2003) Modulation of presynaptic store calcium induces release of glutamate and postsynaptic firing. Neuron 38(6):929–939

Shi SH, Hayashi Y, Petralia RS, Zaman SH, Wenthold RJ, Svoboda K, Malinow R (1999) Rapid spine delivery and redistribution of AMPA receptors after synaptic NMDA receptor activation. Science 284(5421):1811–1816

Staras K, Branco T (2010) Sharing vesicles between central presynaptic terminals: implications for synaptic function. Front Synaptic Neurosci 2:20

Staras K, Branco T, Burden JJ, Pozo K, Darcy K, Marra V, Ratnayaka A, Goda Y (2010) A vesicle superpool spans multiple presynaptic terminals in hippocampal neurons. Neuron 66(1):37–44

Sutton MA, Wall NR, Aakalu GN, Schuman EM (2004) Regulation of dendritic protein synthesis by miniature synaptic events. Science 304(5679):1979–1983

Sutton MA, Ito HT, Cressy P, Kempf C, Woo JC, Schuman EM (2006) Miniature neurotransmission stabilizes synaptic function via tonic suppression of local dendritic protein synthesis. Cell 125(4):785–799

Sutton MA, Taylor AM, Ito HT, Pham A, Schuman EM (2007) Postsynaptic decoding of neural activity: eEF2 as a biochemical sensor coupling miniature synaptic transmission to local protein synthesis. Neuron 55(4):648–661

Szabadics J, Tamás G, Soltesz I (2007) Different transmitter transients underlie presynaptic cell type specificity of GABAA, slow and GABAA, fast. Proc Natl Acad Sci USA 104(37): 14831–14836

Szobota S, Gorostiza P, Del Bene F, Wyart C, Fortin DL, Kolstad KD, Tulyathan O, Volgraf M, Numano R, Aaron HL, Scott EK, Kramer RH, Flannery J, Baier H, Trauner D, Isacoff EY (2007) Remote control of neuronal activity with a light-gated glutamate receptor. Neuron 54 (4):535–545

Tovar KR, Westbrook GL (2002) Mobile NMDA receptors at hippocampal synapses. Neuron 34 (2):255–264

Triller A, Choquet D (2005) Surface trafficking of receptors between synaptic and extrasynaptic membranes: and yet they do move! Trends Neurosci 28(3):133–139

Triller A, Choquet D (2008) New concepts in synaptic biology derived from single-molecule imaging. Neuron 59(3):359–374

Trussell LO, Zhang S, Raman IM (1993) Desensitization of AMPA receptors upon multiquantal neurotransmitter release. Neuron 10(6):1185–1196

Valente P, Casagrande S, Nieus T, Verstegen AM, Valtorta F, Benfenati F, Baldelli P (2012) Site-specific synapsin I phosphorylation participates in the expression of post-tetanic potentiation and its enhancement by BDNF. J Neurosci 32(17):5868–5879

Ventriglia F, Maio VD (2003) Synaptic fusion pore structure and AMPA receptor activation according to Brownian simulation of glutamate diffusion. Biol Cybern 88(3):201–209

Vogt KE, Nicoll RA (1999) Glutamate and gamma-aminobutyric acid mediate a heterosynaptic depression at mossy fiber synapses in the hippocampus. Proc Natl Acad Sci USA 96(3): 1118–1122

von Gersdorff H, Matthews G (1997) Depletion and replenishment of vesicle pools at a ribbon-type synaptic terminal. J Neurosci 17(6):1919–1927

Wahl LM, Pouzat C, Stratford KJ (1996) Monte Carlo simulation of fast excitatory synaptic transmission at a hippocampal synapse. J Neurophysiol 75(2):597–608

Walter AM, Groffen AJ, Sørensen JB, Verhage M (2011) Multiple Ca^{2+} sensors in secretion: teammates, competitors or autocrats? Trends Neurosci 34(9):487–497

Wang Q, Liu L, Pei L, Ju W, Ahmadian G, Lu J, Wang Y, Liu F, Wang YT (2003) Control of synaptic strength, a novel function of Akt. Neuron 38(6):915–928

Westphal V, Rizzoli SO, Lauterbach MA, Kamin D, Jahn R, Hell SW (2008) Video-rate far-field optical nanoscopy dissects synaptic vesicle movement. Science 320(5873):246–249

Xu W, Morishita W, Buckmaster PS, Pang ZP, Malenka RC, Südhof TC (2012) Distinct neuronal coding schemes in memory revealed by selective erasure of fast synchronous synaptic transmission. Neuron 73(5):990–1001

Yao J, Gaffaney JD, Kwon SE, Chapman ER (2011) Doc2 is a Ca^{2+} sensor required for asynchronous neurotransmitter release. Cell 147(3):666–677

Zucker RS, Regehr WG (2002) Short-term synaptic plasticity. Annu Rev Physiol 64:355–405

Chapter 10
Brain Function: Novel Technologies Driving Novel Understanding

John A. Assad, Luca Berdondini, Laura Cancedda, Francesco De Angelis, Alberto Diaspro, Michele Dipalo, Tommaso Fellin, Alessandro Maccione, Stefano Panzeri, and Leonardo Sileo

The central nervous system of mammals is among the most elaborate structures in nature. For example, the cerebral cortex, which is involved in perception, motor control, attention, and memory, is organized in horizontal layers, each of astonishing complexity (Jones and Peters 1990). One cubic millimeter of mammalian neocortex contains about 100,000 neurons (Meyer et al. 2010). Each neuron receives on the order of 20,000 synapses and communicates with tens to hundreds of other cells in an extraordinarily complex and highly interwoven cellular network. Moreover, neurons are remarkably diverse in terms of their morphology, electrical properties, connectivity, and neurotransmitter phenotype.

Given this daunting complexity, the cellular and network mechanisms generating higher brain functions are still poorly understood. There are immense challenges in elucidating how information coming from the outside world is encoded in the form of electrical signals in neurons and how activities in cellular subpopulations and networks give rise to sensation, perception, memory, and complex behaviors. To address these fundamental issues—with an eye toward ultimately developing brain-mimetic artificial devices—we envision at least three essential experimental and technical tasks. First, we need to generate high-resolution maps of the electrical activity of large numbers of cells within the intact brain during complex behavior. Although this is a *correlative* analysis, it provides the initial information about *where* and *when* electrical activities are generated during specific behaviors and *what* information these activities carry. Second, we need to *causally* test the role of identified neurons in specific brain circuits and the role of specific brain circuits in behaviors. By using various types of cell-type-specific actuators, it is now possible to generate or suppress electrical activity in identified neurons and

J.A. Assad (✉) • L. Berdondini • L. Cancedda • F. De Angelis • A. Diaspro • M. Dipalo • T. Fellin • A. Maccione • L. Sileo
Central Research Laboratory, Istituto Italiano di Tecnologia, Genova, Italy
e-mail: John.Assad@iit.it

S. Panzeri
Center for Neuroscience and Cognitive Systems, Istituto Italiano di Tecnologia, Rovereto, Italy

R. Cingolani (ed.), *Bioinspired Approaches for Human-Centric Technologies*,
DOI 10.1007/978-3-319-04924-3_10,

thus to test their sufficiency and necessity for a given behavior in living organisms. Third, because so much of the adaptability and plasticity of the brain appears to reside in synapses, we need to better characterize synaptic mechanisms and dynamics over broad timescales. All these goals require the development of innovative new experimental tools. Finally, collecting the experimental data is only the initial step: mathematical models are needed to truly "understand" brain function, to integrate descriptions at different levels of experimental inquiry, to reduce dimensionality, to devise testable hypotheses, and ultimately to provide the essential computational framework for brain-mimetic artificial devices.

This chapter presents a glimpse of the multidisciplinary approaches that IIT scientists are applying to the fundamental challenge of understanding neural circuits and computations and illustrates how advanced technology and analysis at IIT are driving discovery in neuroscience. Examples include novel optical methods to probe neural circuits and subcellular elements, innovative micro- and nanoscale devices to measure electrical and chemical signaling by neurons, and advanced analytical techniques to make sense of the dizzying multi-scale complexity of the brain. Our overarching view is that the brain overcomes the limitations of its biological hardware by the brilliance of its *architecture*. If we could develop the right tools to deduce that architecture, we could begin to meaningfully mimic the functionality of the brain.

10.1 Mapping Brain Electrical Activity at Cellular Resolution with Light

A prerequisite to understand the function of specific brain areas is to describe how specific cells in a brain area respond in space and time in a given behavioral context. As discussed in Chap. 9, electrophysiology has long been the preferred method for studying the central nervous system because of its excellent temporal resolution and because of its ability to capture a wide range of neural phenomena, from the millisecond-precision spiking activity of individual neurons and small populations to slower network oscillations (see later in this chapter for innovative new approaches for massively parallel electrophysiological techniques). However, the use of fluorescent indicators in combination with two-photon microscopy is now recognized as an equally fundamental tool for brain circuit analysis in vivo. For example, the development of fluorescent calcium indicators (Tsien 1980, 1981) not only revealed the roles of calcium ion as a second messenger but also allowed the monitoring of the activity of neurons, using the entry of calcium ions as proxy for electrical activity. In neurons, the depolarization that underlies an action potential opens voltage-gated calcium channels, leading to significant calcium accumulation in the intracellular space (Helmchen et al. 1996; Svoboda et al. 1997; Borst and Helmchen 1998). Intracellular calcium concentration can thus be used as an indirect measure of the suprathreshold activity of neurons. Moreover, fluorescence calcium imaging is useful for investigating the activity of nonneuronal cells, in particular astrocytes, which are a subtype of glial cells that play important modulatory roles in the brain (Haydon 2001; Volterra and Meldolesi 2005; Fellin 2009). Thus, by using a combination of two-photon microscopy and calcium imaging, it is now possible to monitor the excitability of both neurons and glia in the intact central nervous system.

The value of this optical approach in studying the functional properties of cellular networks is easy to appreciate. Because the interactions between different cells generate the complex ensemble dynamics that must form the basis of brain function, preserving the structure and function of the network circuitry is critical. Because light penetrates the tissue without causing mechanical disturbances, fluorescence calcium imaging allows the investigation of the function of brain cells and their interactions with the external world with minimal invasiveness. Furthermore, in vivo fluorescence microscopy allows simultaneous visualization of the function and *structure* of hundreds of cells with single-cell resolution (Stosiek et al. 2003; Gobel et al. 2007), which is not possible with current electrophysiological approaches.

From an optical point of view, however, recording fluorescent signals generated deep within the brain is not a trivial task. The presence of many molecules and compartments with different optical properties renders the brain optically nonhomogeneous, with large variations in its refractive index (Helmchen and Denk 2005). These differences in optical homogeneity cause the deflection of light rays from their original path, a phenomenon termed scattering. Light scattering plays a fundamental role in the progressive degradation of fluorescence imaging at increasing depths below the brain surface, which renders the signal generally impossible to detect in regions deeper than 1 mm (Helmchen and Denk 2005). Most importantly, light scattering is inversely related to the wavelength of the light that is used; thus, blue-shifted light (of a shorter wavelength) is highly scattered, whereas red-shifted light (of a longer wavelength) is scattered to a lesser extent. The success of two-photon microscopy for in vivo fluorescence imaging relies heavily on using infrared-shifted light to significantly decrease light scattering compared to imaging using the visible wavelength range (Denk et al. 1990; Denk and Svoboda 1997; Zipfel et al. 2003; Svoboda and Yasuda 2006). This approach permits the detection of fluorescent signals from deeper (up to 900–1,000 mm) regions of the brain (Theer et al. 2003) compared to imaging using single-photon excitation (up to 50–100 mm) while providing sufficient spatial resolution to monitor cellular and subcellular structures. Two-photon microscopy is increasingly combined with the use of genetically encoded calcium indicators (Looger and Griesbeck 2012). Compared to synthetic calcium dyes, the genetically encoded indicators have the advantage that they can be targeted to either specific cells in the brain or specific subcellular compartments, thus facilitating the identification of the cellular source of the signal. Moreover, since their expression is stable, functional imaging of calcium signals over extended periods of time (from weeks to months) is possible.

10.2 Manipulating Brain Electrical Activity at Cellular Resolution with Light

The recent advent of optogenetics has brought a revolution in neuroscience by allowing *causal* manipulation of electrical activity in identified neuronal subtypes. Optogenetics is based on the use of light-sensitive, plasma membrane molecules, called opsins (Zhang et al. 2007). At present, three major classes of opsins have been developed for brain studies: light-gated ion channels, such as channelrhodopsin (Boyden et al. 2005); light-gated chloride pumps, such as halorhodopsin (Gradinaru et al. 2008); and light-gated proton pumps, such as archeorhodopsin (Chow et al. 2010). When ChR absorbs a photon, a channel is opened and mainly Na^+ ions enter the cells, leading to cell depolarization. In contrast, when halorhodopsin absorbs a photon, it pumps Cl^- anions into the cell, leading to cell hyperpolarization. Archeorhodopsin is a light-gated outward proton pump that can mediate strong neuronal hyperpolarization when illuminated. A key advantage of the optogenetic actuators is that excitatory and inhibitory opsins have distinct absorption spectra, and thus, one can think of co-expressing different opsins in the same cell to generate or inhibit electrical activity by simply exciting with light of different wavelengths. Thus, optogenetics represents a tremendous tool to remotely control the electrical activity of neurons with light. Moreover, one of the major strengths of this technique is that the actuators (the light-sensitive molecules) are proteins. Thus, by exploiting the cell-specific transcription of genes, it is thus possible to express opsins in a cell-type-specific manner (Gradinaru et al. 2010). This is extremely important for investigating brain circuits: because cellular networks are highly interwoven, finding a technique to *selectively* excite/inhibit *specific* cells within a densely packed tissue has been a long-standing challenge in neuroscience. Optogenetics provides an elegant solution to this problem. Importantly, optogenetics also allows a high-resolution temporal control of the electrical activity of cells, because opsins can generate electrical signal with millisecond precision (Zhang et al. 2007).

10.3 Optogenetic Dissection of the Cellular Determinants of Cortical Network Dynamics

Since the work of Golgi and Cajal, it has been clear that the neocortex contains a large variety of cells with various morphology and different anatomical localization. Cells are organized in horizontal layers, named I through VI, which comprise neurons with specific morphological and functional properties. For example, layer II/III and layer V excitatory cells comprise two of the major output neuronal subtypes of the cortex. However, while layer II/III cells project their axons to deep cortical layers as well as to adjacent cortical areas, layer V neurons project to many cortical and extracortical regions, including the thalamus, striatum,

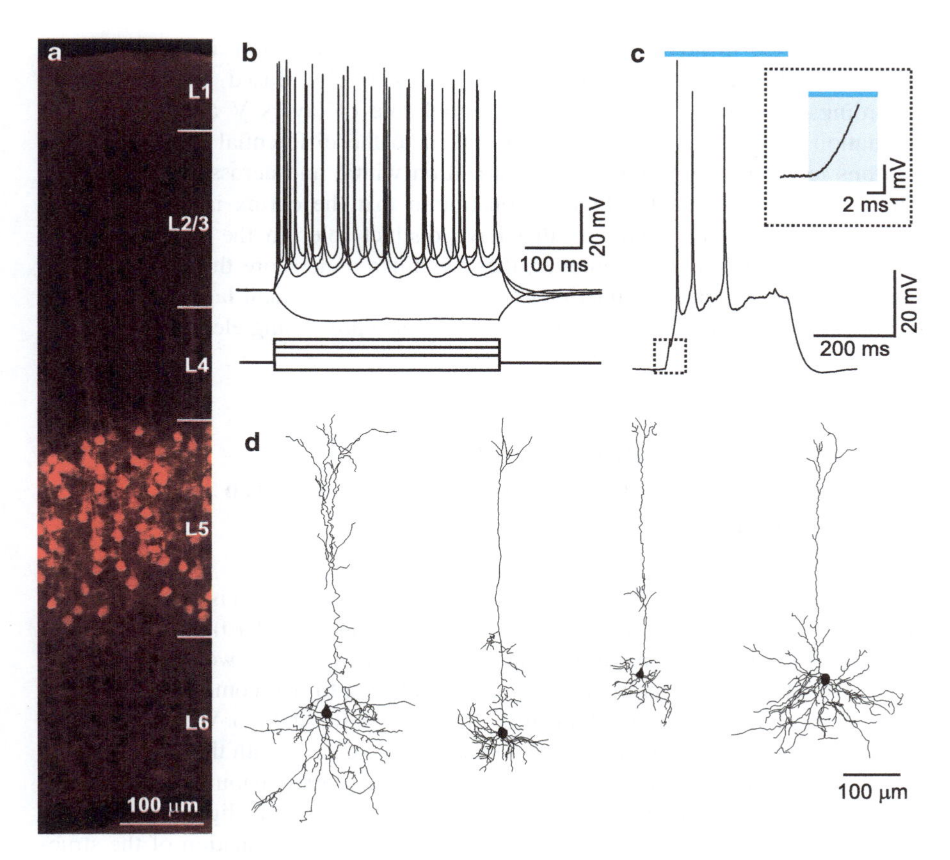

Fig. 10.1 Manipulating the electrical activity of layer V cortical neurons. (**a**) Opsins were selectively expressed in layer V neurons combining the use of the Rbp4-Cre mouse line with viral injections of adeno-associated viruses. (**b–d**) Cells expressing the transgenes (ChR2) were regular firing cells (**b**), display sub-millisecond membrane depolarizations when illuminated with blue light (**c**), and have the typical morphology of pyramidal neurons (**d**). Modified from Beltramo et al. Nature Neuroscience (2013)

superior colliculus, and trigeminal nuclei. It has long been recognized that this anatomical and functional specialization among cortical cells in different layers could serve different functional roles in cortical circuit dynamics. However, a *direct* and *causal* demonstration of this hypothesis has long been prevented due to the lack of tools to manipulate the activity of *specific* cellular subpopulations in vivo. IIT neuroscientists have used optogenetics, which allows the remote control of cellular excitability with light, to investigate the role of excitatory neurons located in layers II/III and V in the propagation of cortical network dynamics, using slow oscillations as an experimental model (Beltramo et al. 2013; Fig. 10.1).

By combining selective expression of excitatory and inhibitory opsins in layer V and layer II/III pyramidal neurons with electrophysiological recordings in anesthetized mice in vivo, we showed that activation/inactivation of a subset of pyramidal neurons located in layer V, but not layer II/III, was sufficient and necessary to generate and attenuate slow oscillations, respectively. Based on patch-clamp recordings, we proposed that the differential role of layers V and II/III in the regulation of slow network activity is linked to the differential ability of these neurons to propagate prolonged depolarization within and across cortical layers. These results represent the first demonstration that the cortex is endowed with *layer-specific* excitatory circuits that have distinct roles in the coordination of ongoing cortical activity. Moreover, these findings underscore the importance of understanding the specific functional microcircuitry of cortical layers, rather than considering the entire cortical column as a uniform processing element.

10.4 New Optical Approaches for Imaging and Manipulating Neuronal Activity In Vivo with Light

Structured light or "wavefront engineering" by phase modulation is a powerful new technique developed in the last few years (Dal Maschio et al. 2010). In combination with fluorescent activity reporters, opsin-based actuators, and two-photon illumination, this technique represents a promising solution to overcome current limitations of fluorescence functional imaging and optogenetics in vivo. We designed and built a "structured light module," a compact, simple optical path that can be easily implemented with commercial scan heads to allow spatial shaping of laser light. The structured light module is based on phase modulation of the light wavefront by liquid crystal spatial light modulators (LC-SLMs). The combination of the structured light module with the scan head provides simultaneous two-photon imaging and stimulation using two independent laser sources at different wavelengths. The optical design allows us to combine the intrinsic three-dimensional spatial resolution of a nonlinear imaging system with simultaneous access of arbitrary regions of the sample in time and space. We validated this approach for calcium imaging at high frame rates (up to 70 frames/s) from multiple cells simultaneously. We also demonstrate that this technique can be used for photo-uncaging MNI glutamate in arbitrary 2D patterns in cultured neurons (Fig. 10.2).

This system can be used for simultaneous scanning imaging of Ca^{2+} dyes and holographic photostimulation of opsins, caged compounds, or photoswitchable proteins leading to fundamental advancements in our understanding of neuronal network function at cellular and subcellular resolution. At the same time, this technique will allow fast, fluorescence imaging with two-photon excitation in user-defined regions of interest and in combination with spot uncaging. These applications, together with the observation that two-photon light penetrates deeper in biological tissue and that some opsins can be excited with two-photon processes, open new perspectives in the use of the present technology for in vivo studies.

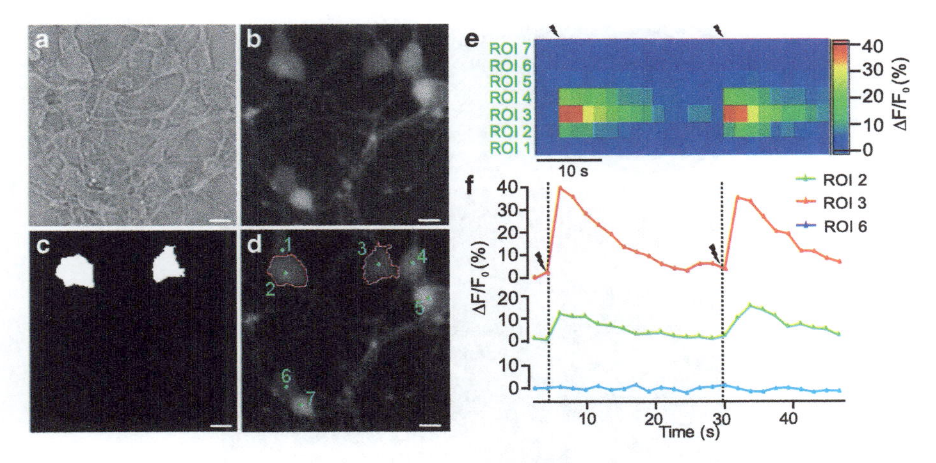

Fig. 10.2 Photostimulating neurons with structured light illumination. (**a–d**) Bright field (**a**) and fluorescence (**b**) images of cerebellar neurons in culture. Scale bar: 10 μm. Neurons are loaded with the fluorescent calcium indicator Fluo-4. Based on this image, an image mask (**c**) is generated and used to photostimulate only two cells [delimited by *red lines* in (**d**)]. (**e**, **f**) Time course of DF/F0 values of Fluo-4 fluorescence in the seven regions of interest (ROIs) displayed in (**d**). The *arrows* indicate the time of delivery of the photolysis stimulus. Modified from Dal Maschio et al. Optics Express (2010)

Phase-modulation approaches have been considered by a number of labs and validated for photostimulation and imaging exclusively with in vitro applications. In Dal Maschio et al. (2011), we reported the first application of this optical setup for in vivo experimental conditions, using wavefront modulation to provide inertia-free focus control—dynamically focusing in depth while keeping the objective in a *fixed* position (Fig. 10.3). As proof of principle, we showed how this system could be used to image functional reporters and cellular markers in different layers of the mouse neocortex with high switching rates (up to 50 Hz).

Our inertia-free focus system not only overcomes the limitations related to the mechanical movements of the objective but also paves the way to decouple the plane of light shaping from the plane of imaging, meaning that in principle neurons in a specific layer can be photostimulated while imaging other cellular populations functionally connected to these but located at a different depth within the sample volume.

10.5 Advanced Optical Methods for Super-resolution

While we have heretofore emphasized the function of large-scale neural networks, a great deal of sophisticated computation also takes place at the *subcellular* scale in neurons. For example, synapses and synaptic spines are complex processing devices in their own right, but are too small to be accessed by conventional

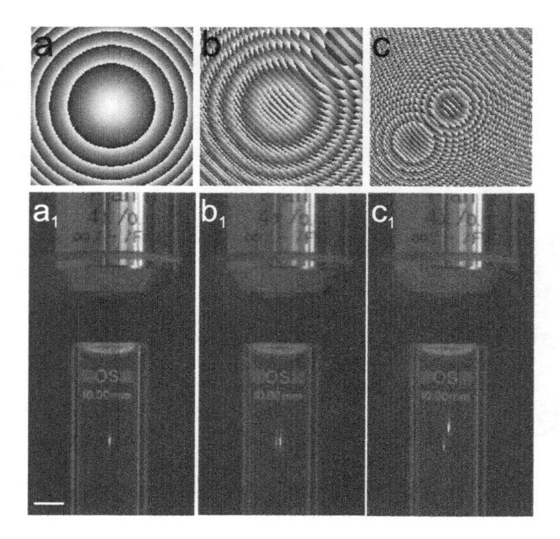

Fig. 10.3 Inertia-free focus control with wavefront engineering. (**a-a**$_1$) The image in **a**$_1$ shows a cuvette of fluorescein excited by a two-photon ($l = 800$ nm) illumination spot generated by the phase hologram shown in (**a**). Scale bar: 5 mm. (**b-b**$_1$) and (**c-c**$_1$) show the same as in (**a-a**$_1$) for structured light illumination patterns generating two spots in the same plane (**b-b**$_1$) and two simultaneous spots at different axial positions (**c-c**$_1$). Modified from Dal Maschio et al. "Optical investigation of brain networks using structured illumination," in "Cellular Imaging Techniques in Neuroscience and Beyond" (2012) Elsevier

electrophysiology, and generally lie beyond the signal limits of conventional optical approaches. A revolution in optical imaging arrived with the development of two-photon excitation (2PE), which, by virtue of minimizing out-of-plane fluorescence and reducing scattering through the use of long-wavelength excitation, allowed unprecedented resolution of submicron structures (Helmchen and Denk 2005). Yet another revolution has occurred in optical microscopy with the advent of *super-resolution* microscopy and optical nanoscopy (Diaspro 2001, 2010a, b), which have opened new vistas on the submicron scale.

Ultimately, spatial resolution is governed by diffraction. However, since fluorescence is so often used as a mechanism of contrast, it is possible to establish an effective "partnership" with the photophysics of fluorescent molecules to beat the diffraction barrier (Hell 2007). When spectrally identical emitting fluorescent molecules are observed through an objective lens of numerical aperture NA $= 2n$ sin α, their emission patterns are spatially confounded when the molecules are closer than $\lambda_{em}/(2\text{NA})$ together. Likewise, diffraction makes it impossible to focus excitation light of wavelength $\lambda_{ex} < \lambda_{em}$ more sharply than a spot of $\lambda_{ex}/(2\text{NA})$ in size. As a result, features that are spectrally identical and closer than the diffraction limit, say $\lambda/(2\text{NA})$, are difficult to distinctly resolve. However, this limitation can be overcome by avoiding the simultaneous emission of adjacent spectrally identical fluorophores: by imaging fluorescent molecules one or a few at the time, it is possible to get a better resolution than when fluorophores emit simultaneously

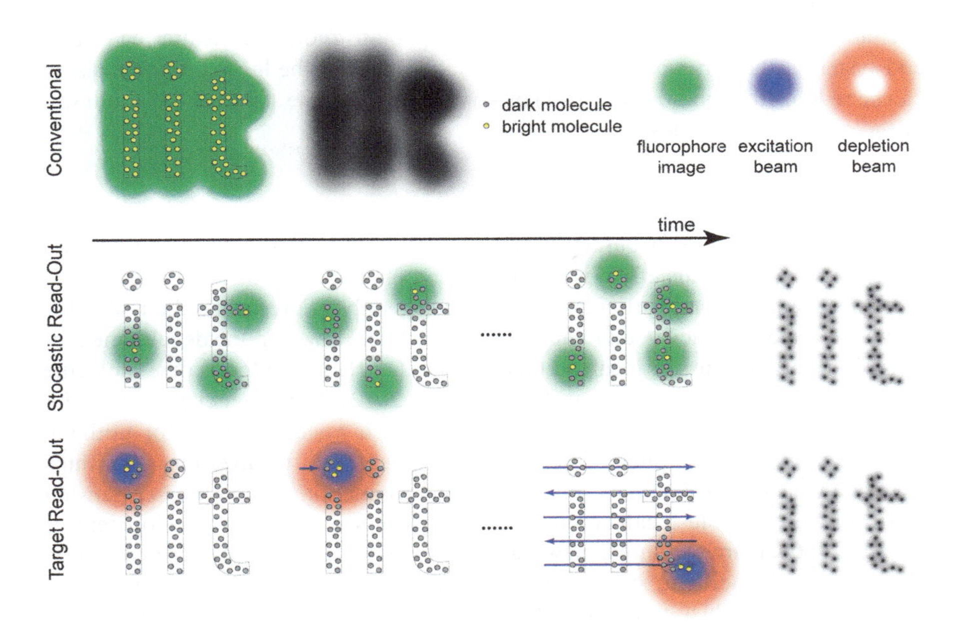

Fig. 10.4 Vignetting super-resolution approaches—targeted and stochastic readout versus conventional imaging. Fluorescent molecule distribution as it appears in conventional imaging, diffraction limited, and as it can be spatially super-resolved (Credit: G. Vicidomini)

(Fig. 10.4). Stochastic readout is related to individual molecule localization methods like PALM (Betzig et al. 2006), FPALM (Hess et al. 2006), STORM (Rust et al. 2006), GSDIM (Folling et al. 2008), or 3D IML-SPIM (Cella Zanacchi et al. 2011). These approaches create a sparse distribution of point-like emitters, single molecules, and localize the emitters with precision of ~20 nm in the *x–y* dimensions and 50 nm along the z dimension. Photoactivatable or photoswitchable molecules are used, and the incident light intensity is reduced to lower the probability of the photoactivation process, thus creating a sparse distribution of fluorescently activated single molecules. Sparse refers to the fact that activated individual molecules are, with high probability, separated by distances larger than the diffraction limit. Data collection is wide field, requiring the collection of hundreds to thousands of frames, and the spatial localization is typically realized off-line by statistical analysis (Thompson et al. 2002; Mortensen et al. 2010).

As long as the number of photons collected for each emitter (N) is sufficient, the fluorophore position can be determined with ten times higher precision than with conventional imaging.

The general relationship is given by

$$s = s_0/\sqrt{N}$$

where s is the localization precision, s_0 is the size of the diffraction-limited excitation/emission spot, and N the number of photons/molecule. Scattering effects and system instabilities can induce additional errors, and the localization precision can be redefined (Aquino et al. 2011) by considering also the standard deviation s_{inst} of the overall instabilities:

$$s_{eff} = \sqrt{(s \cdot s_{inst})}$$

The real localization accuracy is strongly affected by low light conditions and background signal. This effect is stronger when photons are collected deep within biological samples, and particular attention needs to be addressed to the real value of the effective accuracy (Cella Zanacchi et al. 2011). However, the development of new robust algorithms for localization (Starr et al. 2012), able to localize molecule positions within high-density samples (Zhu et al. 2012) (Mukamel et al. 2012) with high background (Smith et al. 2010), has provided a step forward for utilizing super-resolution in complicated and dense samples. New localization algorithms based on Gaussian fitting, maximum likelihood estimation, or compressed sensing allow single-molecule localization in highly dense samples. The development of suitable optical architectures, new far-red or IR dyes, and robust localization algorithms will facilitate super-resolution imaging of thicker samples or tissues. Figure 10.5 shows dual-color STORM images that we made of postsynaptic density protein 95 (PSD95) and extracellular matrix protein LGI1 taken at a lateral spatial resolution of 20–30 nm.

STED, utilizing the general concept of RESOLFT (REversible Saturable OpticaL Fluorescence Transitions), was the first technique to fundamentally break the diffraction barrier (Hell and Wichmann 1994). In a STED microscope, a focused excitation beam shares the focus with a second beam (usually called STED beam) able to de-excite the fluorophores via stimulated emission. Since the STED beam usually forms an annular shape with zero intensity in the center, all the fluorophores located in the excitation spot are kept dark, except those in the proximity of the zero intensity point, which spontaneously emit. By increasing the intensity of the STED beam, the probability of de-exciting the fluorescence by stimulated emission saturates at the outer part of the excitation spot and the volume from which the fluorophores spontaneously emit decreases to sub-diffraction size. Scanning the two co-aligned beams across the sample and recording the spontaneously emitted fluorescence yield the final image, whose spatial resolution can be tuned by adjusting the STED beam intensity. In this manner, the area where molecules reside in a bright state can be made infinitesimally small, despite the diffraction limit. As a consequence, the fluorescence signal available for readout originates from a very small sample region, allowing very sharp images.

The distance (Δd) at which two undistinguishable point-like emitters can be distinguished is given by

$$\Delta d = \lambda / 2n \sin \alpha \sqrt{1 + I/I_{sat}}$$

which can be regarded as an extension of Abbe's equation, which approximates the

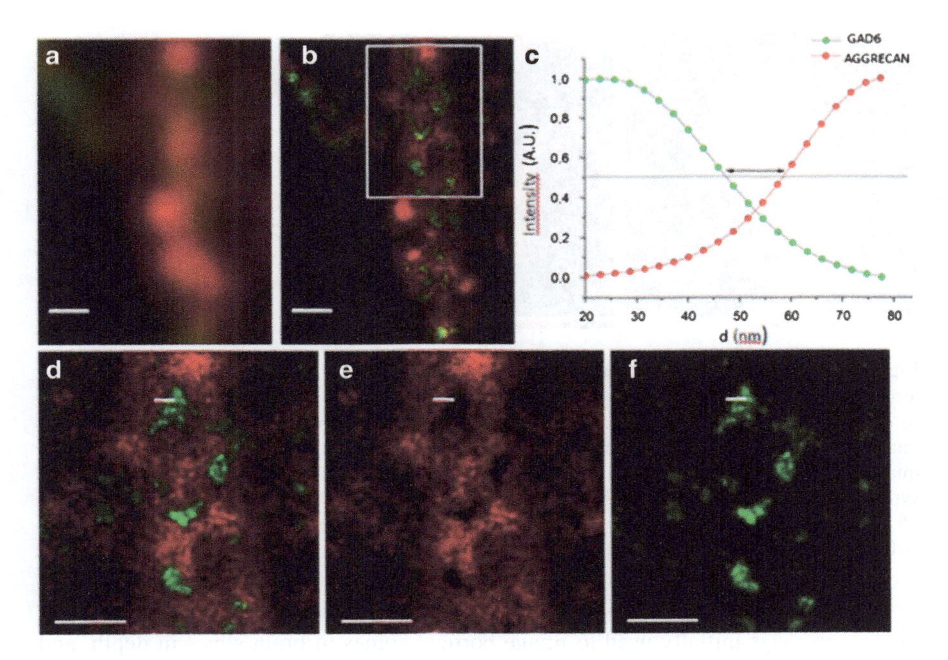

Fig. 10.5 Two-color STORM imaging of GAD65-immunopositive presynaptic GABAergic terminals and aggrecan-rich ECM of perineuronal nets. (**a**) Widefield image of perineuronal nets. (**b**) STORM image of a perineuronal net. (**c**) Intensity profiles at the synaptic boundaries (as example, see the *white line* in (**d–f**)). The intensity-profile analysis provides information about the spatial distribution of the two proteins (after median filtering, the intensity decay can be fitted by a 4th order polynomial distribution and the shift between the FWHM of the distributions is estimated to be 13±7 nm (measurements have been performed over 20 samples to get statistical information). (**d–f**) *Lower panels* show the distribution within a zoomed-in region of interest of aggrecan (*red*) and GAD65 (*green*). Unspecific signal can be removed after a cross-talk subtraction procedure to separate the signal from GAD65 in the *green channel* (**f**) and aggrecan in the *red channel* (**e**). The lateral resolution obtained is approximately 20–30 nm. The objective used is Plan Apo VC 100X 1.40 Oil. Exposure time is 20 ms for each frame. Scale bars: 1 μm. Super-resolution images are reconstructed after the acquisition of 10,000 images. After Korotchenko et al. (2014) (Credit: Francesca Cella Zanacchi)

diffraction limit. In accordance with the RESOLFT concept, I_{sat} is the intensity required for saturating the transition (half of the molecules in the bright state and half in the dark state), which is a photophysical property of the fluorescent molecule in use, and I is the intensity applied to deplete the signal. When the intensity ratio goes to infinite, Δd can reach zero: unlimited resolution. Figure 10.6 shows our imaging of synaptic vesicles in GABAergic terminals of hippocampal neurons labeled with VGAT, as revealed by STED microscopy with resolution enhancement down to 40 nm.

Coupling super-resolution with two-photon excitation provides an unprecedented opportunity to improve imaging depth capabilities and of far-field super-resolution techniques (Ding et al. 2009; Moneron and Hell 2009; Moneron et al. 2010; Bianchini

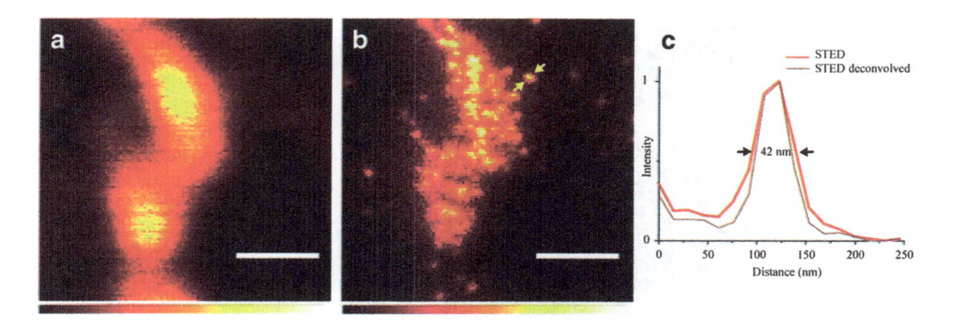

Fig. 10.6 Resolution enhancement with STED microscopy. Synaptic vesicles in GABAergic terminals of hippocampal neurons labeled with VGAT observed in standard confocal mode (**a**). In contrast, STED (**b**) reveals details of single vesicles which are unobservable in the confocal image. Both images show raw data. (**c**) Profile along the line indicated by arrows in the STED image reveals a resolution around 40 nm (*red*), corresponding to the average size of individual synaptic vesicles. Excitation 572/15 nm. Detection 641/75 nm. Depletion 720/20 nm. Pixel size 15 nm. Excitation average power ~4 μW; STED average power ~4.2 mW. Scale bar of 0.5 μm. After Galiani et al. (2012) (Credit: P. Bianchini and S.Galiani)

et al. 2012; Cella Zanacchi et al. 2013; Takasaki et al. 2013). In fact, STED microscopy was initially used to image cortical spines in brain slices in depth, and combining STED with two-photon excitation represents an optimal opportunity for multicolor imaging in living brain tissue (Bethge et al. 2013). Two-photon excitation can also be used to improve localization-based techniques by confining the photoactivation process to increase imaging depth. More recently, 2PE and temporal focusing have been also used to confine the activation process, to perform 3D super-resolution at the whole cell level (York et al. 2011).

Combining STED with two-photon microscopy was realized with continuous-wave STED beams (Ding et al. 2009; Moneron and Hell 2009), a solution that simplifies the combination of 2PE and STED. A new approach that allows performing 2PE-STED imaging using a single wavelength (SW) and, consequently, the very same laser source for 2PE and depletion (Bianchini et al. 2012), SW 2PE-STED, simplifies the image-formation scheme, especially for thick samples and deep-penetration imaging. It is important to note that even if stimulated emission is a one-photon process, scattering of stimulating photons will not increase background, because in most cases, their wavelength is far away from the absorption spectral window of the dye. However, even in the worst scenario, the fluorescence signal induced by the STED beam can be subtracted by lock-in technique (Vicidomini et al. 2013; Ronzitti et al. 2013) to get super-resolved images. Gould et al. (2012) showed that using spatial light modulators in both the excitation and STED beam can compensate sample-induced aberration in a three-dimensional STED implementation. Super-resolution techniques are still in their infancy, yet improvements are rapidly being implemented as demand for possible applications increase, especially in neuroscience.

10.6 Targeting Transgene Expression with Refined In Utero Electroporation

Genetic approaches to control DNA expression in different brain areas and cell types are a fundamental approach for interfering and investigating neural network formation and function in animal models. For example, the optogenetic approaches described above require the exogenous expression of genes in vivo. Typically, exogenous upregulation and downregulation of genes are achieved by introducing nucleic acids (cDNAs and short hairpin RNAs) into neurons. However, it is often important to introduce exogenous genes at precise times, for example, to preserve neural circuit integrity during the development of the brain. In this perspective, in utero electroporation of exogenous nucleic acids presents several advantages compared to more common techniques such as the generation of genetically modified mice or virus-mediated DNA delivery. These advantages include an almost complete lack of cellular toxicity and a straightforward and expeditious approach.

In utero electroporation is based on the direct injection of exogenous DNA into brain ventricles in embryos, followed by the application of an electric field properly addressed by two extrauterine forceps-type electrodes. The electric field induced by the electrodes generates transient pores in the cell membrane. The generation of these pores, in turn, allows negatively charged DNA molecules to flow into the cell driven by the electric field. If applied at embryonic stages, the technique can target cellular progenitors of specific populations of neurons committed to migrate to definite brain areas. However, with standard in utero electroporation, the regions of the brain that can be reliably accessed are very limited (mainly the somatosensory cortex), and the effective temporal window for the procedure is restricted. The main reason for this is not the physiology of the brain: in theory one could address all brain regions by simply targeting the appropriate neuronal progenitors lying at different locations on the surface of the ventricular system. Rather, the main limitations are the technical constraints of reliably placing the electrodes on the embryo's heads inside the uterus and the relatively crude physics behind proper targeting of the electric field by two parallel electrodes.

To extend the spatiotemporal window for in utero electroporation, a multidisciplinary effort was made between IIT departments to develop enhanced electroporation based on a full 3D model of the embryonic brain that took into account the geometric and dielectric properties of the system. This enabled a better understanding of the distribution of the electric field according to the brain morphology and also guided the design of a new hardware to optimize the electroporation (Dal Maschio et al. 2012). In particular, the electric field could be finely tuned to target specific brain regions by the proper placement of a spare third electrode in addition to the standard forceps-type electrodes. By reorientating the three electrodes' positions and polarities, the new configuration allows a more efficient electric field distribution. The application of the new in utero electroporation technique to both rat and mouse embryos consistently resulted in reliable transfection of excitatory neurons of the hippocampus, visual cortex, and motor cortex (Dal Maschio et al. 2012; Szczurkowska et al. 2013). Moreover, the efficient distribution of the electric field by the tripolar configuration extended the time window for efficient electroporation, allowing transfection of the Purkinje cells of the cerebellum in rat (Dal Maschio et al. 2012). Finally, as revealed by mathematical simulation, the symmetry of the electric field generated by the placement of the third electrode allowed for the first time *bilateral* transfection of both brain hemispheres by a single electroporation, an extremely valuable feature for electrophysiological as well as behavioral studies (Dal Maschio et al. 2012).

10.7 Cracking the Neuronal Network Code: Mathematical Tools

The development of advanced optical and electrophysiological tools for massively parallel recording of neuronal activity requires concomitant development of mathematical tools for making sense of the coding strategies of neurons as well as the interaction among neurons. Electrophysiological signals typically consist of time-varying spatial distributions of spikes superimposed on relatively slow varying field potentials, which relate well to subthreshold integrative processes in areas such as dendrites that are otherwise inaccessible (Buzsaki et al. 2012). Different components can be to some extent studied distinctly by using band-separation techniques. Spiking activity of small populations or of single neurons can be detected and classified by examining variations of the signal in the high-frequency range (typically 400–3,000 Hz), whereas subthreshold activity and network fluctuations are computed by the power variation of the so-called local field potential (LFP), defined as the low-frequency range (e.g., 1–150 Hz) of neural activity (Buzsaki et al. 2012). Moreover, biophysical computational models can be used to try to separate out the different neural processing pathways (such as sensory pathways or neuromodulation) captured by electrophysiological recordings (Einevoll et al. 2013).

Computational methods can be used to quantify what specific information is carried by the brain activity and when and where this information is present in this neural activity. Tools developed from information theory (the most rigorous and comprehensive theory of communication) provide a framework to quantify the information carried by any type of neural responses in a single trial, with minimal and largely unrestricting assumptions (Quian Quiroga and Panzeri 2009).

10.8 Determining the Information Content of the Spectrum of Extracellular Signals

Neuronal responses evolve over time over a wide range of timescales. Extracellular recordings from a cortical sensory area show a very rich structure that ranges from oscillations (in the range of approximately 0.1–100 Hz) captured by the LFP to millisecond-scale spiking activity. While many authors have speculated that the time structure of cortical activity plays a role in sensory-related computations, it has been difficult to characterize how it contributes to the representation of the natural sensory environment.

As an example of these approaches, IIT investigators used an information-theoretic formalism to analyze neural activity recorded from the primary visual cortex of monkeys during visual stimulation with naturalistic color movies (Belitski et al. 2008; Montemurro et al. 2008). This revealed how information about the naturalistic sensory environment is spread over the wide range of frequencies expressed by cortical activity. Although the broadband nature of the spectrum might suggest a contribution to coding from many frequency regions, we found that only two separate frequency regions contribute to coding: the low-frequency range (1–12 Hz) and the high-frequency range (from 60 to 120 Hz LFP oscillations to millisecond-scale spikes). Interestingly, low- and high-frequency signals acted as perfectly complementary or "orthogonal" information channels: they share neither signal (i.e., stimulus information) nor "noise" (i.e., trial to trial variability for a fixed stimulus). The existence of low- and high-frequency independent information channels has been later confirmed in auditory cortex of awake animals (Kayser et al. 2009, 2012). This finding has several implications. First, it shows that, despite the broadband spectrum, only a small number of privileged frequency scales are involved in stimulus coding. Second, it suggests that high-frequency and low-frequency activities are generated by different stimulus-processing neural pathways. Third, it suggests that the cortex may use an encoding strategy that engineers call "multiplexing" (i.e., encoding different information along the same physical communication line but using different timescales for each information stream). A clear computational advantage of this "cortical multiplexing" is that it provides a neural population with a means to increase its information capacity, for example, by simultaneously encoding several different stimulus attributes at different timescales.

To study the neural bases of this cortical multiplexing, we mathematically investigated the dynamics of interconnected model network of excitatory and inhibitory neurons receiving slowly varying naturalistic inputs, and we determined how the LFPs generated by these networks encode information about such inputs (Mazzoni et al. 2008). These network model studies reproduced very well and in quantitative detail how the real sensory cortical networks encoded naturalistic information and suggested that (1) high-frequency oscillations are generated by the recurrent dynamics of excitatory–inhibitory loops and encode the overall strength of the input from the sensory periphery and (2) the low-frequency information channel is generated by stimulus–neural interactions (entrainment of thalamic activity to the slow dynamics of naturalistic stimuli) and encodes information about the temporal structure (rather than the strength) of slow stimulus variations.

Advanced mathematical methodologies at IIT are also generating hypotheses about neural circuit function that can be addressed by innovative new experimental techniques, and reciprocally, new experimental approaches are demanding innovative analytical approaches. For example, the ability to "causally" manipulate neuronal circuits calls for better mathematical techniques to chart the flow of information within the brain, going beyond classic correlative measures. Moreover, specific predictions of computational models can be tested for the first time with controlled activation of specific neuronal populations. For example, we are in a position to test whether the low- and high-frequency independent information channels are generated by different neuronal subtypes or by neuronal populations in different cortical laminae. These fundamental questions will require an intimate union of theory and experiment.

10.9 Multi-scale Neuroelectronic Brain Interfacing: Challenges and Approaches

Current brain-interfacing technologies generally do not provide adequate spatial and temporal resolution to access the activity of both single neurons and large neuronal ensembles. Imaging techniques such as electroencephalography, electrocorticography, magnetoencephalography, and functional magnetic resonance provide real-time maps of the collective activity of large groups of neurons, but all are coarsely limited in their temporal and/or spatial resolution. Optical methods, described above, are a promising new method but likewise are still restricted with respect to accessible spatial scale. Complementary approaches must be generated to fill in the current spatiotemporal void in our understanding of brain function.

Microelectrodes remain the most precise transducers of electrophysiological signals from single neurons, with the resolution to detect spiking neural activity (~1 kHz) and low-frequency field potentials (LFPs, <500 Hz). Classic microelectrodes allow recording from one neuron at a time, but modern multielectrode probes allow recording from many neurons simultaneously. An archetypical multielectrode probe includes a structured and implantable substrate to place electrodes in the target brain areas as well as the electrical wiring that connects each electrode to electronic circuits for signal conditioning, transmission, and acquisition. These components advanced dramatically with the advent of microfabrication processes on silicon substrates in the 1970s. Current multielectrode probes are used in a wide range of basic studies of brain function as well as for clinical and neuroprosthetic applications. However, there is still a stringent need for increased sampling capabilities beyond the few tens or hundreds of neurons that can be currently measured simultaneously (Buzsaki 2004; Stevenson and Kording 2011) as well for improved signal quality (Spira and Hai 2013). Recent achievements in nanostructuring capabilities and microelectronic circuits applied to large-scale neural recordings open new perspectives that have the potential to dramatically scale-up the performance of multielectrode devices.

Conventional multielectrode probes are realized using microfabrication processes to integrate tens of microelectrodes on structured substrates (typically silicon) and to embed the electrical wires on-probe to connect each electrode to on-chip or off-chip signal conditioning and acquisition circuits. Currently, two major types of probes are commercially available, using either "in-plane" fabrication approaches with micron-scale photolithography (Wise et al. 2004, 2008), compatible with on-probe integration for signal conditioning and multiplexing (Sodagar et al. 2009) or "out-of-plane" processing from a single block of silicon, using etching, doping, and heat treatments to realize a three-dimensional array of "needlelike" electrodes (Maynard et al. 1997; Rousche and Normann 1998; Nordhausen et al. 1994). Current technologies allow access to tens to hundreds of neurons simultaneously, but multielectrode recording must be dramatically scaled up to measure signals from thousands of neurons. This requires novel array architectures to individually address each electrode while spatially constraining the geometry and size of the probe.

10.10 Large-Scale CMOS Multielectrode Arrays

IIT scientists have contributed to developing novel generations of dense active multielectrode arrays with several thousand micro-/nanoelectrodes (Berdondini et al. 2009; Hierlemann et al. 2011). These arrays are realized with standard complementary metal–oxide–semiconductor (CMOS) technologies. The adoption of CMOS technology and the development of microelectronic circuits for multielectrode-array recordings have drastically increased during the last decade (Jochum et al. 2009). Circuits have been developed to provide signal conditioning close to the microelectrodes, to multiplex signals to reduce output wires, and to wirelessly transmit data (Perlin and Wise 2010), but CMOS circuits are increasingly used to record from a larger number of electrodes simultaneously. Hybrid architectures of application-specific integrated circuits (ASICs) realized in CMOS technology and connected to *passive* electrode arrays have been developed (Dabrowski et al. 2004; Blum et al. 2007; Bottino et al. 2009; Grybos et al. 2011) and used to record from hundreds of retinal ganglion cells in ex vivo retina, with single-cell resolution (Field et al. 2010). However, *active* multielectrode-array architectures could dramatically increase the number and density of microelectrodes (Berdondini et al. 2009; Eversmann et al. 2003; Heer et al. 2004). Berdondini and collaborators introduced the first high-resolution active MEA, in 2001, incorporating 4,096 electrodes (Berdondini et al. 2001). In this device (today also commercially available by 3Brian GmbH), the electrode connectivity is managed using an architecture based on the active-pixel sensor (APS) array originally applied for high-speed light-imaging sensors. The original in-pixel circuitry for light sensing was entirely redesigned to provide sensitivity to small extracellular charge variations resulting from cellular electrical activity. This concept for electrophysiological recordings provides a modular, scalable circuit architecture.

To enable simultaneous recordings from thousands of electrodes, the experimental platform was developed based on two concepts derived from the field of imaging sensors (Fig. 10.7). The first was to integrate APS technology, as described above. The second was to acquire and manage the massive datasets as *image sequences*, rather than acquiring and visualizing single voltage traces as conventionally done in electrophysiology. These concepts are integrated in an experimental platform (Fig. 10.8) including the CMOS chips and hardware platform and a software tool designed to enable recordings from the whole active area at 7.8 kHz or from selected regions of interest at higher sampling frequencies.

The chips are solid-state CMOS integrated circuits (IC) fabricated in a standard 5-metal layer technology (0.5 μm in the early generations and 0.35 μm successively). To resolve single action potentials, a sampling rate of >~6 kHz is required, and an early version able to record from the whole array at 7.8 kHz/electrode was presented in 2008 (Imfeld et al. 2008). The active area of each chip includes an array of pixels, each integrating a microelectrode and a circuit for the first stage amplifier and low-pass filtering. Different generations of these chips provide recording areas up to ~25 mm^2, with a density of electrodes up to 520 electrodes/mm^2.

The electrodes themselves are square, are 21 μm × 21 μm in size, and have a recessed morphology into a top insulation layer of ~2 μm (Fig. 10.8a). The electrode pitches are 42–84 μm and can thus finely map propagating electrical activity. On-chip circuitry includes three stages of amplification with a total programmable gain of 52–76 dB as well as addressing and multiplexing circuits to read out the 4,096 electrode signals on 16 analog output lines. Recently, new chips were generated with 16 on-chip electrical stimulation electrodes interlaced within an array of 64 × 64 recording sites. The metal electrodes were initially made of silicon–aluminum alloy (layer of the CMOS process) but more recently are post-processed with Au or Pt by electrodeposition. The hardware architecture of the platform is also a field-programmable gate array (FPGA) board used for the real-time control and acquisition of the data. The FPGA comprises a module of 16 analog-to-digital converters (ADCs), a processor unit for operation and addressing of the CMOS chip and for real-time signal filtering, and a serializer for high-speed communication through a camera-link standard protocol (data rate of ~60 Mbyte/s). A host computer equipped with a high-speed frame grabber and with hard drives configured for fast data storage is used to control the devices and for managing the recorded data. Finally, an important component of the platform is the custom software application that was developed to manage the critical issues related to large datasets acquired from these devices. The software integrates solutions to manage the fast data stream of ~62 Mbyte/s, algorithms for event

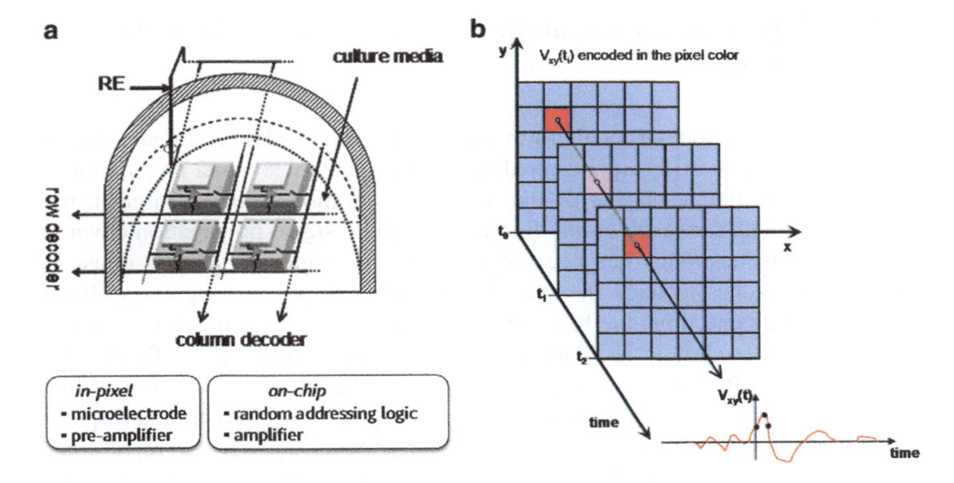

Fig. 10.7 Concepts derived from the light-imaging sensor field and adapted to manage large-scale electrode array recordings. (**a**) Active-pixel sensor concept used to implement arrays of pixels with in-pixel electrodes and local amplifiers. (**b**) Electrode signals are acquired from the entire array as image sequences by encoding the extracellular signal of each electrode in each frame

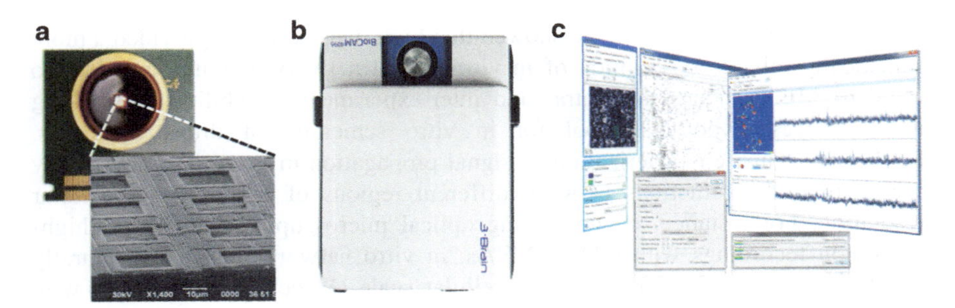

Fig. 10.8 Overview of the components of the 4096 electrode array platform. (**a**) View of a CMOS APS-MEA chip mounted on its printed circuit board and SEM close-up on the square electrodes and electronics integrated underneath. (**b**) View of the real-time hardware. (**c**) Screenshots of the software developed for managing the experiments

detection, tools to visualize the spatiotemporal distribution of the activity, and data-mining tools to extract information from the acquired data.

10.11 Experimental Capabilities of Large-Scale Electrode Arrays

The APS multielectrode-array platform was initially validated on cultured neuronal networks, ex vivo cortico-hippocampal brain slices, and mice retina preparations.

The high spatial resolution of the device allows monitoring of large neural networks yet with the resolution to finely track spatial signal propagation down to cellular dimensions. This has necessitated the development of a new range of analysis approaches to track the spatial distribution of propagating extracellular signals. At the same time, the high-sampling frequency allows monitoring of fast spiking activity and slow oscillations, such as LFPs in brain slices. Recordings performed on different types of preparations are illustrated in Fig. 10.9. While high-quality extracellular voltage traces can be acquired for conventional displays of single-unit activity, spatial propagations of neuronal activity are represented as image sequences of the 64×64 multielectrode-array area, incorporating extracellular signals sensed over the entire array. The CMOS Multielectrode Arrays (CMOS-MEAs) are able to sense both fast oscillations in the band of 700–6,000 Hz and local field potentials or multiunit activity in the frequency band of 10–100 Hz. The noise of the system is low enough to allow reliable spike detections from single units.

In Maccione et al. (2010), we showed that high-density arrays provided a more statistically reliable description of in vitro neural network activity compared to standard MEAs, decreasing intra- and inter-experiment variability and making these devices a potential tool for in vitro screening of drugs or toxins. Furthermore, fine characterization of signal propagation in networks can identify spatiotemporal interactions between different regions of a network at cellular resolution. For instance, by combining optical microscopy imaging with high-resolution recordings with CMOS-MEAs, in vitro networks can be structurally and functionally characterized at the cellular scale (Maccione et al. 2012) with respect to the activity of specific neural populations in the network (e.g., GABAergic vs. non-GABAergic) or by quantifying changes in functional connectivity estimates. We have also developed adaptive algorithms to track and quantify neural activity propagations: trajectories of spatiotemporal propagations in networks (Fig. 10.10a) can be estimated based on the "center of activity trajectory" analysis presented in Garofalo et al. (2009). We used a similar approach to characterize chemically induced interictal events in cortico-hippocampal brain slices (Fig. 10.10b), by recording field potentials with high-density MEAs (Ferrea et al. 2012). Such events were successively classified by generating maps of activity based on clustering of LFP shapes recorded by multiple electrodes. This approach has the potential to provide screens for novel neuropharmacological and neurotoxicologal targets.

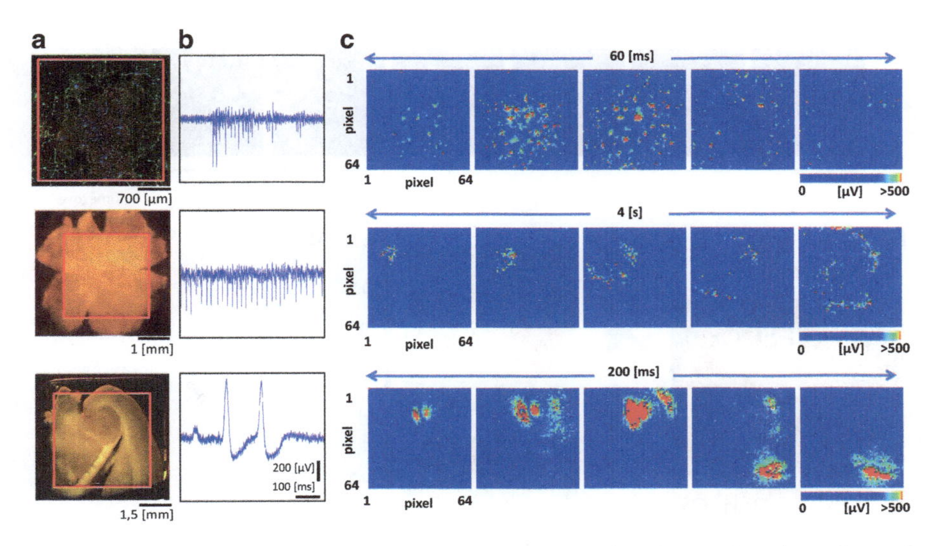

Fig. 10.9 High-resolution recordings with CMOS-MEAs in cultured networks, mice retina, and cortico-hippocampal brain slices. (**a**) In vitro models on CMOS-MEA chips. *From top to bottom*: immunofluorescence image of a network of hippocampal rat neurons at 21DIV, explanted mice retina (P5), and cortico-hippocampal brain slice of a 3-week-old mouse; the *red square* represents the active recording area of the CMOS chip. (**b**) Examples of recorded signals by an electrode selected over the 4096 and (**c**) illustration of the corresponding spatial propagations over the entire 4096 electrode array. *From top to the bottom*: activity during a burst event propagating in the culture; tonic firing of a ganglion cell in the retina during a retinal wave propagation; field potential (FP) occurring in the hippocampus of a brain slice. Each frame is a 64 × 64 image representing in false colors the maximal signal variation in a time window of 10 m/s for the culture and 50 m/s for the tissues for each electrode

10.12 Nanostructuring and Nanofabrication for Neuroscientific Application

In addition to advances in optical and microelectronic approaches for neuroscience, nanotechnology offers tremendous promise for monitoring and interacting with the nervous system. Nanotechnology could offer novel ways to monitor or actuate neuronal activity with cellular and subcellular resolution and to measure neuroactive chemicals in real time in vivo. IIT scientists are exploring nanotechnological applications for neuroscience in a broad, multidisciplinary effort.

Many techniques used today for nanotechnology come from advancements in nanofabrication technologies developed for the semiconductor industry. Overall, these techniques can be distinguished as *top-down* or *bottom-up* approaches. Briefly, in the top-down approach, a bulk material is structured at the nanoscale to obtain the desired properties and geometries. In the bottom-up approach, the molecular constituents are assembled together in order to “grow” a complex nanostructure. The main processes used in the top-down approach are lithography, deposition and etching methods, nanoimprinting, and ion milling. Bottom-up

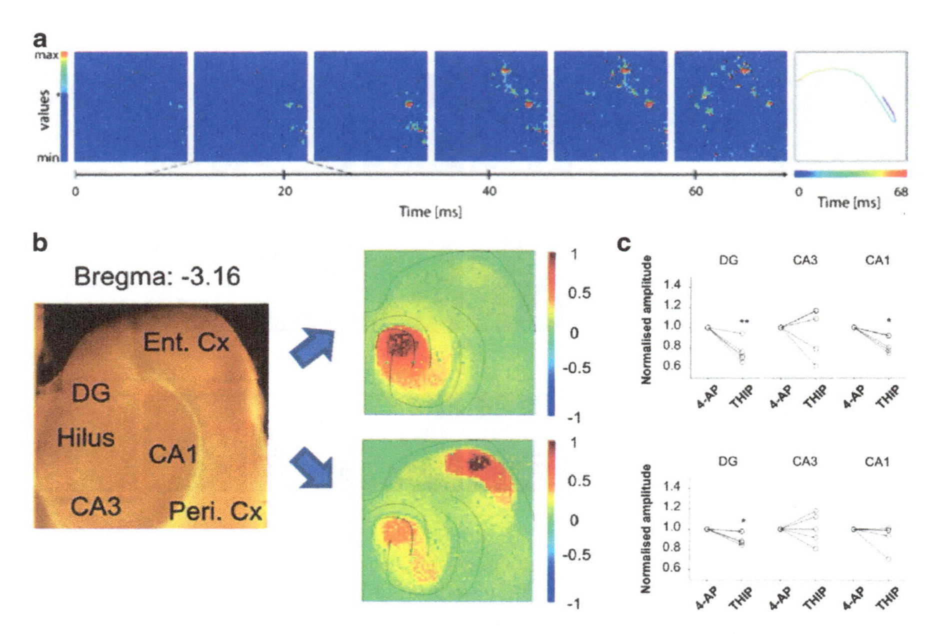

Fig. 10.10 Spatiotemporal analysis of high-resolution electrophysiological signals acquired from (**a**) cultured network (adapted from Garofalo et al. 2009) and (**b**) cortico-hippocampal brain slices (adapted from Ferrea et al. 2012). In (**a**) the trajectory (*last inset on the right*) was calculated with the "center of activity trajectory" analysis of a burst event. In (**b**) the position of a cortico-hippocampal slice on the electrode array is shown in correspondence with false color maps of the activity recorded during two interictal propagating patterns. (**c**) Identification of the effects of THIP on interictal event amplitudes with respect to specific brain regions (dentate gyrus, CA3, and CA1) and by distinguishing the two main propagating classes of events. This methodology could be applied for neuropharmacological and neurotoxicological screenings

approaches include chemical vapor deposition, with variants of electron beam-induced and/or ion beam-induced deposition. IIT scientists are employing both general approaches in developing innovative biosensors. Several examples are presented below to provide a sense of the depth and versatility of nanofabrication innovation at IIT.

10.13 Innovative Electrophysiological Approaches Through Nanostructuring

One area of application for nanotechnology is in devising novel methods for monitoring electrical activity in neurons. Extracellular electrodes capacitively transduce the voltage drop caused by ionic transmembrane currents in the surrounding extracellular medium. However, the reduced invasiveness of extracellular recordings comes at the price of a reduced signal-to-noise ratio (SNR), which is usually insufficient to resolve subthreshold potentials arising from synaptic activity. Miniaturization of the electrode size helps to avoid signal overlap from multiple neurons, although the consequent increase of the electrode impedance negatively affects the SNR. In general, the SNR of extracellular recordings could be increased by (1) achieving a closer apposition between the electrode and the cell membrane and (2) increasing the surface area of the cell/electrode junction. Close apposition increases the resistance to ionic currents in the cleft between the electrode and the cell, thus increasing the extracellular potential, while a more extended junction leads to a higher total current in the cleft together with a higher resistance of the cleft itself. Classical approaches for enhancing the cell-to-substrate interaction rely on protein coatings (Cai et al. 2008; Wrobel et al. 2008) or topographical patterning of the electrode surface (Sniadecki et al. 2006; Spatz and Geiger 2007), the latter also increasing the effective surface area of the junction.

A recent method to achieve both a closer apposition to the membrane and a larger contact surface was based on fabricating mushroom-shaped electrodes that are effectively engulfed by cells (REFs), leading to SNR orders of magnitude higher than with standard extracellular recording. The method exploits the tendency of cells to engulf three-dimensional microprotrusions in a phagocytosis-like fashion (Hai et al. 2010, 2009, 2010; Hai and Spira 2012; Spira et al. 2007a, b; Fendyur and Spira 2012; Van Meerbergen et al. 2008). Analysis of the interface revealed a lower average distance of the cell membrane from the structured electrode surface than for flat surfaces. Thus, 3D nanostructures offer a promising approach to extend the capabilities of microelectrode recording.

An emerging fabrication technique for realizing 3D nanostructures is the focused ion beam (FIB), a top-down nanofabrication technique. As the name implies, the method consists of a focused beam of accelerated ions directed toward the substrate of interest. Due to the large mass of the ion beams, a physical sputtering of the substrate material occurs on the spot hit by the beam. This technique can shape materials in three dimensions with great precision. The FIB can be scanned on the surface with a predefined pattern to generate the desired planar structure, akin to electron beam lithography. The dwell time of the beam on the same spot determines the depth of the etching in the area, so that three-dimensional structures can be created.

While FIB has low throughput, for neuroscience applications, it offers the advantage of rapid and versatile prototyping as well as the ability to combine nanostructuring with other technologies, such as novel microelectrode arrays. For example, we have examined the use of different nanostructured protrusions to enhance microelectrode–neuron interactions for electrophysiological recording. FIB allows the fabrication of nanostructures of different shapes and sizes on the same substrate, allowing direct comparisons in neurophysiological experiments. At IIT, Martiradonna et al. (2012) fabricated straight nanopillars and nail-headed and sphere-headed pillars on top of the recording electrodes of a multielectrode-array substrate (Fig. 10.11). Hippocampal neurons were cultured on the modified chip after functionalization of the chip surface with poly-L-lysine (PLL). After 7 days of culturing, cells were found to adhere to the nanostructured electrodes. Pillars were

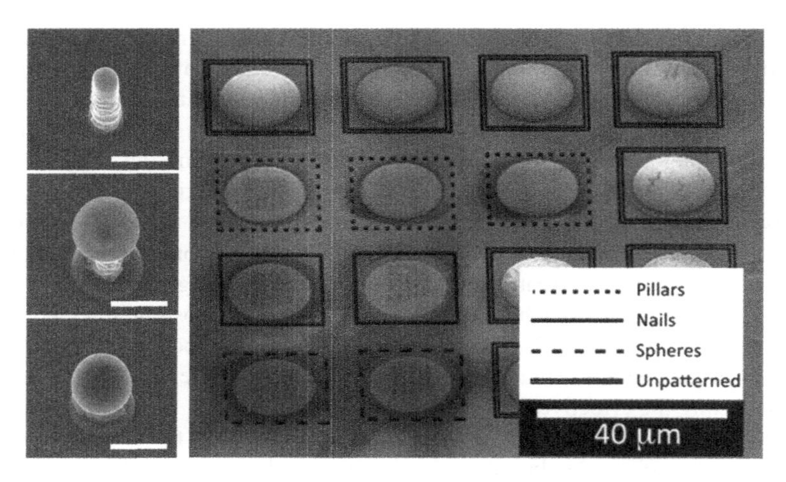

Fig. 10.11 Focused ion beam deposition of nanoprotrusions with different shapes and sizes on top of a MEA substrate for comparative analysis on the mechanisms of interaction with cultured neurons. On the *left-hand side, from top to bottom*, SEM pictures of nanopillar, nail-headed, and sphere-headed nanoprotrusions (scale bar of 1 μm). *On the right-hand side*, 5 × 5 arrays of different nanoprotrusions as fabricated on targeted pads of the MEA. Figure adapted from Martiradonna et al. (2012)

wrapped by neurites extending from neurons attached on the flat insulating layer between the electrodes (Fig. 10.12), and all three kinds of nanostructures readily sustained cellular projections. In particular, a guiding effect was observed in the case of straight nanopillars (Fig. 10.12b). Sometimes, neurites were seen to form suspended bridges between adjacent pillars, while in other cases, they contacted the underlying gold pad and were only partially guided by the nanostructures. In contrast, nail-headed and sphere-headed pillars promoted the formation of a dense network completely detached from the substrate.

This tendency of cells to engulf nanoprotrusions could be used to enhance correspondence between neurons and the recording sites of a MEA. For example, we fabricated 2 × 2 arrays (2.5 μm pitch) of either straight or nail-headed nanopillars on an active-pixel sensor microelectrode array (Fig. 10.13). Nanostructures were made of both conductive platinum and low-conducting silicon dioxide to distinguish the contributions to the neuron/electrode electrical coupling of the tight attachment and of the reduced electrode impedance. Rat hippocampal neurons were cultured on the substrate after functionalization with PLL. Cells readily engulfed all types of FIB-fabricated nanostructures (Fig. 10.14) (Sileo et al. 2013). The figure also highlights the use of the dual-beam system to also visualize the fine structure of the cell-probe interface.

Another nanostructure morphology with considerable potential for neuroscience applications is 3D *hollow* nanocylinders (De Angelis et al. 2013), which could allow novel ways to interface with neurons. At IIT, hollow nanostructures were fabricated using common polymers and with a novel FIB technique applied on

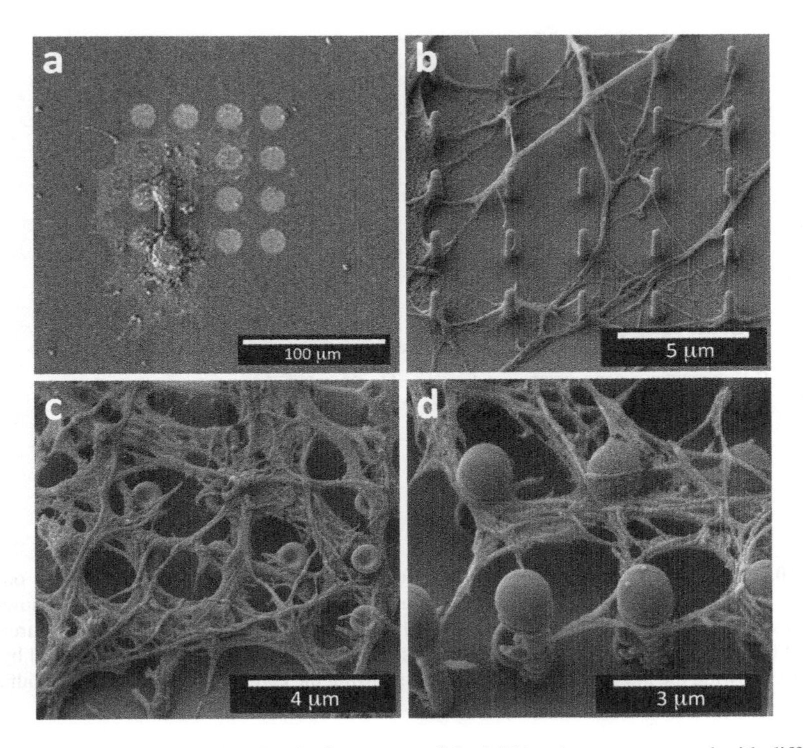

Fig. 10.12 Results of neural cell culturing on top of the MEA substrate processed with different nanoelectrode morphologies. (**a**) Top view showing the neurons agglomerating in the flat region between the processed pads and extending neurites toward the nanoprotrusions. The interaction of neuritis with the different nanoprotrusions resulted in a guiding effect in the case of (**a**) straight nanopillars and in the formation of denser networks detached from the substrate in the case of both (**b**) nail-headed and (**c**) sphere-headed pillars. Figure from Martiradonna et al. (2012)

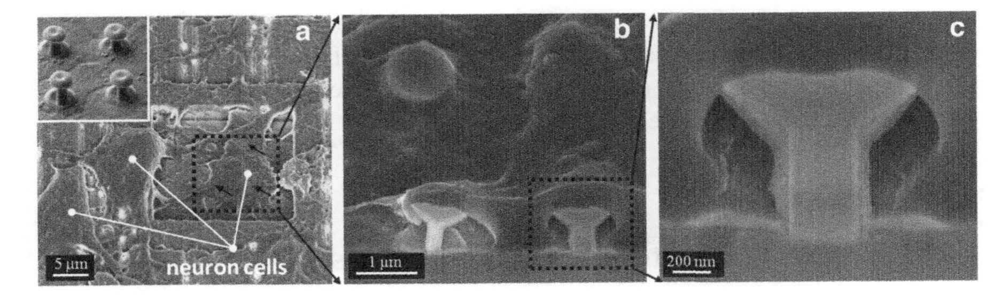

Fig. 10.13 FIB-fabricated nanoelectrodes on an active-pixel sensor multielectrode array. (**a**) 2×2 arrays of nanoprotrusions. Both (**b**) pillars and (**c**) nail-like nanoprotrusions were deposited on the same substrate

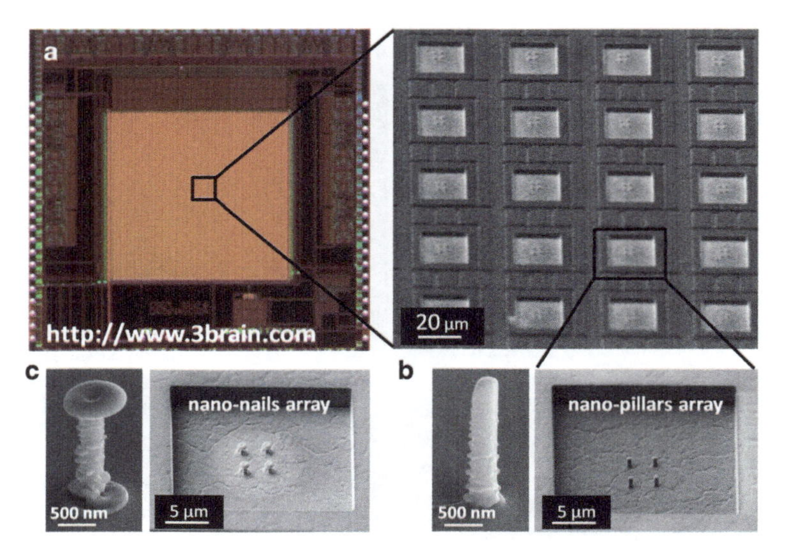

Fig. 10.14 The nanoelectrode–neuron interface. (**a**) SEM image of neurons attached on the surface of an APS-MEA microelectrode with a 2 × 2 array of nanonails (the *inset* shows an array as fabricated), the *arrows* indicating the hidden nanonails. One of the visible neurons is pinned by the nanoprotrusions on the electrode site. (**b**) Section of the same cell, realized by ion milling, showing the attachment sites. (**c**) Detail showing the cell membrane partially engulfing a nanonail. Figure from Sileo et al. (2013)

silicon nitride membranes to produce multiple complex nanostructures in parallel. The technique allows fabrication of hollow nanocylinders with extremely high aspect ratio at the nanoscale, with heights up to 4–5 μm and with internal diameter and wall thicknesses from 20 to 100 nm (Fig. 10.15). Hollow nanocylinders could potentially combine many advantages of 3D nanostructures. For example, they could have potential for intracellular recordings and drug delivery and, if metalized with noble metals, could allow optical/plasmonic spectroscopy (see below) and cell poration with the same 3D transducer. Moreover, since these nanostructures can be fabricated in large quantity on planar substrates, they could interact in principle with multiple cells simultaneously.

10.14 Optical Nanostructured Transducers

By providing the capability to transduce biological signals at the nanoscale, optical and plasmonic nanostructures have tremendous potential for applications in neuroscience. Sensors based on optics and plasmonics work by measuring light absorbed, emitted, or reflected by an analyte or by the active elements of the sensors when they are affected by the analyte. Optical-based biosensors have the advantage of being relatively noninvasive for living systems as they mainly passively detect

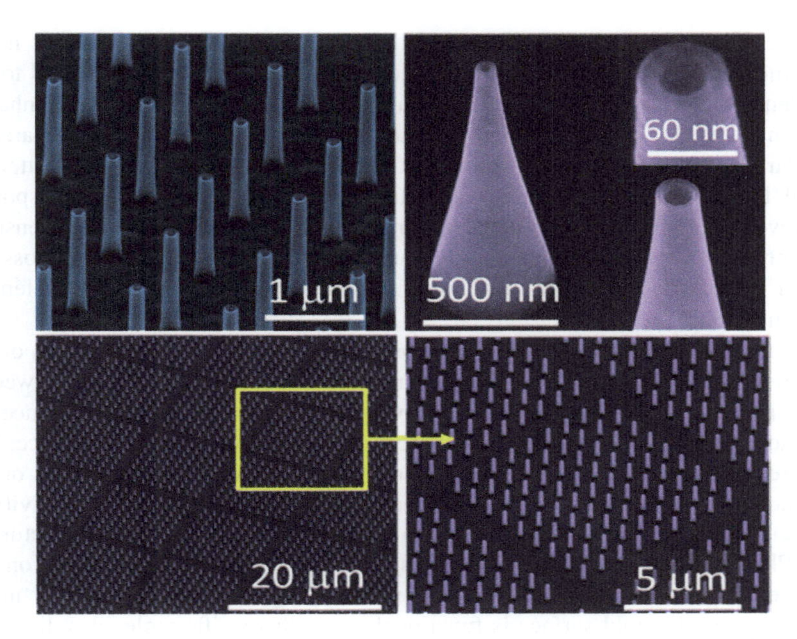

Fig. 10.15 3D hollow nanocylinders fabricated as arrays for advanced neural interfacing and spectroscopy applications (De Angelis et al. 2013)

light, with light stimulation performed at power levels below the threshold of damage.

An example of an optical transducer is Raman spectroscopy cell-based biosensors. Raman signals are inelastic scattering events of the incoming photons with vibrating molecules of the bio-system. Consequently, the spectrum of scattered Raman signals at different wavelengths represents a comprehensive map of the biochemical environment of the system. Each molecular species found in cells, like proteins, DNA, and lipids, has characteristic Raman peaks that can be used to measure the presence and quantity of this species. Moreover, by acquiring Raman spectra in time, it is possible to measure the dynamics of various molecular species by tracking the positions and intensities of peaks as a function of time. The sensitivity of Raman spectroscopy can be greatly improved by exploiting nanostructures as functional interfaces to the biological analyte. These improvements are due to the "field enhancement" generated by surface plasmons on the nanostructure surface that is excited with light. Surface plasmons are coherent oscillations of electrons generated by photon excitation at the interface between a dielectric medium and a metal. If the metal surface has spatial extensions in the nanometer range, the surface plasmon frequency has a resonance when excited with light in the visible and near-infrared range. Biosensing techniques such as surface-enhanced Raman spectroscopy (SERS) exploit these phenomena. SERS is a Raman spectroscopy technique in which the Raman signals of biomolecules are enormously enhanced by the presence of metallic nanostructures on the sensor's surface. The nanostructures can be in the form of surface roughness or nano-patterned metal thin layers; these metallic elements on the surface respond to the incident light with the generation of localized surface plasmons that can enhance Raman signals by factors up to 10^{11}, greatly enhancing the sensitivity compared to standard Raman biosensors. In comparison to roughened surfaces, nano-patterned metal layers offer a more controlled, tunable, and narrow frequency response. However, due to the enormous field enhancement factors, Raman signal intensities are very sensitive to small geometric variations of the nanostructures across the sensor's surface, which can lead to inaccurate measurements of bio-element concentration.

Surface plasmon resonance (SPR) biosensors are based on the detection of the variation of the resonance frequency of surface plasmons at the interface between a noble metal and the wet environment in which the analyte is immersed. Since the plasmons are confined at the metal surface, any small change at the interface, like the presence of ligands or active biomolecules, results in a large variation of the plasmon resonance frequency. This effect leads to extremely high sensitivity at molecular level, which is the workhorse of SPR biosensors. The typical structure of an SPR biosensor includes a glass substrate with a gold film deposited on the surface in contact with the liquid buffer containing the target molecules under investigation; the gold surface is functionalized with specific molecules, like proteins or DNA, which will bind to or interact with the target molecules, thus changing the gold surface's response in terms of plasmon resonance. From the other side of the glass substrate, light of tunable wavelength can be directed to the gold/electrolyte interface at various incident angles with the aid of a prism. Light reflected from the gold film goes again through the glass substrate and through the prism to a detector.

For optical transducers, the morphology and geometry of the nanostructures plays a crucial role. While two 2D nanostructures were initially proposed (e.g., metallic optical nanoantennas and quantum dots), recent advances in nanostructuring technologies are enabling a wide range of submicron three-dimensional morphologies that include nanowires, cones, and cylinders. Cone-like or nose-cone-like shapes are particularly interesting for optical/plasmonic biosensing applications in which spectroscopy techniques are employed for detection. If such nanostructures are made of noble metals and have the correct size in the nanoscale, they act as nanoantennas or nano-waveguides that can confine optical electromagnetic fields well below their diffraction limit, augmenting field intensities up to a factor of 10^3. The confinement effect is generated by the surface plasmon polaritons (SPPs) that are produced by light excitement and that travel along the metal/dielectric interface of the cone surface. In fact theoretical calculations predict an effect of adiabatic compression of SPPs at the tip of perfectly conical shapes with tip radius of few nanometers (Ropers et al. 2007; Stockman 2004). At IIT, De Angelis et al. (2008) reported the fabrication of such nanostructures and their use for Raman detection of very few molecules with sub-wavelength spatial confinement. The reported 3D structure was a gold-coated nanoantenna with a pointed tip fabricated with electron beam-induced deposition

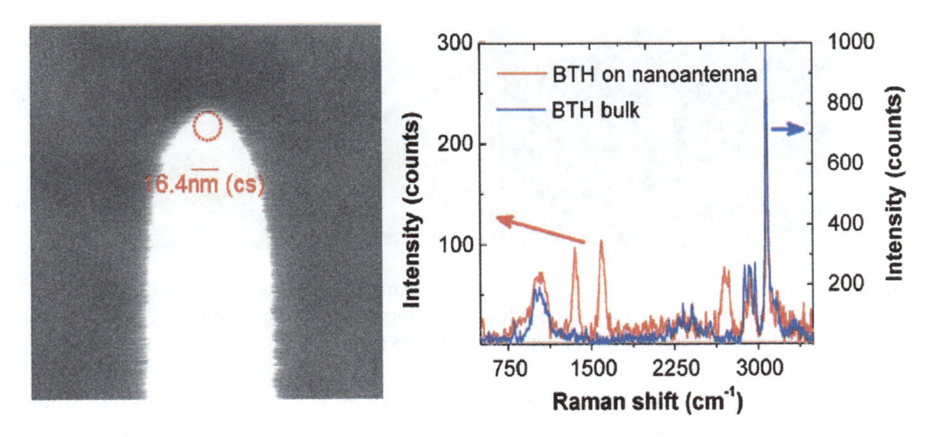

Fig. 10.16 Gold nanoantenna with tip radius below 17 nm and Raman spectroscopy of a benzenethiol (BTH) monolayer chemisorbed on the gold nanoantenna (*red*) compared with a spectrum of bulk BTH

(EBID; see below), a bottom-up nanofabrication technique (Fig. 10.16). The coupling between incident light and SPPs on the nanoantenna was achieved by means of a photonic crystal produced on the substrate on which the nanoantenna was fabricated. The authors performed far-field Raman spectroscopy of a benzenethiol (BTH) monolayer chemisorbed on the gold nanoantenna, acquiring signals from an estimate of about 200 molecules deposited on the nanoantenna tip. The spectrum of these few BTH molecules presents the same characteristic peaks and shift positions as spectra acquired with bulk BTH.

The previous paragraph introduced the use of EBID, which is a specific variant of chemical vapor deposition (CVD), in which thin and thick layers are grown using molecular precursors from the gas phase. In CVD the molecular precursors are decomposed in proximity of the substrate by providing either thermal energy (thermal CVD) or radiofrequency plasma energy (plasma-enhanced CVD). Once decomposed, the free radicals may combine with other different radicals to form new nonvolatile molecules that deposit on the substrate. Alternatively, in the presence of only one type of molecular precursor, some atoms from the decomposed molecules deposit directly on the substrate and bind to the preexisting structure. By carefully adjusting the gas mixture, energy, and pressure/temperature conditions, several materials can be grown by CVD techniques, including crystalline, polycrystalline, and amorphous silicon; silicon compounds (SiO_2 and Si_3N_4); diamond; gallium arsenide; and gallium nitride. Variants of CVD, such as EBID and ion beam-induced deposition (IBID), make use of electron or ion beams for locally decomposing the gas molecular precursors on the substrate spot where they are illuminating; by decomposing the precursors, constituent atoms are deposited on the substrate surface. An interesting property of EBID and IBID techniques is that the deposition process takes place in the vertical direction as long as the beam is illuminating the spot. This combined with the fact that electron and ion beam can be

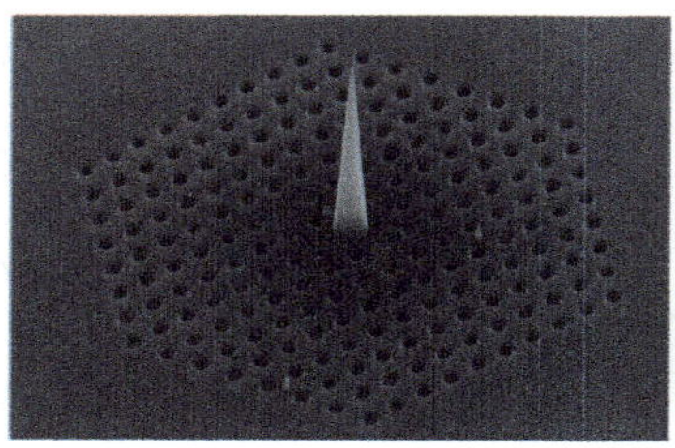

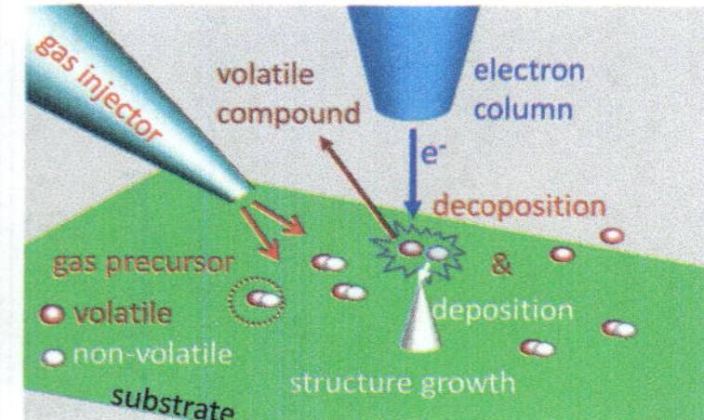

Fig. 10.17 Nanostructures fabricated using electron beam-induced deposition (EBID). (**a**) Silver coated nano-cone fabricated on a silicon nitride photonic crystal using EBID (De Angelis et al. 2010). (**b**) EBID fabrication-process scheme (De Angelis et al. 2011)

focused to nanometer size allows the fabrication of very precise tridimensional nanostructures, like cones and cylinders. As an example, De Angelis et al. (2010) reported on the fabrication of nanoscale cones using EBID (Fig. 10.17). The cone had a tip radius below 5 nm, which allows adiabatic compression of polaritons for enhanced Raman spectroscopy.

EBID and IBID are limited in terms of throughput because the deposition occurs on spot, and the beam must thus be scanned on the substrate. However, the techniques are ideal for prototyping novel devices, especially for neuroscience applications. For example, IIT scientists have used EBID to fabricate plasmonic 3D nanostructures directly on the electrode contacts of multielectrode devices, to potentially provide multimodal sensors for neuroscience. The presence of nanostructures on the electrode surface could merge of electrical recordings with optical/plasmonic spectroscopy to identify and measure local levels of local of neurotransmitters or metabolites. This concept is being actively pursued at IIT. Figure 10.18 illustrates possible approaches for the fabrication of plasmonic 3D nanostructures directly on MEAs. The SEM picture on the left depicts gold-coated platinum–carbon cones fabricated directly on the CMOS-MEA electrode by EBID, as proof of concept. The SEM image in the right is of a CMOS-MEA electrode structured with a dense array of gold-coated nanocylinders fabricated with the novel FIB-based technique. FIB has the capability of large-area parallel processing and is therefore promising for the future integration of 3D nanostructures on CMOS-MEA devices.

10.15 Summary and Broad Future Perspectives

Major new research programs in Europe and the USA have been established to map the connectivity of the brain ("connectomics"), in analogy to how the Human Genome Project mapped the sequence of human DNA in the genome. The Human Genome Project was propelled by rapid improvements in DNA sequencing technology and by general innovation in molecular biology. However, developing analogous technological advancements in neuroscience has proven more

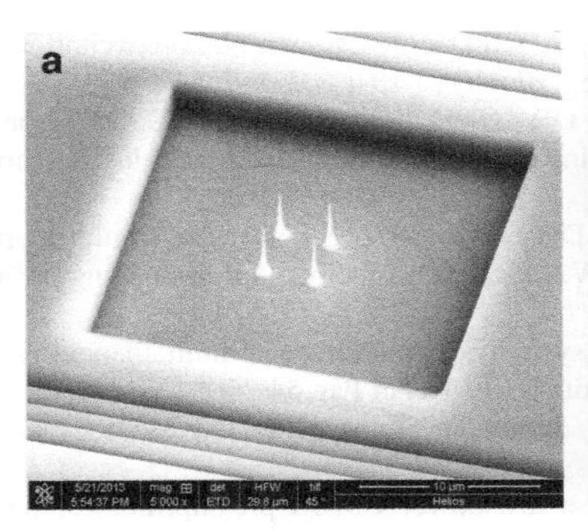

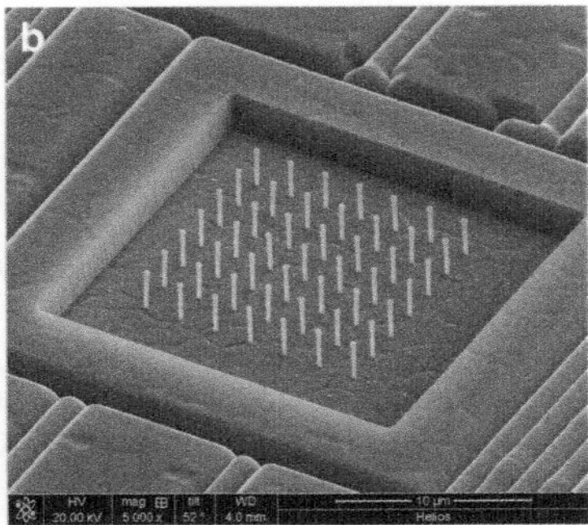

Fig. 10.18 Plasmonic nanostructure fabricated on CMOS-MEA. (**a**) Gold-coated platinum–carbon nanocones deposited with EBID. (**b**) Gold-coated hollow nanocylinders fabricated with polymer structured with FIB

challenging. IIT's goal is exactly to address these challenges, using a multidisciplinary approach to generate novel ideas and apply novel technology. Technical challenges include simultaneously monitoring and manipulating thousands of neurons with high-spatiotemporal resolution, exploiting the power of gene transfer and molecular biology to probe and perturb specific neuronal populations, developing nanoscale materials and structures to allow novel ways to interrogate and interact with neurons, and developing analytical tools to make sense of the daunting complexity of the brain. Data-driven models of brain function will in turn shed light on the function of the normal and diseased brain and will guide the development of truly brain-mimetic artificial devices.

References

Aquino D, Schönle A, Geisler C, Middendorff CV, Wurm CA, Okamura Y et al (2011) Two-color nanoscopy of three-dimensional volumes by 4Pi detection of stochastically switched fluorophores. Nat Methods 8:353–359

Belitski A, Gretton A, Magri C, Murayama Y, Montemurro MA, Logothetis NK, Panzeri S (2008) Low-frequency local field potentials and spikes in primary visual cortex convey independent visual information. J Neurosci 28:5696–5709

Beltramo R, D'Urso G, Dal Maschio M, Farisello P, Bovetti S, Clovis Y, Lassi G, Tucci V, De Pietri Tonelli D, Fellin T (2013) Layer-specific excitatory circuits differentially control recurrent network dynamics in the neocortex. Nat Neurosci 16:227–234

Berdondini L, Overstolz T et al (2001) High-density microelectrode arrays for electrophysiological activity imaging of neuronal networks. In: ICECS: The 8th IEEE international conference on electronics, circuits and systems, Malta

Berdondini L, Imfeld K et al (2009) Active pixel sensor array for high spatio-temporal resolution electrophysiological recordings from single cell to large scale neuronal networks. Lab Chip 9:2644–2651

Bethge P, Chéreau R, Avignone E, Marsicano G, Nägerl UV (2013) Two-photon excitation STED microscopy in two colors in acute brain slices. Biophys J 104(4):778–785

Betzig E, Patterson GH, Sougrat R, Lindwasser OW, Olenych S, Bonifacino JS, Davidson MW, Lippincott-Schwartz J, Hess HF (2006) Imaging intracellular fluorescent proteins at nanometer resolution. Science 313(5793):1642–1645

Bianchini P, Harke B, Galiani S, Vicidomini G, Diaspro A (2012) Single-wavelength two-photon excitation-stimulated emission depletion (SW2PE-STED) superresolution imaging. Proc Natl Acad Sci USA 109(17):6390–6393

Blum RA, Ross JD et al (2007) An integrated system for simultaneous, multichannel neuronal stimulation and recording. IEEE Trans Circuits Syst I Regul Pap 54:2608–2618

Borst JG, Helmchen F (1998) Calcium influx during an action potential. Methods Enzymol 293:352–371

Bottino E, Massobrio P et al (2009) Low-noise low-power CMOS preamplifier for multisite extracellular neuronal recordings. Microelectron J 40:1779–1787

Boyden ES, Zhang F, Bamberg E, Nagel G, Deisseroth K (2005) Millisecond-timescale, genetically targeted optical control of neural activity. Nat Neurosci 8(9):1263–8

Buzsaki G (2004) Large-scale recording of neuronal ensembles. Nat Neurosci 7:446–451

Buzsaki G, Anastassiou CA, Koch C (2012) The origin of extracellular fields and currents — EEG, ECoG, LFP and spikes. Nat Rev Neurosci 13:407–420

Cai N, Gong Y et al (2008) Adhesion dynamics of porcine esophageal fibroblasts on extracellular matrix protein-functionalized poly(lactic acid). Biomed Mater 3:015014

Cella Zanacchi F, Lavagnino Z, Perrone Donnorso M, Del Bue A, Furia L, Faretta M, Diaspro A (2011) Live-cell 3D super-resolution imaging in thick biological samples. Nat Methods 8:1047–1049

Cella Zanacchi F, Lavagnino Z, Faretta M, Furia L, Diaspro A (2013) Light-sheet confined super-resolution using two-photon photoactivation. PLoS One 8:e67667. doi:10.1371/journal.pone.0067667

Chow BY, Han X, Dobry AS, Qian X, Chuong AS, Li M, Henninger MA, Belfort GM, Lin Y, Monahan PE, Boyden ES (2010) High-performance genetically targetable optical neural silencing by light-driven proton pumps. Nature 463:98–102

Dabrowski W, Grybos P et al (2004) A low noise multichannel integrated circuit for recording neuronal signals using microelectrode arrays. Biosens Bioelectron 19:749–761

Dal Maschio M, Difato F, Beltramo R, Blau A, Benfenati F, Fellin T (2010) Simultaneous two-photon imaging and photo-stimulation with structured light illumination. Opt Express 18:18720–18731

Dal Maschio M, De Stasi AM, Benfenati F, Fellin T (2011) Three dimensional in vivo scanning microscopy with inertia-free focus control. Opt Lett 36:3503–05

Dal Maschio M, Ghezzi D, Bony G, Alabastri A, Deidda G, Brondi M, Sato SS, Zaccaria RP, Di Fabrizio E, Ratto GM, Cancedda L (2012) High-performance and site-directed in utero electroporation by a triple-electrode probe. Nat Commun 3:960

De Angelis F, Patrini M et al (2008) A hybrid plasmonic-photonic nanodevice for label-free detection of a few molecules. Nano Lett 8:2321–2327

De Angelis F, Das G et al (2010) Nanoscale chemical mapping using three-dimensional adiabatic compression of surface plasmon polaritons. Nat Nano 5:67–72

De Angelis F, Liberale C et al (2011) Emerging fabrication techniques for 3D nano-structuring in plasmonics and single molecule studies. Nanoscale 3:2689–2696

De Angelis F, Malerba M et al (2013) 3D hollow nanostructures as building blocks for multifunctional plasmonics. Nano Lett 13:3553–3558

Denk W, Svoboda K (1997) Photon upmanship: why multiphoton imaging is more than a gimmick. Neuron 18:351–357

Denk W, Strickler JH, Webb WW (1990) Two-photon laser scanning fluorescence microscopy. Science 248:73–76

Diaspro A (2001) Confocal and two-photon microscopy: foundations, applications, and advances. Wiley-Liss, New York
Diaspro A (2010a) Optical fluorescence microscopy: from the spectral to the nano dimension. Springer, Heidelberg, pp 1–244
Diaspro A (2010b) Nanoscopy and multidimensional optical fluorescence microscopy. Chapman and Hall/CRC, London
Ding J, Takasaki K, Sabatini B (2009) Supraresolution imaging in brain slices using stimulated-emission depletion two-photon laser scanning microscopy. Neuron 63:429–437
Einevoll GT, Kayser C, Logothetis NK, Panzeri S (2013) Modelling and analysis of local field potential for studying the function of cortical circuits. Nat Rev Neurosci 14:770–785
Eversmann B, Jenkner M et al (2003) A 128x128 CMOS biosensor array for extracellular recording of neural activity. IEEE J Solid State Circuits 38:2306–2317
Fellin T (2009) Communication between neurons and astrocytes: relevance to the modulation of synaptic and network activity. J Neurochem 108:533–544
Fendyur A, Spira ME (2012) Toward on-chip, in-cell recordings from cultured cardiomyocytes by arrays of gold mushroom-shaped microelectrodes. Front Neuroeng 5:21
Ferrea E, Maccione A et al (2012) Large-scale, high-resolution electrophysiological imaging of field potentials in brain slices with microelectronic multielectrode arrays. Front Neural Circuits 6:80
Field GD, Gauthier JL et al (2010) Functional connectivity in the retina at the resolution of photoreceptors. Nature 467:673–654
Folling J, Bossi M, Bock H, Medda R, Wurm CA, Hein B, Jakobs S, Eggeling C, Hell SW (2008) Fluorescence nanoscopy by ground-state depletion and single-molecule return. Nat Methods 11:943–945
Galiani S, Harke B, Vicidomini G, Lignani G, Benfenati F, Diaspro A, Bianchini P (2012) Strategies to maximize the performance of a STED microscope. Opt Express 20(7):7362–7374
Garofalo M, Nieus T et al (2009) Evaluation of the performance of information theory-based methods and cross-correlation to estimate the functional connectivity in cortical networks. PLoS One 4:e6482
Gobel W, Kampa BM, Helmchen F (2007) Imaging cellular network dynamics in three dimensions using fast 3D laser scanning. Nat Methods 4:73–79
Gould TJ, Burke D, Bewersdorf J, Booth MJ (2012) Adaptive optics enables 3D STED microscopy in aberrating specimens. Opt Express 20(19):20998–21009
Gradinaru V, Thompson KR, Deisseroth K (2008) eNpHR: a Natronomonas halorhodopsin enhanced for optogenetic applications. Brain Cell Biol 36:129–139
Gradinaru V, Zhang F, Ramakrishnan C, Mattis J, Prakash R, Diester I, Goshen I, Thompson KR, Deisseroth K (2010) Molecular and cellular approaches for diversifying and extending optogenetics. Cell 141:154–165
Grybos P, Kmon P et al (2011) 64 Channel neural recording amplifier with tunable bandwidth in 180 nm CMOS technology. Metrol Meas Syst 18:631–643
Hai A, Spira ME (2012) On-chip electroporation, membrane repair dynamics and transient in-cell recordings by arrays of gold mushroom-shaped microelectrodes. Lab Chip 12:2865–2873
Hai A, Kamber D et al (2009) Changing gears from chemical adhesion of cells to flat substrata toward engulfment of micro-protrusions by active mechanisms. J Neural Eng 6:066009
Hai A, Shappir J et al (2010) In-cell recordings by extracellular microelectrodes. Nat Methods 7:200–250
Haydon PG (2001) GLIA: listening and talking to the synapse. Nat Rev Neurosci 2:185–193
Heer F, Franks W et al (2004) CMOS microelectrode array for the monitoring of electrogenic cells. Biosens Bioelectron 20:358–366
Hell SW (2007) Far-field optical nanoscopy. Science 316(5828):1153–1158
Hell SW, Wichmann J (1994) Breaking the diffraction resolution limit by stimulated emission: stimulated-emission-depletion fluorescence microscopy. Opt Lett 19(11):780–782
Helmchen F, Denk W (2005) Deep tissue two-photon microscopy. Nat Methods 2:932–940

Helmchen F, Imoto K, Sakmann B (1996) Ca^{2+} buffering and action potential-evoked Ca^{2+} signaling in dendrites of pyramidal neurons. Biophys J 70:1069–1081

Hess ST, Girirajan TP, Mason MD (2006) Ultra-high resolution imaging by fluorescence photoactivation localization microscopy. Biophys J 91:4258–4272

Hierlemann A, Frey U et al (2011) Growing cells atop microelectronic chips: interfacing electrogenic cells in vitro with CMOS-based microelectrode arrays. Proc IEEE 99:252–284

Imfeld K, Neukom S et al (2008) Large-scale, high-resolution data acquisition system for extracellular recording of electrophysiological activity. IEEE Trans Biomed Eng 55:2064–2073

Jochum T, Denison T et al (2009) Integrated circuit amplifiers for multi-electrode intracortical recording. J Neural Eng 6(1):012001

Jones EG, Peters A (eds) (1990) Cerebral cortex. Comparative structure and evolution of cerebral cortex, vol 8A. Plenum, New York, pp 269–283

Kayser C, Montemurro MA, Logothetis NK, Panzeri S (2009) Auditory information coding is boosted by nested spike-phase and spike-pattern codes. Neuron 61:597–608

Kayser C, Ince RAA, Panzeri S (2012) Analysis of slow (theta) oscillations as a potential temporal reference frame for information coding in sensory cortices. PLoS Comput Biol 8(10):e1002717

Korotchenko S, Cella F, Diaspro A, Dityatev A (2014) Zooming in on the (peri)synaptic extracellular matrix. In: Antoine T, Valentine N (eds) Nanoscale imaging of synapses, vol 84. Humana, Totowa, NJ, pp 220–230

Looger LL, Griesbeck O (2012) Genetically encoded neural activity indicators. Curr Opin Neurobiol 22:18–23

Maccione A, Gandolfo M et al (2010) Experimental investigation on spontaneously active hippocampal cultures recorded by means of high-density MEAs: analysis of the spatial resolution effects. Front Neuroeng 3:4

Maccione A, Garofalo M et al (2012) Multiscale functional connectivity estimation on low-density neuronal cultures recorded by high-density CMOS micro electrode arrays. J Neurosci Methods 207:161–171

Martiradonna L, Quarta L, Sileo L, Schertel A, Maccione A, Simi A, Dante S, Scarpellini A, Berdondini L, De Vittorio M (2012) Beam induced deposition of 3D electrodes to improve coupling to cells. Microelectron Eng 97:365–368

Maynard EM, Nordhausen CT et al (1997) The Utah intracortical electrode array: a recording structure for potential brain-computer interfaces. Electroencephalogr Clin Neurophysiol 102:228–239

Mazzoni A, Panzeri S, Logothetis NK, Brunel N (2008) Encoding of naturalistic stimuli by local field potential spectra in networks of excitatory and inhibitory neurons. PLoS Comput Biol 4: e1000239

Meyer HS, Wimmer VC, Oberlaender M, de Kock CP, Sakmann B, Helmstaedter M (2010) Number and laminar distribution of neurons in a thalamocortical projection column of rat vibrissal cortex. Cereb Cortex 20:2277–2286

Moneron G, Hell S (2009) Two-photon excitation STED microscopy. Opt Express 17(17):14567–14573

Moneron G, Medda R, Hein B, Giske A, Westphal V, Hell SW (2010) Fast STED microscopy with continuous wave fiber lasers. Opt Express 18:1302–1309

Montemurro MA, Rasch MJ, Murayama Y, Logothetis NK, Panzeri S (2008) Phase of firing coding of natural visual stimuli in primary visual cortex. Curr Biol 18:375–380

Mortensen KI, Churchman LS, Spudich JA, Flyvbjerg H (2010) Optimized localization analysis for single-molecule tracking and super-resolution microscopy. Nat Methods 7(5):377–381

Mukamel EA, Babcock H, Zhuang X (2012) Statistical deconvolution for superresolution fluorescence microscopy. Biophys J 102(10):2391–2400

Nordhausen CT, Rousche PJ et al (1994) Optimizing recording capabilities of the Utah-intracortical-electrode-array. Brain Res 637:27–36

Perlin GE, Wise KD (2010) An ultra compact integrated front end for wireless neural recording microsystems. J Microelectromech Syst 19:1409–1421
Quian Quiroga R, Panzeri S (2009) Extracting information from neuronal populations: information theory and decoding approaches. Nat Rev Neurosci 10:173–185
Ronzitti E, Harke B, Diaspro A (2013) Frequency dependent detection in a STED microscope using modulated excitation light. Opt Express 21(1):210–219
Ropers C, Neacsu CC et al (2007) Grating-coupling of surface plasmons onto metallic tips: a nanoconfined light source. Nano Lett 7:2784–2788
Rousche PJ, Normann RA (1998) Chronic recording capability of the Utah intracortical electrode array in cat sensory cortex. J Neurosci Methods 82:1–15
Rust MJ, Bates M, Zhuang X (2006) Sub-diffraction-limit imaging by stochastic optical reconstruction microscopy (STORM). Nat Methods 3(10):793–795
Sileo L, Pisanello F et al (2013) Electrical coupling of mammalian neurons to microelectrodes with 3D nanoprotrusions. Microelectron Eng 111:384–390
Smith CS, Joseph N, Rieger B, Lidke KA (2010) Fast, single-molecule localization that achieves theoretically minimum uncertainty. Nat Methods 7(5):373–375
Sniadecki NJ, Desai RA et al (2006) Nanotechnology for cell-substrate interactions. Ann Biomed Eng 34:59–74
Sodagar AM, Perlin GE et al (2009) An implantable 64-channel wireless microsystem for single-unit neural recording. IEEE J Solid State Circuits 44:2591–2604
Spatz JP, Geiger B (2007) Molecular engineering of cellular environments: cell adhesion to nano-digital surfaces. Methods Cell Biol 83:89–111
Spira ME, Hai A (2013) Multi-electrode array technologies for neuroscience and cardiology. Nat Nanotechnol 8:83–94
Spira ME, Kamber D et al (2007) Improved neuronal adhesion to the surface of electronic device by engulfment of protruding micro-nails fabricated on the chip surface. In: Solid-state sensors, actuators and microsystems conference, 2007. Transducers 2007 International
Spira ME, Kamber D et al (2007) Engulfment of protruding micro-nails fabricated on chip surface by cultured neurons improve their adhesion to the electronic device. MRS Online Proceedings Library 1004:null-null M3.doi:10.1557/PROC-1004-P1502-1505
Starr R, Stahlheber S, Small A (2012) Fast maximum likelihood algorithm for localization of fluorescent molecules. Opt Lett 37(3):413–415
Stevenson IH, Kording KP (2011) How advances in neural recording affect data analysis. Nat Neurosci 14:139–142
Stockman MI (2004) Nanofocusing of optical energy in tapered plasmonic waveguides. Phys Rev Lett 93:137404
Stosiek C, Garaschuk O, Holthoff K, Konnerth A (2003) In vivo two-photon calcium imaging of neuronal networks. Proc Natl Acad Sci USA 100:7319–7324
Svoboda K, Yasuda R (2006) Principles of two-photon excitation microscopy and its applications to neuroscience. Neuron 50:823–839
Svoboda K, Denk W, Kleinfeld D, Tank DW (1997) In vivo dendritic calcium dynamics in neocortical pyramidal neurons. Nature 385:161–165
Szczurkowska J, dal Maschio M, Cwetsch AW, Ghezzi D, Bony G, Alabastri A, Zaccaria RP, di Fabrizio E, Ratto GM, Cancedda L (2013) Increased performance in genetic manipulation by modeling the dielectric properties of the rodent brain. Conf Proc IEEE Eng Med Biol Soc 2013:1615–1618
Takasaki KT, Ding JB, Sabatini BL (2013) Live-cell superresolution imaging by pulsed STED two-photon excitation microscopy. Biophys J 104(4):770–777
Theer P, Hasan MT, Denk W (2003) Two-photon imaging to a depth of 1000 micron in living brains by use of a Ti:Al_2O_3 regenerative amplifier. Opt Lett 28:1022–1024
Thompson RE, Larson DR, Webb WW (2002) Precise nanometer localization analysis for individual fluorescent probes. Biophys J 82(5):2775–2783

Tsien RY (1980) New calcium indicators and buffers with high selectivity against magnesium and protons: design, synthesis, and properties of prototype structures. Biochemistry 19:2396–2404
Tsien RY (1981) A non-disruptive technique for loading calcium buffers and indicators into cells. Nature 290:527–528
Van Meerbergen B, Jans K et al (2008) Peptide-functionalized microfabricated structures for improved on-chip neuronal adhesion. Conf Proc IEEE Eng Med Biol Soc 2008:1833–1836
Vicidomini G, Coto Hernández I, d'Amora M, Cella Zanacchi F, Bianchini P, Diaspro A (2013) Gated CW-STED microscopy: a versatile tool for biological nanometer scale investigation. Methods pii: S1046-2023(13)00241-7. doi: 10.1016/j.ymeth.2013.06.029
Volterra A, Meldolesi J (2005) Astrocytes, from brain glue to communication elements: the revolution continues. Nat Rev Neurosci 6:626–640
Wise KD, Anderson DJ et al (2004) Wireless implantable microsystems: high-density electronic interfaces to the nervous system. Proc IEEE 92:76–97
Wise KD, Sodagar AM et al (2008) Microelectrodes, microelectronics, and implantable neural microsystems. Proc IEEE 96:1184–1202
Wrobel G, Holler M et al (2008) Transmission electron microscopy study of the cell-sensor interface. J R Soc Interface 5:213–222
York AG, Ghitani A, Vaziri A, Davidson MW, Shroff H (2011) Confined activation and subdiffractive localization enables whole-cell PALM with genetically expressed probes. Nat Methods 8:327–333
Zhang F, Aravanis AM, Adamantidis A, de Lecea L, Deisseroth K (2007) Circuit-breakers: optical technologies for probing neural signals and systems. Nat Rev Neurosci 8:577–581
Zhu L, Zhang W, Elnatan D, Huang B (2012) Faster STORM using compressed sensing. Nat Methods 9(7):721–723
Zipfel WR, Williams RM, Webb WW (2003) Nonlinear magic: multiphoton microscopy in the biosciences. Nat Biotechnol 21:1369–1377

Lightning Source UK Ltd.
Milton Keynes UK
UKOW06n2042270616

277168UK00002B/26/P

9 783319 049236